Y0-CLB-401

THE BERKELEY SCHOOL GUIDE TO

Beauty · Charm · Poise

THE BERKELEY SCHOOL

EAST ORANGE, NEW JERSEY   RIDGEWOOD, NEW JERSEY

HICKSVILLE, NEW YORK   WHITE PLAINS, NEW YORK

NEW YORK, NEW YORK

© Copyright 1962-1963-1967-1969
Milady Publishing Corp.
Bronx, N. Y.

All rights reserved. No part of this book may be reproduced in any form, by mimeograph or any other means, without permission in writing from the publishers.

Printed in the United States of America

FOREWORD

THE IMPORTANCE OF CHARM IN TODAY'S BUSINESS WORLD

A survey conducted by Glamour Magazine indicates that two-thirds of all job dismissals are due to personality difficulties and not to a lack of technical know-how. A charm course can pave the way for smoother human relations by teaching the techniques for getting along with others. The thing referred to as "It" in personality can be acquired.

A private and vocational school survey shows that the majority of dropouts are those students who have not developed the correct set of success traits such as perseverance and dependability. A charm course can provide the desire to see ahead and to overcome the traits of personality and appearance that stand in the way of reaching your own "Land of Heart's Desire."

For those students who already have the necessary physical, mental and personality resources for success, a charm course will give that "plus" quality that is usually found in the successful person, not in the beginner.

The proof of the value of charm training is evident in the success stories written up almost daily in the newspapers. It is difficult to think of anyone prominent in public life who has not undergone a concentrated course in "charm." Likewise, it is difficult to think of truly successful personalities who are not the embodiments of all that is charming.

How is a charm course going to help you? Well, let's assume that you are among the majority. That, first of all, you want to have a full life outside your career with, perhaps, a husband and children. Then let us examine for a moment the feminine traits that will attract and hold a man.

A man selects his mate on a more or less emotional evaluation of her qualities. He enjoys looking, so he is attracted to a girl who is good looking from his personal standpoint. Today, his idea of beauty requires a well-rounded but not fat figure. Many overweight girls sit at home frustrated because they are not getting dates, eating because they are frustrated and frustrated because they are eating—too much.

A man enjoys being accepted. His ego is much more vulnerable than a woman's, so he is attracted to the girl who seems to be happy and self-confident. This is precisely why the wall flower is left sitting in the corner. A girl then, needs self-confidence to attract a man.

A man is more conservative and idealistic than a woman so he wants a girl whom he can put on a pedestal. This leads him to select a girl who meets his idealization of womankind. He wants a girl who is feminine in that she is kind, tender, thoughtful, gentle and morally stable.

A man enjoys comfort so he wants a woman who can put him at his ease. This calls for poise in a woman which simply means that she is able to handle unexpected or embarrassing circumstances with equanimity (balance). She doesn't get flustered.

A man wants to protect so he selects a woman who gives him the opportunity to show off his masculinity by taking care of her in little ways. He wants her to be mentally alert, but he doesn't want her to wear her knowledge on her sleeve. He wants her to be physically able but he wants her to wait until he can pull the chair out for her, help her into her coat and in other ways assist her.

A man has a more sensitive sense of smell than a woman and this leads him to be attracted to the girl who makes the most of her attractiveness by being scrubbed and polished. Her hair is clean and sweet smelling as is her entire person. She is well-groomed.

A woman then, *to attract a man,* should:
  Be easy on the eyes;
  Be happy and self-confident;
  Be feminine, tender, kind and thoughtful;
  Be poised;
  Be dependent;
  Be well-groomed;

All these things might be summed up by saying that a man looks for a woman who has "sex appeal." And what is "sex appeal"? It is a womanliness expressed in a *happy face, a modulated voice* and *graceful movements*. It can be acquired and it is a woman's best advertisement.

Your charm course can impart all these virtues. And more, it can place you among the working elite who are making from $50.00 to $100.00 more per month because of their charming ways. A Government survey discloses that women who have had charm training earn more than those who have a comparable business background but no such training.

Whatever field you have chosen for your career, charm training will give you the added advantages of greater self-confidence, amplified beauty and personality "plus".

CONTENTS

UNIT ONE

Skin Care, Cosmetic Application and Hair Beautification

CHAPTER 1—SKIN CARE 3
Skin conditions; skin types classified; steps in skin care; lubricating oils; lubrication for normal or dry skin, oily skin and problem skin; stimulation for all skin types; facial massage; massage techniques to erase wrinkles; stimulation for problem skin; protection for all skin types; an anti-wrinkle campaign for ageing skins.

CHAPTER 2—COSMETIC APPLICATION AND CORRECTIVE MAKE-UP 15
Introduction; the illusion of beauty; facial shapes; typical proportions of facial types; magic of corrective make-up; do's and don'ts for facial shapes; classification of complexions; complexion coloring; enhancing the complexion with subtle cosmetic colors; cosmetic inventory; the eyebrows; plucking the brows; brow shapes for correcting facial features; lips; complete make-up application; hints for corrective make-up; rouge; corrective make-up for the eyes; effects of artificial light; a glossary of cleansers and creams.

CHAPTER 3—HAND CARE AND MANICURING 49
Introduction; manicuring equipment and materials; manicuring procedure; corrective nail polish; beauty tips for hands and nails.

CHAPTER 4—LEG CARE AND PEDICURING 55
Introduction; leg care; pedicuring; foot care.

CHAPTER 5—HAIR CARE, SHAMPOOING AND COIFFURE ARRANGEMENTS 57
Introduction; brushing the hair; shampooing; hair protection; coiffure arrangements for various hair colors; selecting a hairstyle; height; neck length; profiles; facial shapes; setting pin curls; the finishing touches.

UNIT TWO

Visual Poise

CHAPTER 6—STANDING 70
 Basic stance; legs classified; the pedestal stance; five hand-hip positions; additional hand positions; three rules for beautiful hands; review.

CHAPTER 7—WALKING 79
 Introduction; learning to walk correctly; the five-step practice walk; variation for five-step practice walk; techniques for a graceful walk; hand coordination with the feet; review; ten rules for a beautiful walk; you must practice.

CHAPTER 8—SITTING 87
 Introduction; learning to sit correctly; the "T" sitting position; the "S" sitting position; sitting-pretty principles for feet, legs and hands; don'ts for sitting; getting in and out of cars; do's and don'ts for getting in and out of a car.

CHAPTER 9—SOCIAL POSTURES 97
 Introduction; the arch; greeting people; the hand shake; the open doorway; the picture pose; leaving through an open doorway; the closed doorway; crossing in front of and standing before a group; stair techniques; stair rules.

CHAPTER 10—HANDLING PERSONAL BELONGINGS 105
 Introduction; wraps; coats; when your escort assists you; stoles; cigarettes; gloves; handbags.

CHAPTER 11—VISUAL POISE FOR SOCIAL AFFAIRS 119
 Introduction; our changing customs; let's go to the theatre; let's go to a party; refreshments; new contacts; going to dinner; time to eat; time to dance; repairing your lipstick; removing an unmasticable object; serving dessert; unforgivable manners.

UNIT THREE

Wardrobe Planning

CHAPTER 12—WARDROBE PLANNING 132
 Introduction; your clothing inventory; your clothing upkeep; how well do you care for your clothes?; types of fabric; avoid inferior fabrics.

CHAPTER 13—PLANNING PURCHASES **139**
>Plan to combine your ensembles; the order of purchase; imaginary shopping tour; selecting a store; intelligent purchase; buying by brand; match colors; hosiery shopping; personality and purchases; good shopping habits; appropriate dress for shopping; how to find the right foundation; buying bras and girdles.

CHAPTER 14—THE BASIC WARDROBE **149**
>Introduction; what is a basic wardrobe?; basic clothes; purchases for basic wardrobe; dress-up, dress-down accessories; seasonal items; fabrics for summertime only; fabrics for wintertime only; ingenious ways to get by; fabric combinations.

CHAPTER 15—LINES FOR FIGURE FLATTERY **161**
>Introduction; optical illusions in dress; illusions caused by lines; selecting flattering silhouette lines; what's your line?; how does your figure look?; the three hip lines; chart your figure foibles; style selector for figure types.

CHAPTER 16—THE PSYCHOLOGY OF COLOR AND COLOR MAGIC **177**
>Introduction; significance of color; the color wheel; color harmonies; color and personality; color magic; skin colors and their compliments; when your hair has turned to silver; colors in cosmetics; summary on color selection.

CHAPTER 17—ACCESSORIES **187**
>Introduction; hats; jewelry; earrings; necklaces and chokers; gloves; beautiful bags; shoes; scarf arrangements; boutonnieres; handkerchiefs; eyeglasses.

CHAPTER 18—THE TWELVE PERSONALITY TYPES IN DRESS **201**
>Introduction; dressing to type; analysis of personality types.

CHAPTER 19—FRAGRANCE **215**
>Introduction; where to apply; which is your type?; have your scents make sense.

UNIT FOUR

Personality Development

CHAPTER 20—PERSONALITY IS PREFERRED **220**
>Introduction; scientific approach to personality; the three major trait areas; the top nine traits; develop a positive slant; test of your friend-making skill; increasing your friend-making skill; seven keys to popularity for women; seven keys to popularity for men; the cornerstones to success.

CHAPTER 21—THE ART OF GRACIOUSNESS **231**

Introduction; a story to illustrate limited vision; be persuasive; how persuasive are you?; graciousness and manners; introductions; the handshake; when to make introductions; remembering names; additional hints on good manners; good manners quiz.

CHAPTER 22—SOCIABILITY AND PERSONALITY MEASUREMENTS **249**

Introduction; personality measurement; seven personality dimensions; chart your personality dimensions; what are your interests?; interests in the world of work; develop your interests; overcoming harmful personality traits.

UNIT FIVE

Your Voice and You

CHAPTER 23—VOICE IMPROVEMENT **258**

Introduction; achieving a satisfactory speaking voice; setting goals for voice improvement; develop your most attractive voice; qualities to develop; expressions to be avoided; words frequently misused; pronunciation; voice improvement.

CHAPTER 24—CONVERSATIONAL CHARM **267**

Introduction; the ten commandments for conversational charm; try to understand the other fellow's viewpoint; fit your mood to the mood of the occasion; learn to guide the conversation; don't be silent; don't monopolize the conversation; use simple language that all can understand; find out how people spend their leisure; don't become personal; talk about ideas rather than people; select entertaining rather than argumentative subjects; leadership through conversation; assignment for rewording questions.

CHAPTER 25—PUBLIC SPEAKING—PLATFORM TECHNIQUE **275**

Introduction; how to overcome stage fright; component parts of a speech; the importance of planning; selecting and developing the subject; have something worthwhile to say; applying the "seven-fold plan"; giving your subject life; a sample outline; bodily action; facial expression; twelve steps to success in public speaking.

UNIT SIX

Being Successful on The Job

CHAPTER 26—THE PSYCHOLOGY OF SUCCESS **286**
Introduction; what do you want?; motives; what is blocking your path?; how do you usually meet such barriers?; the direct approach; the positive attitude; summary.

CHAPTER 27—PERSONALITY POTENTIAL **293**
Introduction; twelve steps to a winning personality; promotion; leaving the job; plan your exit; winning confidence.

CHAPTER 28—CHARM IN THE OFFICE **299**
Introduction; rules of office etiquette; loyalty is important; cooperating with your co-workers; observe common courtesies; making office introductions; making special requests; your business manners in action; business etiquette away from the office; appropriate dress and grooming; dating after work; persons and pitfalls to avoid; sex appeal.

CHAPTER 29—THE BUSINESS TELEPHONE **317**
Introduction; answering the phone; telephone etiquette and technique; handling telephone complaints; telephone speech habits; personality-plus; good business practice; the tools of the telephone; rate your telephone manners.

CHAPTER 30—APPLYING FOR A JOB **323**
Introduction; preparing for a job interview; know your qualifications; dress correctly; last-minute suggestions; the resumé; the interview; acknowledging an interview.

CHAPTER 31—HOW TO CONDUCT A MEETING **331**
Introduction; parliamentary procedure; meaning of parliamentary procedures; basic principles of parliamentary procedure; definitions; duties of the officers; elections and voting; the order of business; duties of a good chairman; a dramatized exercise for "order of business"; committees; function of committees; special committees.

UNIT SEVEN
Body Perfection

CHAPTER 32—POSTURE FOR BODY PERFECTION 348
The spine; good posture; posture correction; posture exercises; causes of bad posture; correct standing and sitting postures; correct reaching technique; correct stooping technique.

CHAPTER 33—EXERCISES FOR BODY PERFECTION 357
Introduction; take your measurements; measurement chart; your daily exercise program; the exercises; general strength exercises; bustline building exercises; facial exercises; exercises for a firm neck and chin; for a beautiful back, arms and shoulders; for diaphragm and waistline; hipline trimmers; stomach exercises for the flat look; leg exercises; calf beautifiers; exercises for underweight; for over-developed calves; for over forty; for firming thighs.

CHAPTER 34—NUTRITION FOR BODY PERFECTION 391
Introduction; nutrition through balanced meals; fresh foods; cooked foods; devitalized foods; good digestion; impaired digestion; good circulation; good elimination; normal weight; losing weight; a calorie; carbohydrate-rich foods; fats and oils; protein-rich foods; alkaline mineral-rich foods; fresh fruits; liquids; rules for weight reduction; gaining weight; cleansing diet; maintaining normal weight; variety in balanced meals.

CHAPTER 35—RELAXATION FOR BODY PERFECTION 409
Introduction; barriers to relaxation; for tired feet; foot exercises; check your arches; bunions; for tired legs; for tired shoulders, neck and arms; for tense and tired torso; for headache and eye strain; massage for relaxation; Yoga exercises; ten commandments for happiness; time counts.

INDEX 425

UNIT ONE

SKIN CARE, COSMETIC APPLICATION AND HAIR BEAUTIFICATION

Introduction

Since the dawn of history, women have used beauty aids to add to their natural attractiveness. According to legend and written history, women of ancient times applied cosmetics with a deft hand and a great deal of results. Just think for a moment of Cleopatra's famed beauty that was due, in no small measure, to her beauty rituals. She used every artifice, including perfumed oils, to capture the hearts of Julius Caesar and Marc Anthony. Her success undoubtedly changed the course of history.

Perhaps you don't want to set the world on fire, but you probably wish to be as attractive as nature and the cosmetic industry will allow. There is no reason you can't be. Authorities believe that there are no unattractive women, only lazy ones and those who are uninformed.

CHAPTER 1

SKIN CARE

Be that as it may, you are going to enjoy being initiated into the mystic order of make-up artists. These are the girls who enhance their natural loveliness until they look glamorous. Webster defines glamour as "magic; a spell or charm." Glamour is something we can put on and take off, it is not permanent like natural beauty and should never be used as a substitute. No cosmetic in the world can take the place of a healthy, glowing complexion. To insure the beauty of your complexion, do you:

1. Eat a balanced diet?
2. Have regular elimination?
3. Drink plenty of water?
4. Get enough fresh air?
5. Get eight hours of sleep each night?
6. Exercise daily?
7. Avoid frowning and squinting?

SKIN CONDITIONS

The condition of your skin is affected by both internal and external factors. Among the *internal factors* are heredity, age, state of health, presence of disease, nutritional habits and glandular changes as during pregnancy or adolescence. Among the *external factors* are the weather; the temperature and humidity of the air indoors; sun exposure; contact with chemicals; friction that causes blisters, callouses and corns; and simply soap and water.

Our objective here is to teach the *steps in external skin care*. The first four include *cleansing, lubrication, stimulation* and *protection*. The next step is *beautification*. It is the glamourizing step and comes after, not before the other steps.

SKIN CARE

A dermatologist (*skin specialist*) can help you with extreme skin problems, but there are beauty rituals you can perform for yourself to guarantee "the skin you love to touch."

Keep in mind that your face can never be really attractive without a lovely complexion. Work toward having the type of skin that we call "normal" which is neither oily, dry, nor blemished.

Inasmuch as different skin conditions require different care (beauty rituals), we have devised five classifications. For you to discover into which one your skin fits, scrutinize your complexion with a magnifying mirror in bright light.

SKIN TYPES CLASSIFIED

Into which classification does your skin fall?

NORMAL SKIN Soft, supple, smooth. It is neither greasy nor dry in appearance; the texture is fine and even; the color is pink and softly glowing.

DRY SKIN Rough and scaly, feels "tight" and drawn, has fine lines at mouth and corners of eyes.

OILY SKIN Has oily shine, predisposition to blackheads, pimples, enlarged pores.

COMBINATION SKIN A combination of two or more types.

Combination skin needs to be treated as though it were world's apart. If you are wondering why you have enlarged pores on your forehead, nose or chin and not elsewhere, it is because of what make-up artists call the "T" Zone which is prone to oiliness.

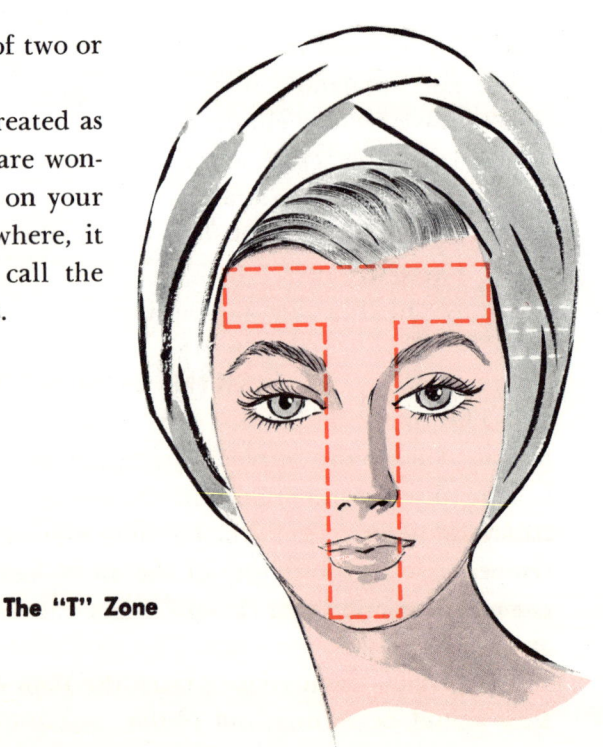

The "T" Zone

SKIN CARE

PROBLEM SKIN   Requires the assistance of a doctor if the problem is serious. If you have allergies or acne, do not proceed without a medical OK. The oiliness and acne of adolescence responds nine times out of ten to a program of controlled diet and external skin care. This condition is aggravated by sweets, pastries, chocolate, fried foods, fat meats, rich gravies, salad dressing and cream; consequently, these foods should be limited or eliminated.

Scrupulous cleansing and consistent daily care as outlined for "Oily Skin" should prove immensely beneficial. See pages 46-48, the glossaries on cleansers and creams for products that have been especially formulated for your condition.

STEP ONE IN SKIN CARE
"Cleansing is the foundation of a clear and glowing complexion."

CLEANSING FOR NORMAL SKIN   Use a mild soap twice a day, or if you prefer, use one of the new, wonderful cleansing lotions. Hollywood stars use cold cream to remove heavy make-up. This is an inexpensive cream and is not drying to the skin.

Scrub a rub dub, get in the tub;
don't go to bed with your make-up on.

You lucky one with the normal skin, keep in mind that your skin can change with the seasons and the passing of years. Keep a watchful eye on your lovely complexion to make sure it is not tipping the balance toward either oiliness or dryness. It is more likely to tip toward dryness because as we get older the oil glands become less active. Be particularly watchful after age twenty-five.

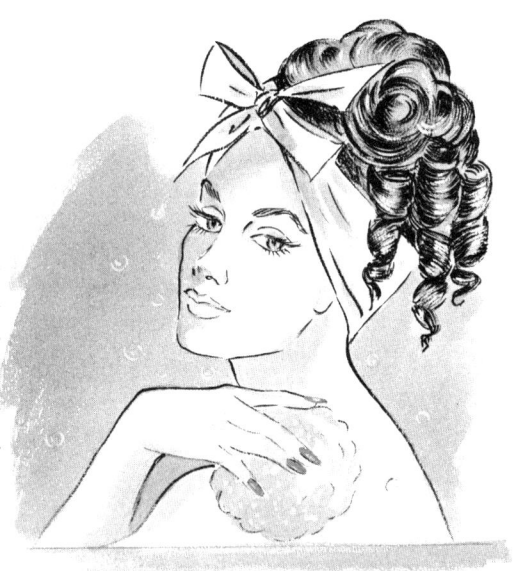

Don't sit on your laurels and assume that what's perfect today will be good tomorrow. But for now, congratulations! Keep up the good work.

CLEANSING FOR DRY SKIN   Dry skin needs soap and water too in moderate amounts, but washing should always be followed by the application of a good lubricating cream. If applied just before going to bed it can be left on the face during the night. The excess will be absorbed by the skin.

Dry skins usually fare best when they are cleansed only once a day. This would be at night, of course, to remove all make-up.

If you are not a soap and water gal because you have found that cleansing in this way makes your face feel "tight," use one of the excellent cleansing creams on the market that has been especially concocted for your dry skin.

Once-a-day cleansing is sufficient for you, if you will follow through on the suggestions given for you on *lubricating, stimulating* and *protecting*.

CLEANSING FOR OILY SKIN As you looked at your complexion with the magnifying mirror under good light, you were able to see the pores. They were enlarged and probably filled with oil. If they were black, they were dirty.... You have blackheads. If they were inflamed, they were infected.... You have a problem! It is your skin that needs the most fastidious cleansing. Once a day is not enough and maybe twice won't turn the tide. Cleanse your face often, and if you are inclined to pick at it, carry a small bottle of rubbing alcohol and some sterile cotton so you can dab the itches with this rather than with scratches. Keep your hands away from your face, you are just spreading the infection.

Use a generous amount of soap and water plus cleansing preparations that will:

1. Clean out the pores.
2. Dissolve the oil.
3. Kill bacteria.
4. Close the pores.

Keep your cleansing routine simple so that you will not be tempted to skip a single time, let alone a day.

CLEANSING FOR COMBINATION SKIN Select the simplest possible procedure for each area so that you can get the job done effectively and efficiently. For instance, if your "T" Zone is oily and the rest of your face is dry, wash the oily area with soap and water twice a day and finish off with an astringent. Wash the rest of your face only once a day or use just a cleansing cream on the dry area. Close the pores with cold water. It would be as simple as one, two, three.

1. Wash oily area and let suds remain on while you cream the dry area and wipe the cream off.
2. Rinse the entire face in cold water.
3. Place astringent on oily area.

Decide right now what procedure you are going to follow and do it. As your skin normalizes under your daily care, you can change your cleansing routine to fit its new condition.

CLEANSING FOR PROBLEM SKIN On pages 46-48, you will find a glossary on cleansers and creams. If your condition is mild or has developed because of neglect, you will probably get excellent results by selecting for

SKIN CARE

your personal use, those items on the market that have been made specifically for your problem, whatever it is. *For serious problems, don't do anything without the direction of your doctor.*

Warning: Don't make the mistake of thinking that if one product is good, two will be twice as good. Doctor your skin, don't drown it in unguents, ointments, salves, solvents, soaps, froths, foams and foundations.

STEP TWO IN SKIN CARE—LUBRICATION

The reason for lubricating the skin is to supplement the natural oils that have been removed by soap, weather and time.

LUBRICATING OILS

The oils used to lubricate the skin may be divided into three categories according to their origin.

MINERAL OILS These are taken from the ground and include petroleum jelly, paraffin wax and mineral oil.

VEGETABLE OILS These are extracted from plants and include a long list of seeds, nuts and herbs. The ones most commonly used on the skin are:

almond	palm
avocado	pine
cocoa butter	rose
camphor	sandalwood
lemon	sunflower
olive	wintergreen

ANIMAL OILS These are products of living creatures such as animals and fish. You have undoubtedly heard of:

butter	sperm (whale)
egg	tallow
lanolin	wool oil
lard	wool grease

All of these are used in one way or another on the skin, and lanolin especially has come into great popularity. It is used in a wide variety of beauty products for both skin and hair. It is reputed to be more like **human skin oil** than any other.

LUBRICATION FOR NORMAL OR DRY SKIN

Keeping the skin lubricated so that it isn't rough and tough (leathery) looking is just about half the battle of keeping the skin youthful. Whether your skin is normal or dry, you will want to supplement the natural oils, especially if you are over twenty-five. To prevent wrinkles and premature ageing, it is imperative that you keep your skin supple and smooth with lubrication.

PREVENTING DRY SKIN There are many products on the market for you to consider. There has been so much progress made in the area of prevention for ageing skins through cosmetics that it has been predicted that wrinkling will be unknown in the near future. But for now, *you* should take advantage of the products that are available to keep your skin young.

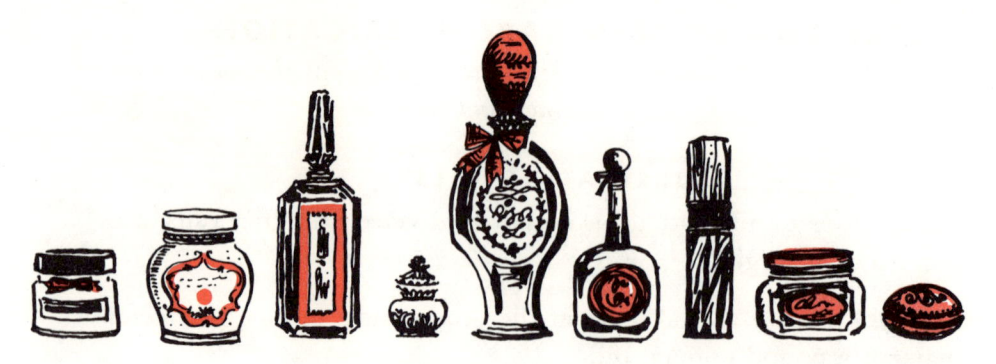

This is the one place we suggest you simply go "hog wild" and buy whatever you need to get results. The glossary on creams at the end of the chapter can serve as a guide. If you can afford several products, you may want to have all of these on your cosmetic shelf:

1. Cleansing cream
2. Lubricating cream or oil
3. Eye oil
4. Hormone or vitamin cream
5. Humectant cream
6. Bath oil
7. Hand and Body lotion

Some products are made to get multiple results. For example, your lubricating cream may contain both vitamins and humectants.

LUBRICATION FOR OILY AND COMBINATION SKIN

Perhaps you skimmed over the "lubricating" section thinking that your skin would need no lubrication because it was already oily. If you have examined it carefully though, you have probably discovered that you have a *combination skin*. Perhaps your face is oily only in the "T" Zone.

But whether it is oily or combination, it will benefit from the manipulations suggested under "Massage." For this, you will need mineral oil at least. For the normal or dry areas, refer to the preceding paragraphs.

LUBRICATION FOR PROBLEM SKIN

If your problem is acne, you will want to use an acne cream for your facial massage. Other than this, skip the step of lubrication in skin care until your face clears.

If your problem is sensitiveness or allergy, select one of the hypo-allergenic creams that is non-irritating. You will find them almost devoid of perfume, but otherwise as pleasant to use as any.

SKIN CARE

STEP THREE IN SKIN CARE—STIMULATION

The purpose of stimulating the skin and its underlying structure is to clear up complexion blemishes and retain or restore youthfulness.

There is a two-fold good to be realized from stimulation of the skin. One is increased circulation to carry away waste products and bring new life-giving nutrients to the cells. The other is the removal of the sloughed off dead cells and debris. Obviously, the younger the individual cells of the skin, the more youthful it will appear.

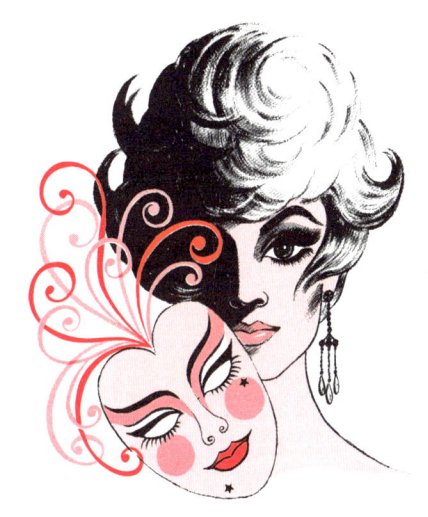

STIMULATION FOR ALL SKIN TYPES

There are a number of methods from which you can choose the ones that are best suited to your skin and your way of life. Just keep in mind that you want your program to stimulate both internally and externally. Also keep in mind that your complexion doesn't mean just your face, although because it is exposed, you give it special care. But any program on skin care that is complete will include the entire surface of the body and not just the face and hands.

Here is a summary of the methods from which you can choose:

1. CHANGES OF TEMPERATURE

    For the *face:*

        Skin freshner after cleansing.

        Splashing with cold water.

    For the *body:*

        Alcohol rubs.

        A warm bath followed by a cold shower.

    For *face* and *body:*

        Rubbing with ice cubes (very invigorating).

        Hot packs alternated with cold.

2. EXERCISING

    For the *face:*

        Doing facial exercises in front of a mirror or using an electric impulse machine designed for this purpose.

    For the *body:*

        Doing general exercises vigorously enough to perspire.

3. CHANGING THE FLOW OF BLOOD

For the *face:*

By putting the head down between the knees.

By assuming the knee-chest position. This is done by kneeling and leaning the torso forward to the floor.

For the *face* and *body:*

By lying with the feet higher than the head in the "beauty slant" position.

By standing on the head like a Yogi.

The Beauty Slant

4. PACKS

For the *face:*

A wonderful variety from which to choose, such as; hot oil, clay, egg, milk, mint, oat meal.

For the *body:*

Professional mud baths, hot packs and wax treatments are given in some massage parlors.

5. MASSAGE

For the *face:*

Facial manipulation with hands or vibrator.

For the *body:*

The brush bath which is done in the tub with a fairly stiff brush and mild soap suds. Brush from the extremities toward the heart. This exercises the tiny muscles in the skin and helps to keep it functioning properly.

FACIAL MASSAGE FOR EVERYONE

Experiments show that women who massage their faces have definitely better complexions than those who do not. Aside from softening the skin, massage stimulates the circulation in the surface blood vessels that bring "life" to the complexion.

Experts on massage have been reluctant to suggest that the average woman attempt to massage her own face because of the damage that can result from stretching the skin. This danger can be avoided by first applying a cream of some sort so that your fingers can slide over the skin rather than pull it. Be sure to use upward and outward motions, don't drag down.

It is suggested that you do your facial massage in the privacy of your bathroom so that you can strip to the waist and thereby avoid the serious mistake of not including your neck and shoulders. Protect your hair with a shower cap, head band, towel or whatever and here we go!

SKIN CARE

MASSAGE TECHNIQUES

Use both hands. Get the elbows up and out, away from the body. Use the thumbs for anchors, massage with the finger tips except where the heel of the thumb is suggested.

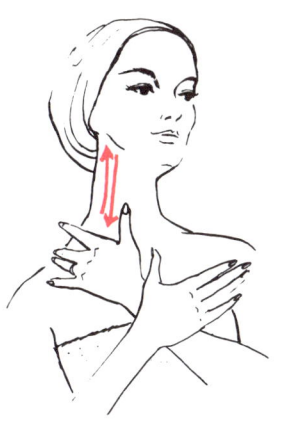

NECK AND CHEST MANIPULATION Massage the right side of the throat with the left hand and vice versa. Stroke up to the hair line and down to the shoulders. Don't neglect the back of the neck.

JAW MANIPULATION To "rub out" jowls and double chins use the heel of the thumb of each hand, the right hand on the right side; alternating hands, make upward, outward circles. Really press the flesh against the bone.

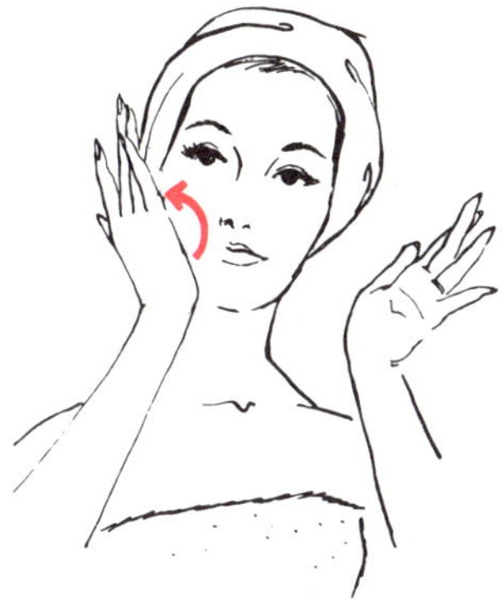

For Neck and Chest

The Jaw

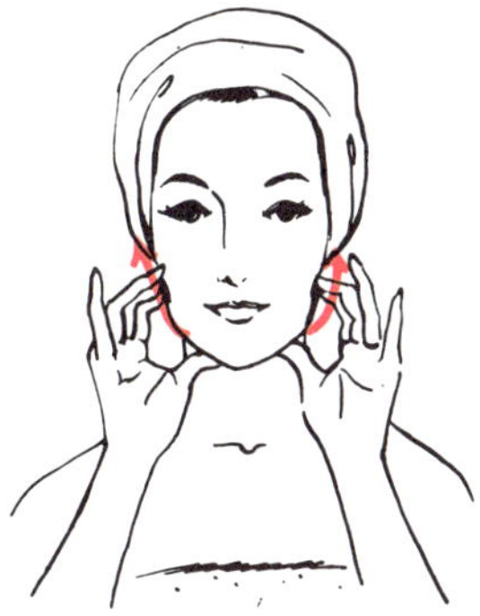

CHEEK MANIPULATION Anchor the thumbs under the jaw, start with the fingers close to the jaw and "walk" them up the cheeks toward the top of the ear. Return and repeat.

EYE AREA MANIPULATION Gently pat, don't rub, the area below and above the eye where there is no underlying bone. This is sensitive, thin skin so use plenty of cream.

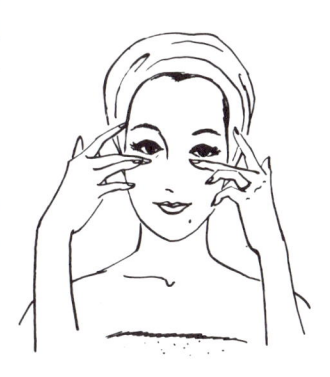

For the Cheeks

Eye Area

FOREHEAD MANIPULATION Anchor the thumbs on the temples. Start at the bridge of the nose and rub upward and outward with alternating hands. Get a move on. Quick, quick, quick!

While your thumbs are anchored to the temples, do the next one.

NOSE MANIPULATION Use the middle finger, alternate hands and rub downward on the nose. Finish off by making circles at the side of each nostril.

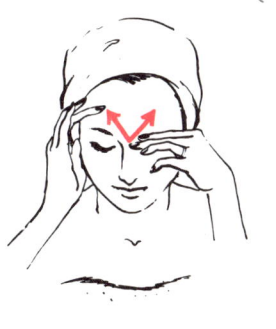

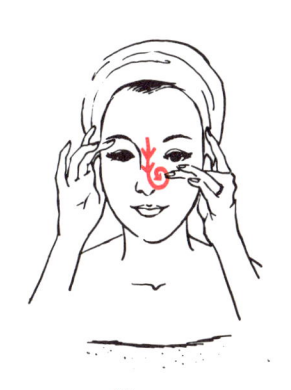

The Forehead

Nose

MASSAGE TECHNIQUES TO ERASE WRINKLES

1. *Laughter lines around the mouth.* Puff up the cheeks with air and gently massage the laughter lines with upward, outward circular motions. Also pat the puff with outward strokes.
2. *Laughter lines at the corners of the eyes.* Manipulation here should be very light. Use the middle and ring finger to make small upward-outward circles.
3. *Frown lines between the eyebrows.* Massage across the lines with horizontal strokes. Alternate hands, but keep both thumbs anchored on temples.
4. *Furrows on the forehead.* A circular motion across the forehead with first one hand and then the other will prove beneficial.

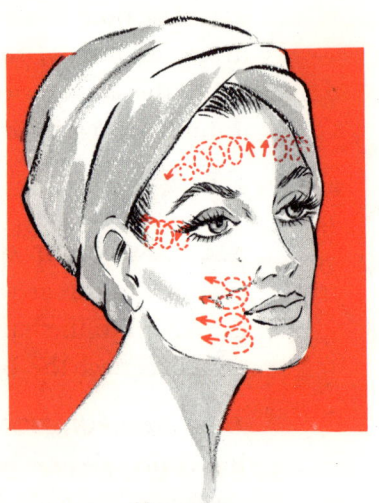

Massage To Erase Wrinkles

"An ounce of prevention is worth a pound of cure," is one adage that holds true. Everytime you are tempted to neglect the daily care of your skin, think about it.

Perhaps you have given some thought as to how you can work out a ritual just before going to bed that will combine several steps. For instance, you can cleanse and cream your face just before your bath; after your bath of warm and cold water, you can place a large towel on the bed and rub your entire body with your favorite lotion or oil. Lie on the towel and swing both legs up in the air where you can reach them with your hands while lying on your back. You will be getting the stimulation of warm and cold temperatures, the stimulation of massage, and the stimulation of changing the flow of blood by having your feet in the air. Besides, you have a towel handy to wipe off any excess oil. Baby your skin if you want it to be soft as a baby's.

TO SUM UP ON MASSAGE

1. Never massage without a lubricant.
2. Be gentle so that you don't stretch the skin or cause irritation.
3. Never drag down on the face but use upward, outward motions.
4. You can be gentle but firm.
5. Massage is beneficial for all types of skin.

STIMULATION FOR PROBLEM SKIN

SUNSHINE AND SUN LAMPS Doses of sunshine will help dry up pimples and eliminate enlarged pores. Many dermatologists suggest the use of a sun lamp for winter months. A sun lamp is an inexpensive investment in health and beauty that requires only five minutes a day.

SKIN CARE

THE SALT RUB Another wonder-worker for oily skin is a salt rub. You simply rub damp salt onto your skin while it is lathered with soap. The salt is very drying and should be used only once or twice a week, maybe less often. Try it.

FACE PACKS There are a number of face "packs" on the market that are excellent. They help to refine the pores and slough off scale and dead tissue. They make the skin look fresher and more youthful.

Warning: Don't try too many things at one time. It is much wiser for you to decide on a particular procedure and stay with it for several weeks rather than trying all suggestions at one time.

The stimulation you accomplish while cleansing your face will aid it toward normalcy.

STEP FOUR IN SKIN CARE—PROTECTION

Protecting the skin is to prevent roughness, dryness and ageing caused by exposure. This again, is that ounce of prevention, worth a pound of cure.

PROTECTION FOR ALL SKIN TYPES

You have undoubtedly observed a woman's face that looked older than her body, or a woman's hands that looked older than she really was. Did you ever wonder why? It is because the skin of the face and hands is not protected from the elements and dirt and grime by clothing as is the rest of the body. You should have learned a lesson. . . . The skin in these areas needs protection too.

You can protect the pores of your face with foundation that is either colored or colorless and the skin of your hands with gloves. You should plan to wear rubber gloves whenever there is rough work to be done. Wear the new "invisible" gloves of protective lotion always.

Your skin continues to grow until death; therefore, it is possible for you to retain a youthful complexion if you will follow the rules for internal and external health.

It seems that women who live in climates that are hot and dry have older looking skins than those who live in more temperate climates. All old looking skins are dry skins. It is dry skin that wrinkles. Keep your skin forever young looking by protecting it and, remember, skins do not take kindly to long sun exposure. Avoid it.

TO SUMMARIZE ON EXTERNAL SKIN CARE

1. There must be consistent daily care.
2. Cleansing is the most important ritual.
3. Lubricating enhances softness which is synonymous with femininity.
4. Stimulating the skin encourages it to produce new cells.
5. Protecting your skin today will beautify it tomorrow.

AN ANTI-WRINKLE CAMPAIGN FOR AGEING SKINS

NUTRITION Any woman seriously interested in wrinkle-resistance must learn her vitamin A.B.C.'s. It's an accepted fact that adequate protein helps tone the muscles and firm the skin. Vitamin B_1 (one) as in wheat germ, brewer's yeast, pork, cereal grains and sunflower seeds helps stabilize nerves. Calcium as in cheese and milk helps the nerves as well as the bones and teeth. Jittery nerves cause facial pleats; calm nerves, smooth face. Vitamin C as in oranges and green vegetables helps skin suppleness. Vitamin E as in butter and wheat germ oil can stave off ageing.

FACIAL EXERCISE Exercise for the face is deeply firming, definitely young-making. Lines can be lifted out when the muscles controlling that portion of the face are properly stimulated and exercised. The most widely available method of achieving a muscular workout for the face is done professionally in passive, high-speed electronic form. The technician knows exactly how to select the muscle that underlies the trouble.

There are a few schools in which "setting up exercises for the face" are routinely taught. Next to plastic surgery, the most dramatic results known are produced by facial exercise.

CREAMS AND LOTIONS Anti-wrinkle creams fall into two groups: one, to alleviate the *external* causes of the skin's ageing; the other, to combat *internal* causes. Into the first group would go the moisturizers and contour creams. Into the second, the preparations with serums, vitamins, placenta or estrogenic hormones. Conducting an anti-wrinkle campaign without these is pointless.

THE "FACIAL" What most salon facial treatments can be expected to do is cleanse, brighten and smooth the face. Such treatments generally concentrate on improving the skin from the connective tissue up. Although the benefits are temporary, they are noticeable immediately. By-product of even one professional treatment is the groundwork laid for the forming of good daily habits by the realization of what just one treatment can do. Some facial treatments are given "in depth." The surface muscles are manipulated to tighten the skin by toning the muscles that lie under the skin.

PLASTIC SURGERY The most spectacular of plastic surgery operations is face lifting, rhytidectomy. An oblique incision is made on either side of the forehead beyond the hairline. Along this planned incision, a strip of superfluous skin, responsible for the wrinkles, is carefully removed. Although this type of surgery is not effective forever and the cost is considerable, it is one solution for the woman who can't be happy with her face as it is.

CHAPTER 2

COSMETIC APPLICATION AND CORRECTIVE MAKE-UP

Introduction

From Nefertiti of ancient Egypt until the present time, women have been using cosmetics to enhance their natural beauty. But until a few short years ago, the beauty secrets of the world's loveliest women belonged to a favored few. It was not until late in the nineteenth century that word leaked out—the common girl could improve on nature with powder, paint and perfume. She could quite literally be a Cinderella who always wins the fella.

Although cosmetics are old, they are new in that great advances have been made in recent years. Today there is a variety of colors available in foundation, rouge, lipstick, powder and eye make-up. The up-to-the-minute beauty takes advantage of this. She carefully selects those colors that will flatter her own natural loveliness to make her look *naturally* lovely.

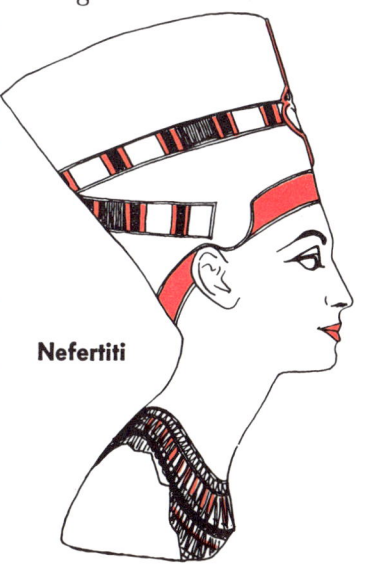

Nefertiti

THE ILLUSION OF BEAUTY

Beauty has many facets all of which contribute to the illusion of a dream ... walking. Two important facets are harmony of color and harmony of line. Before you start creating the illusion of beauty with make-up, you need to ask yourself two questions:

1. What colors should I choose for my make-up to emphasize the best in my hair, eye and skin coloring.
2. What lines should I choose for my face and features to create the ideal oval?

FACIAL SHAPES

The oval is considered the perfect face shape. Everything that you do with make-up should tend to make your face appear more oval. You will be unable to do this until you have carefully studied your face; its lines, planes, angles and shape. Before you can apply the deceptions used by renowned beauties, you must be thoroughly aware of your best features, and your worst.

What is the shape of your face? The best way for you to discover its shape is to be about twelve inches away from a mirror with a head band pulling your hair back exposing the hairline. Look directly into the mirror. Now read the descriptions given for the seven face shapes and see if you can place your own.

TYPICAL PROPORTIONS OF THE FACIAL TYPES

THE OVAL FACE The artistically ideal proportions and features of the oval face are used to form the basis for all corrective make-up application. It is divided into equal thirds lengthwise. The first third is measured from the hairline to the point between the eyebrows where they begin. The second third is measured from here to the end of the nose. The last third is measured from the end of the nose to the bottom of the chin.

The ideal oval face is approximately three-fourths as wide as it is long.

The distance between the eyes is the width of one eye.

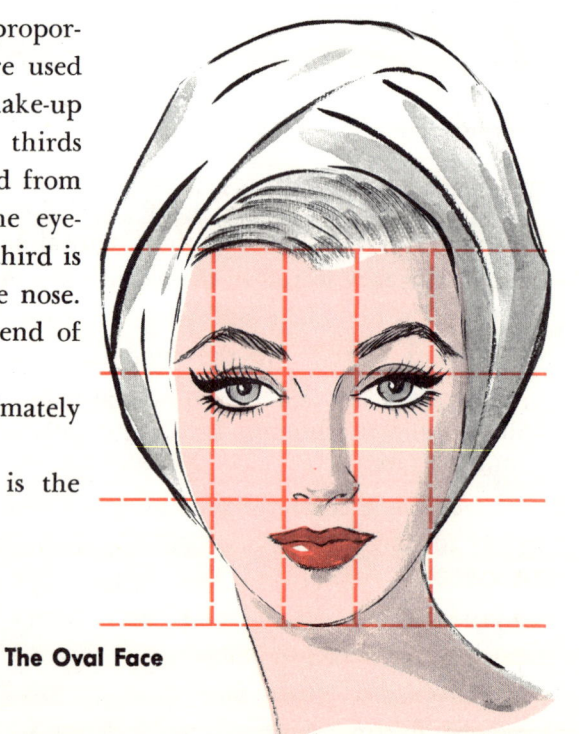

The Oval Face

COSMETIC APPLICATION AND CORRECTIVE MAKE-UP

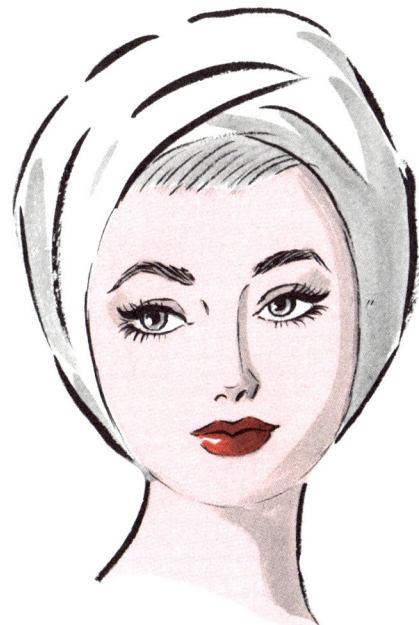

THE ROUND FACE The round face is usually broader in proportion to its length than the oval face. It has a rounding chin and hairline.

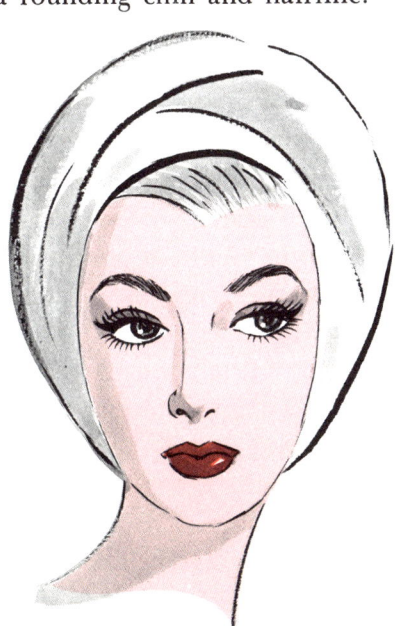

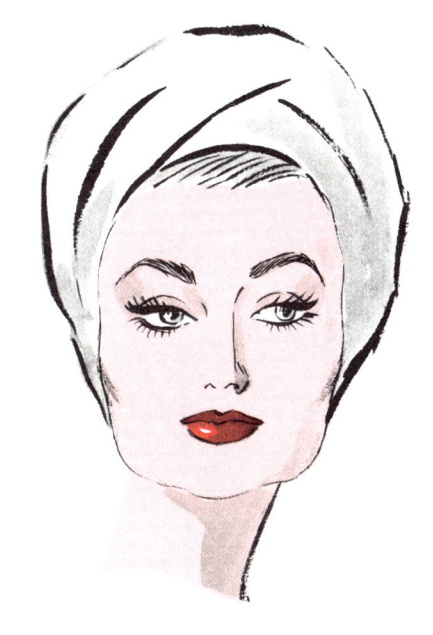

THE SQUARE FACE The square face is composed of comparatively straight lines with a straight forehead hairline and square jawline.

THE OBLONG FACE This face too has fairly straight lines, but it has greater length in proportion to its width than the square face. It is long and narrow.

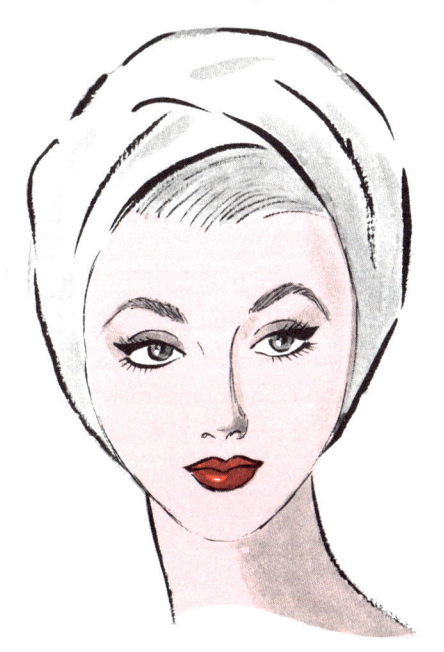

THE HEART-SHAPED FACE This face gets its name from the Valentine heart shape. It has a wide forehead and a pointed, narrow chin.

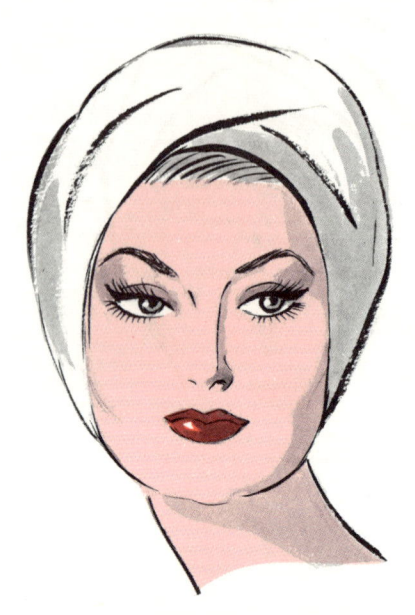

THE TRIANGULAR FACE This face is characterized by a jaw that is wider than the forehead.

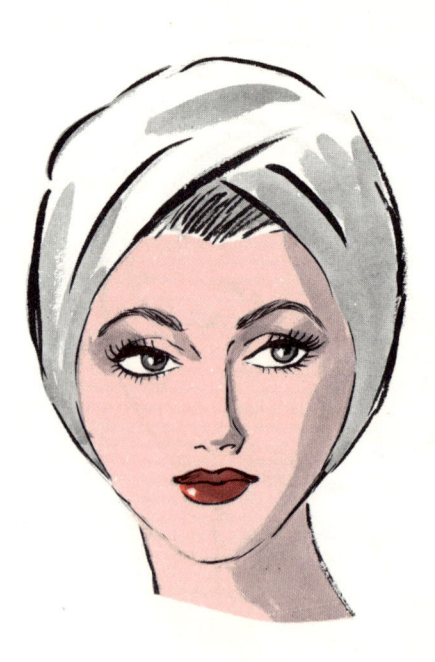

THE DIAMOND FACE This face has a narrow forehead combined with a narrow chin. This creates an appearance of too much width across the cheek bones.

If you have looked and looked and still cannot decide just what shape your face is, enlist the aid of a friend or two. They are bound to look at your face more objectively than you possibly can. Keep in mind too that your face might be a combination of shapes. For instance, it may be a square-oval, oval in shape but angular in appearance. Don't let this discovery throw you. A little time spent in experimentation will tell you the right combination of hair, eyebrow and lip lines that will be most flattering.

Read again, carefully, the description for the ideal oval. Where does your face differ? Apply the rules for giving width, length, softness of whatever is needed to create the illusion of the perfect oval.

Have fun!

COSMETIC APPLICATION AND CORRECTIVE MAKE-UP 19

THE MAGIC OF CORRECTIVE MAKE-UP

Beautifying the face through cosmetic application is the sorcery of enhancing your natural good looks with the corrected lines of eyebrows and lips and the heightening of your complexion and eye coloring. The following rules will serve as a helpful guide in the application of cosmetics.

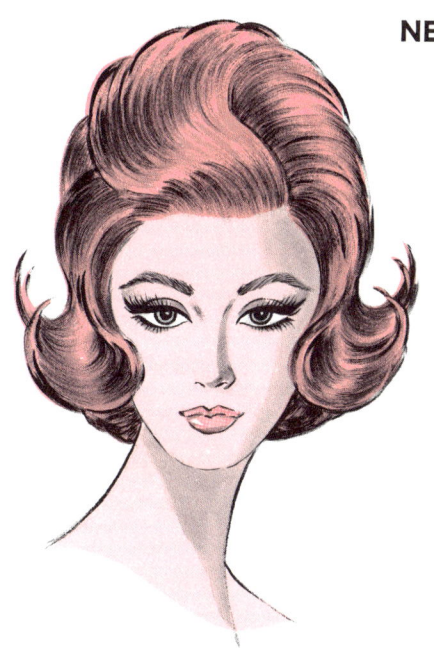

NEW FACES

THE OVAL FACE

Place rouge on your cheek, in the center and then blend it up over the cheekbone toward the temple. If you have dark circles under your eyes you can blend it lightly under the eye area.

Keep your eyebrow line natural and follow the general rules for eyebrows given at the end of the chapter.

Apply eye-shadow to the lid close to the lashes from inner corner to outer corner.

Mascara on the upper lashes only please.

Follow the natural outline for your lips unless they are a problem and then use rules on lip lines on page 39.

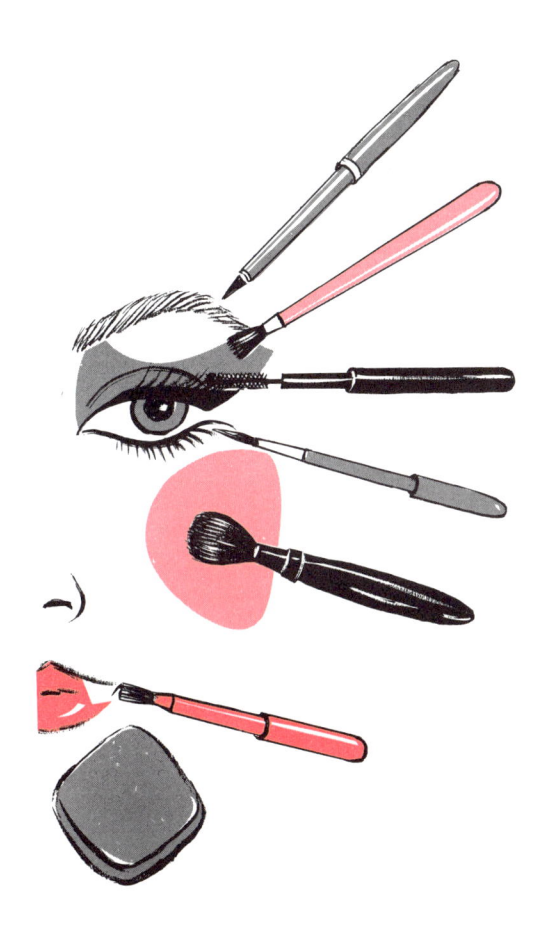

COSMETIC APPLICATION AND CORRECTIVE MAKE-UP

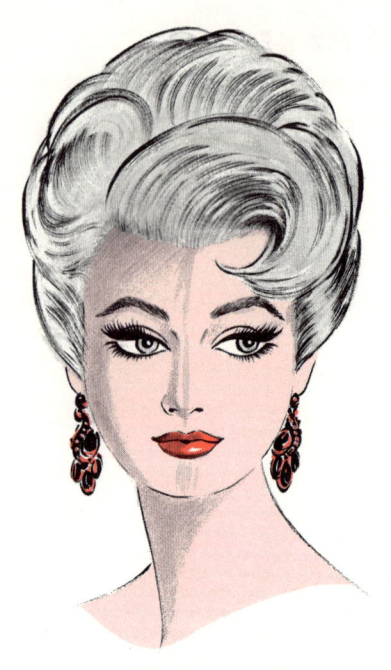

THE ROUND FACE

An inverted V line to the eyebrow will give some much needed angularity.

Because your face doesn't need width, keep your eyebrows fairly short.

For the same reason, angle your eyeshadow toward the end of the brow.

Rouge toward the center of the cheek.

Shade out the roundness of the jaw with a slightly darker foundation.

Make your mouth wide and full. Use straight lines as suggested on page 38, "Lipstick Application."

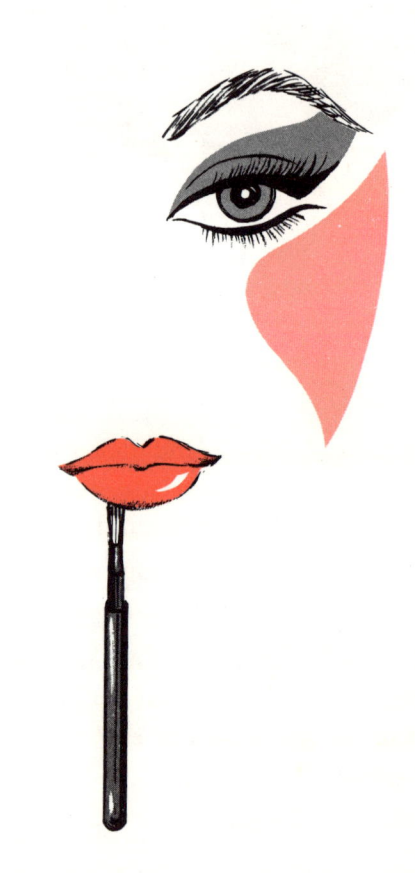

COSMETIC APPLICATION AND CORRECTIVE MAKE-UP 21

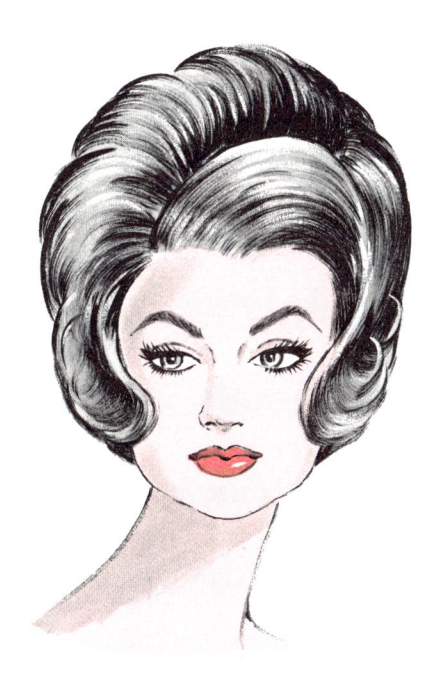

THE SQUARE FACE

Rouge that forms a light V line will lengthen the face and give it more ovalness.

With your eyebrow, remember that length adds width and that a curve will minimize the straight lines of your face.

Eye-shadow can be applied to give the eye an upward slant by applying it close to the eye just above the lashes on the inner eye, but bringing it to the eyebrow by the temples (not too exaggerated now).

You can minimize your square jaw line by darkening it with a shade darker foundation than you use for the rest of your face.

Your mouth must look full and round. The corners should come to a point just below the pupil of the eye.

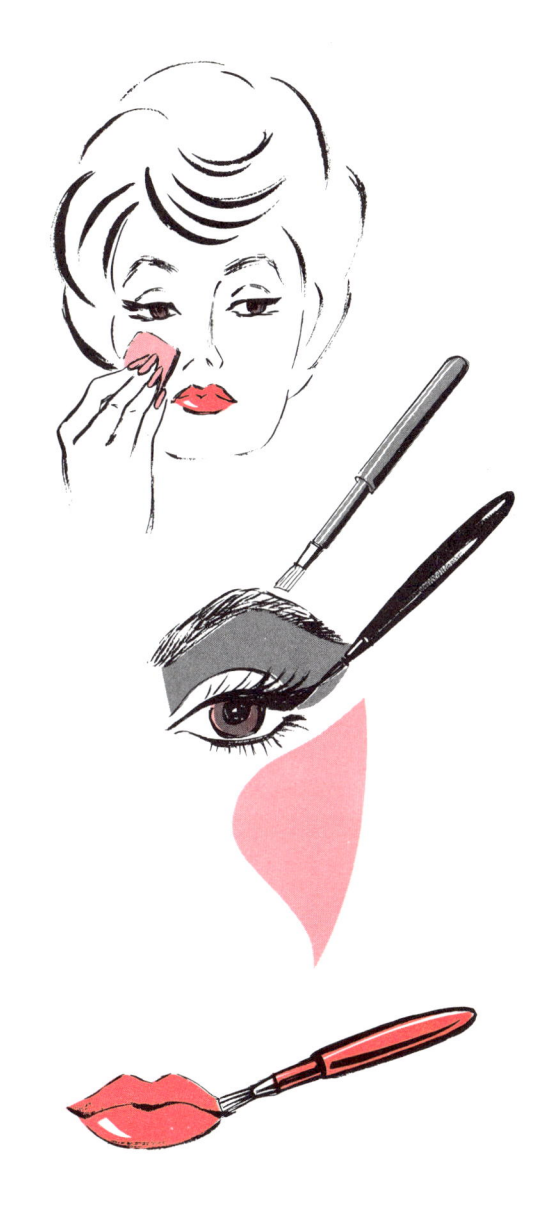

Incidentally your type of face has a look of strength, don't weaken it with too little hair, too thin eyebrows, or a too thin mouth.
Note: Round lines will counteract square ones.

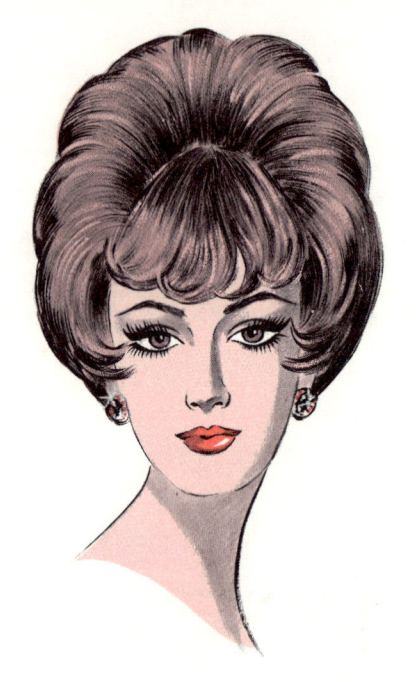

THE OBLONG FACE

A long face can be minimized if the eye area is made as broad as possible. This calls for a nicely curved eyebrow that ends well beyond the outer corner of the eye.

An oblong face calls for rouge applied on the cheek bone and blended out and up on the temple.

Eye-shadow can be applied more heavily on the outer corner as can mascara. The emphasis should be as far away from the nose as possible.

Your mouth should be softly rounded with the lip rouge coming to the natural corners.

Incidentally, you will enjoy having a certain amount of width in your hairstyle right at the temples. Try it and see.

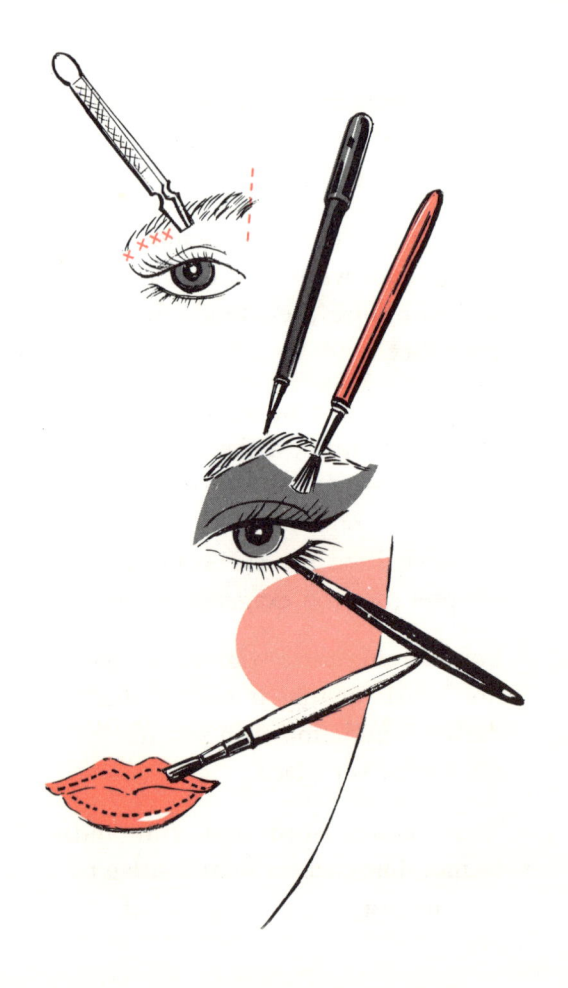

COSMETIC APPLICATION AND CORRECTIVE MAKE-UP

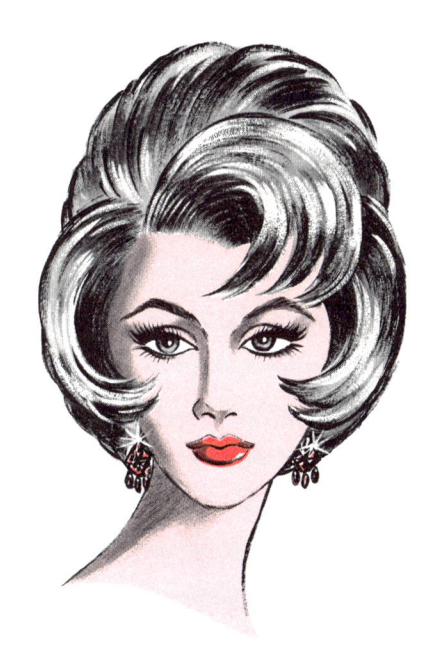

THE HEART-SHAPED FACE

Eyebrows should be rounded in the arch rather than pointed. To point them would be to repeat the pointed chin line and would emphasize it.

Rouge should be applied under the middle of the eye and should be blended out on the cheek bone.

Mascara and eye-shadow should give emphasis to the entire eye.

Use eye liner for evening only. It will be too harsh for your face in the daytime.

The lower lip should have a flat horizontal line across the bottom between the two spots directly below the nostrils. The upper lip should be softly rounded but not exaggerated.

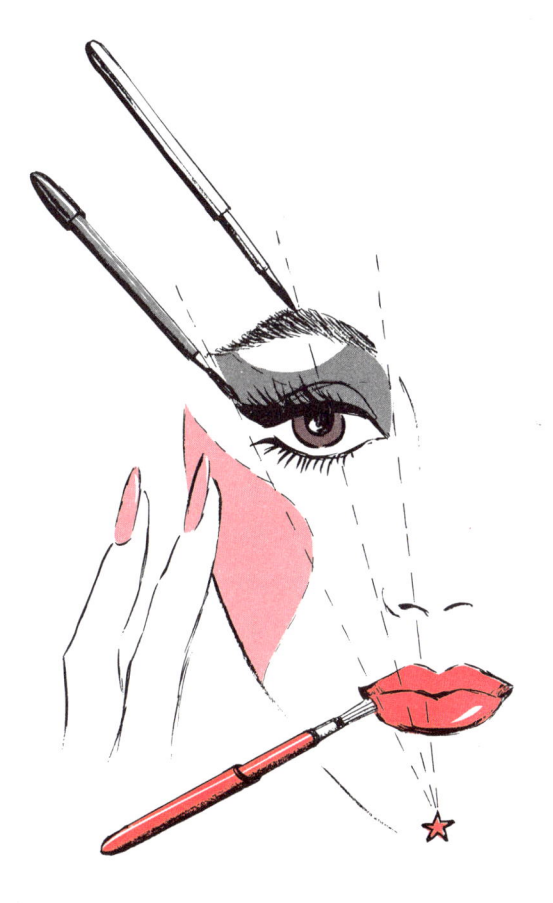

The width of the forehead and temple can be minimized by applying a darker foundation to the temple area from hairline to one-half inch in on the face. If the forehead protrudes, apply to entire forehead.

If the chin is long as well as pointed, apply the darker foundation horizontally across the tip.

COSMETIC APPLICATION AND CORRECTIVE MAKE-UP

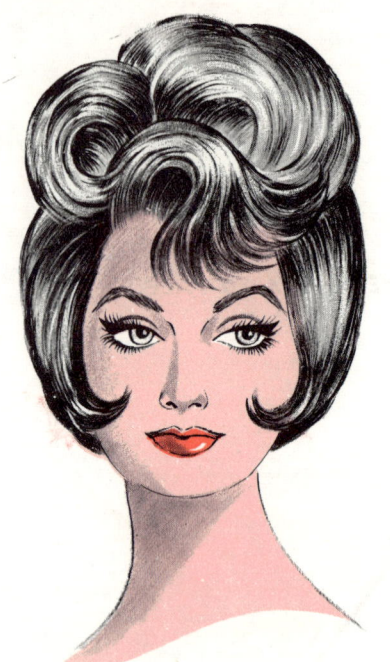

THE TRIANGULAR FACE

An eyebrow that has its highest point slightly out beyond the iris of the eye will give width. So will extending the eyebrow about one-eighth of an inch beyond the imaginary line drawn from the nostril past the corner of the eye.

Rouge application that gives a point of interest wide on the face about one-half inch from the hairline will give width where it is needed to counter-balance the width of the jaw.

Mascara and eye-shadow should be applied as for the square face with most of the interest on the outer one-third of the eye.

Eye make-up is a real boon for you. It draws attention to your eyes and away from the lower part of the face.

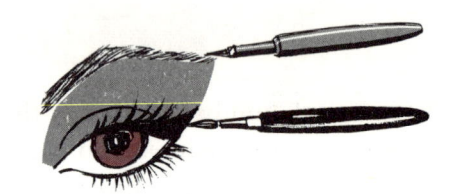

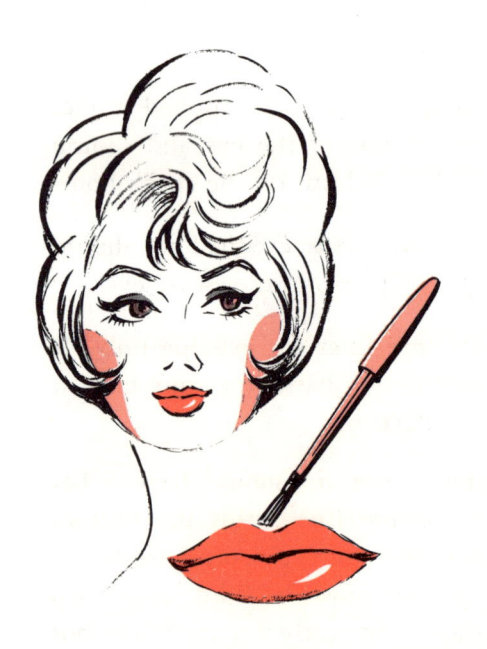

Rounding the lower lip line will minimize the wide jaw line. Making the upper lip slightly full will help too.

Do shade out some of the width of the jaw with a foundation a shade or two darker than that used on the rest of the face.

COSMETIC APPLICATION AND CORRECTIVE MAKE-UP

THE DIAMOND-SHAPED FACE

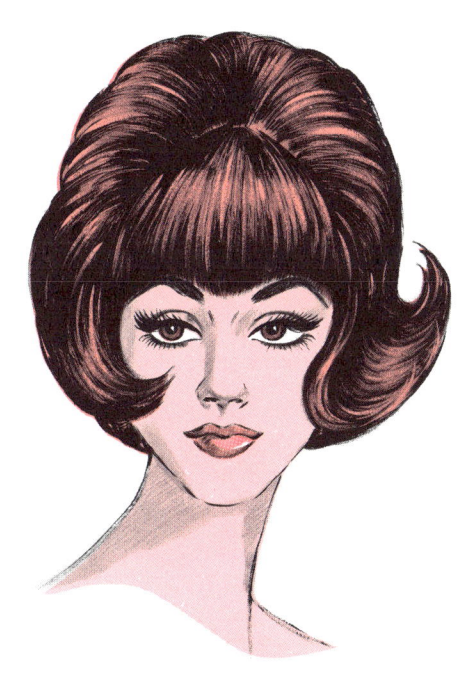

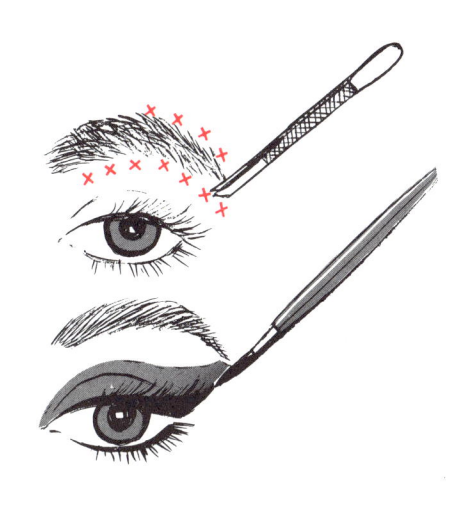

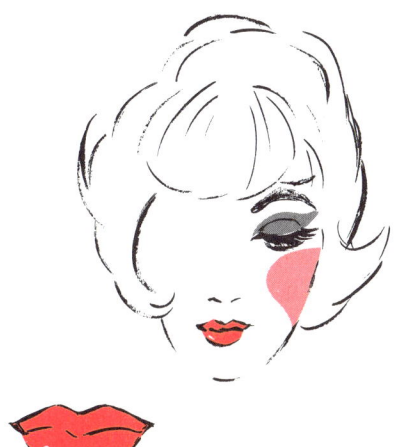

A straight eyebrow will give more width at the forehead.

Rouge applied very high right under the eye and smoothed out almost to the hairline on the temple.

Mascara and eye-shadow should be applied as for the square face. You'll love the "winged" look.

Try for a delicate mouth line that will fit neatly onto your face.

By the way, if your chin is long you can break the line by having some hair shown below the ears.

Let your face be polished, not a diamond in the rough.

CLASSIFICATION OF COMPLEXIONS

The purpose of this section will be to educate you in the selection of *cosmetic colors* so that you can bring your natural good looks to their fullest bloom. The techniques for make-up application will soon be within your reach, in fact, within your hand. This is your golden opportunity to become a conjurer of beauty.

It has been found that the "perfect beauty" is the woman who has learned to give the illusion of perfection. She has achieved this by the *subtle* application of make-up.

Select the shades for your make-up that will compliment your eyes, hair and skin. Choose them so that they seem to be a part of you and not something you have plastered on without rhyme or reason.

COMPLEXION COLORING

"Complexion" is the word that will be employed throughout this section to denote the *color* of the skin. Seven categories ranging from "white" through "ebony" will classify the various complexions according to the predominating color tone.

Assuming that complexions vary in color because of different combinations of red, yellow and brown, which best describes your skin?

WHITE COMPLEXION:

Has very little color. It has a translucent quality like china; is usually associated with blond hair.

CREAM COMPLEXION:

This is the peaches and cream complexion of story and song. It has an equal combination of red and yellow and a varying amount of brown.

PINK COMPLEXION:

Has more red than yellow and is most often combined with red hair. If it is too pink it looks flushed. It is the florid complexion.

GOLDEN COMPLEXION:

Is the so called "sallow" complexion. It has an over-abundance of yellow and varying amounts of brown. It may range from light to medium dark in value.

TAN COMPLEXION:

This skin is medium to dark in value. It has an abundance of red, yellow and especially brown.

COSMETIC APPLICATION AND CORRECTIVE MAKE-UP

OLIVE COMPLEXION:

The cool looking skin that seems to have almost green undertones. It is usually combined with brown eyes and dark hair.

BROWN, COPPER OR EBONY COMPLEXIONS:

The underlying skin tone may be reddish, tan or copper.

Having read through the seven categories, were you able to place your own complexion? If not, ask your teacher to assist you, or you may wish to compare your complexion with several others. The minute you place your face next to another, you will be able to see the subtle differences in coloring.

Your analysis will not be accurate unless you remove all make-up and study your skin in a light that is like daylight. You may even wish to go out-of-doors. There's nothing better than broad daylight to give you a true analysis.

Before we continue with the selection of colors for your make-up, let's get a vocabulary we can use to discuss the qualities we need to know about color.

DEFINITIONS DESCRIBING COLOR:

1. *Value* Indicates the lightness or darkness of a color.
2. *Hue* Indicates the predominant underlying tone i.e., pink hue.
3. *Intensity* Indicates the brightness or dullness of a color. For a color to be more intense, it is brighter.

We also need to understand some of the *terms* used by make-up artists, such as:

TERMS: (used to denote intensity of color)

1. *Emphasize* To make more noticeable, to accent.
2. *Minimize* To make less noticeable, to detract from.
3. *Highlight* To make the lightest portion; to give vivid interest.

Who says you have to follow any prescribed set of rules when selecting your make-up colors? Nobody, that's who. The only thing is, you want your make-up to compliment and enhance, you don't want it to make you look like a Halloween mask. One safe criterion to follow for daytime make-up is: *Let your lipstick be the only obvious cosmetic.* Apply everything else with a light hand. Don't miss the boat of beauty by over-emphasizing.

ENHANCING THE COMPLEXION
WITH SUBTLE COSMETIC COLORS

WHITE COMPLEXION Because this skin has very little pigment, it needs to have a certain amount of color added to enhance its beauty.

Foundation

Slightly darker in value than the skin; pink undertone.

Rouge

Pink or coral, rather than true red or blue-red, will be consistent with the delicacy of the skin tone.

Powder

A shade lighter than foundation, with pink hue.

Eyebrow Pencil

Slightly darker than the hair. Usually light brown.

Eye-Shadow

Pastel colors to compliment the clothing. Light blue, light green, light violet are lovely.

Eye Liner

Please, not in the daytime. A colored eye liner to match your eye-shadow will be more delicate than brown for evening wear. Absolutely no black.

Mascara

Dark brown unless you like the drama of black mascara. Use it on the upper lashes only.

Lipstick

The same hue as rouge. It may be a shade darker.

CREAM COMPLEXION To change the color of this complexion with foundation, is to gild the lily.

Foundation

Colorless, or colored to match the skin tones.

Rouge

Should match the natural coloring of the cheeks. This may be red, pink or coral. If you prefer, match your rouge and lipstick to the dress color when it is in the red range.

Powder

If the complexion is clear, you may prefer to go without powder. Otherwise, just a shade lighter than foundation.

Eyebrow Pencil

If the eyebrows are too light, a shade slightly darker than the hair. Otherwise, the same color as the eyebrows.

Eye-Shadow

Light, bright colors. Experiment. If you can afford only one color, match it to your eyes.

COSMETIC APPLICATION AND CORRECTIVE MAKE-UP

Eye Liner
>May match the eye-shadow in a darker value, or it may be black or brown like your mascara for evening.

Mascara
>Dark brown or black.

Lipstick
>The same as rouge only more intense.

PINK COMPLEXION This is the skin that needs its intensity minimized.

Foundation
>Less pink than the skin but not so different as to make the coloring look unnatural. Success is ofttimes achieved by selecting a color for the foundation that blends with the freckles sometimes found with this type of skin.

Rouge
>An orange rouge and lipstick will do wonders to counteract the pinkness of the complexion.

Powder
>A beigy tone of powder can work its magic of cover-up for the florid complexion. It should not be darker in value than the foundation.

Eyebrow Pencil
>Auburn is the color for the red-headed gal. Otherwise, match the eyebrows as closely as possible.

Eye-Shadow
>Moss green is lovely. Some of the more intense violets may be lovely too.

Eye Liner
>Dark brown.

Mascara
>Dark brown or dark blue, not black unless the complexion is flawless.

Lipstick
>An orange tone that is more yellow than red.

GOLDEN COMPLEXION This skin coloring may be medium to medium-dark in value. The value of the skin is determined by the amount of brown pigment and will have a great deal to do with the intensity of the make-up colors. As a general rule, the *fairer* the complexion, the *less* vivid the cosmetic colors. Conversely, the *darker* the complexion the more vivid the cosmetic colors.

Foundation
>A beige tone that matches the skin in intensity will give a neutral background upon which to "paint" the features and add highlights.

Rouge

Don't be caught without it. Your complexion is so neutral that you can run the gamut of reds. Just be sure your rouge and lipstick colors have enough intensity to counteract the sallowness of your complexion.

Powder

This is the cosmetic to use when you want to add a gentle "flush" to your face. It can be somewhat lighter in value than your foundation and can have a definite peach tone.

Eyebrow Pencil

Slightly darker than the eyebrows if they are light; otherwise, matching.

Eye-Shadow

Intense colors to match the color of your eyes or to match the clothes being worn if they are shades of blue or green. Never wear brown eye shadow.

Eye Liner

Don't wear it in the daytime. For evening use black or one of the exciting irridescent shades.

Lipstick

True red, coral, intense orange-red are usually more flattering than blue-red.

TAN COMPLEXION This is the skin color that has a tendency to look muddy when worn with dark, uninteresting colors such as black, dark brown or navy blue. It needs color and lots of it. The Navajo Indians created bright hues to liven up the desert-tan landscape. Just look at their pottery, blankets and jewelry. You can liven up your face by selecting intense colors.

Foundation

An intense tan foundation that matches your skin tone. For goodness sake, don't try to lighten your skin with foundation.

Rouge

The true reds and corals are the most flattering. Blue-reds are too much the same value as the skin, avoid them.

Powder

Stay with tan powder, you don't want to look as though you have dipped your head in a flour barrel.

Eyebrow Pencil

Sometimes none is needed. If you wish to correct an eyebrow line, match the eyebrow hairs as closely as possible by mixing brown and black. Beware of harsh black.

COSMETIC APPLICATION AND CORRECTIVE MAKE-UP

Eye-Shadow

Intense green or blue is lovely with brown eyes. But no matter what the color of your eyes, avoid brown and violet.

Eye Liner

Use a color to match your eye shadow, not brown or black.

Mascara

Black on the upper lashes only.

Lipstick

Vivid reds and corals.

OLIVE COMPLEXION Hello, exotic one. Do you want to look like a limpid pool or a summer meadow with flowers abloom? Decide what effect you want to achieve with your cosmetics.

Foundation

It is better for you to select a colorless foundation than to drastically change your own coloring. You may need to lighten the area around your eyes.

Rouge

Wear it, always. Select a true red.

Powder

Should have a peach rather than a pink hue in a shade just lighter than the skin.

Eyebrow Pencil

Do you need it? If your hair is black, try ebony or dark gray rather than black.

Eye-Shadow

Lighter, less intense shades of eye shadow will flatter. Avoid dark dingy ones. Try a number of shades before settling for one.

Eye Liner

If your skin is light in value, you may be able to wear black eye liner even in the daytime. It will enhance your exotic look.

Mascara

Black, without a doubt.

Lipstick

True red or a slightly orangy-red.

BROWN, COPPER OR EBONY COMPLEXION Your choice of cosmetic colors will depend upon how much emphasis you wish to give to each individual feature and will also depend upon the underlying color tone of your complexion. Please read through the suggestions given for both "Tan" and "Olive" complexions.

Foundation
    A color to match your complexion.

Rouge
    Study your face to decide whether or not you need it. If so, keep it subtle in a tone to match the underlying tone of the skin in true red, orange-red or coral.

Powder
    Wear it just a shade lighter than your foundation.

Eyebrow Pencil
    Try a shade to match the color of your hair. For instance, dark auburn eyebrows could have their line filled-in with auburn and black pencil . . . A combination of colors will ofttimes look most natural.

Eye-Shadow
    Experiment with various colors until you find the best ones for you. The irridescent ones will lighten and brighten your eyelids.

Eye Liner
    A highlight of white just above black will give definition to the eyes

Mascara
    Black or one of the bright colors.

Lipstick
    To match the rouge.

COSMETIC APPLICATION AND CORRECTIVE MAKE-UP

COSMETIC INVENTORY

You are progressing beautifully toward becoming a sorcerer with make-up, but just as Aladdin had his lamp and ring, so you need certain objects to work your magic. Have you taken an inventory of your cosmetics to see whether or not you have everything necessary? *Check against this list.*

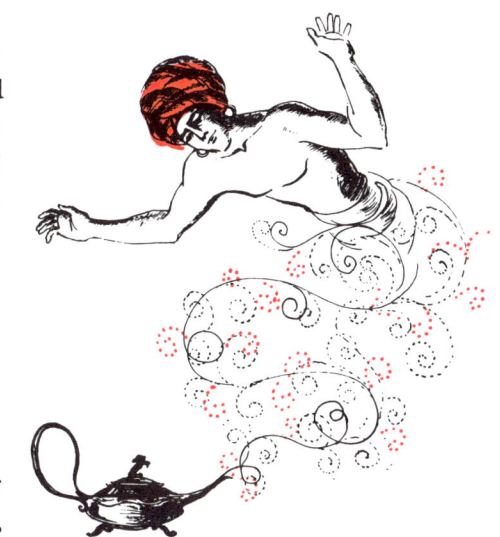

INVENTORY CHECK LIST

- **FOUNDATION:** One of these in the correct color tone. Another for contouring, see in addition, "Hints for Corrective Make-up" on page 41.

    Liquid foundation is easy to apply. It is excellent for normal skin and may be used on dry if it has an oil base. It is not thick enough to be used as a cover-up.

    Cream foundation is thicker in consistency than liquid. It has an oil "creamy" base and is excellent for dry skin.

    Cake foundation is a dry foundation to which water is added for application. It is drying to the skin. Because of its great "staying" power, it is used for the stage and for photography. It is heavy for everyday wear.

    Medicated foundation should be worn by the girl with skin blemishes. Under no circumstances should she be content to simply "cover-up" her problem.

- **ROUGE:** At least one of these in a flattering color.

    Liquid or *cream* rouge is applied after the foundation and before powder.

    Dry rouge is applied after powder. It is the type that should be used with cake foundation or with a dry medicated foundation.

- **POWDER:** Both kinds in the same color.

    Loose powder is the best type for general application. If you have a nice complexion, you may not want to wear powder. In fact, some girls prefer the dewy look. If, however, you have an oily complexion, you will want to cut the "shine" with powder.

    Cake powder is most convenient to carry in a compact for touching up your make-up.

- **EYEBROW PENCIL**

    Whatever type you use, *sharpen it* with a one-edged razor to look like a screwdriver.

☐ **EYEBROW BRUSH**
   This can be a clean mascara brush. It is used to brush the eyebrows into place and to remove powder from the hairline.

☐ **EYE-SHADOW:** At least one of these in a complementary color.
   Cream shadow sometimes "runs" unless powder is applied over it.
   Powdered shadow is gaining favor because it is subtle and stays put.

☐ **EYE LINER:** Either one.
   Pencil eye liner comes in a variety of colors. Powdering the eye shadow before applying the eye liner will make it stay neat looking longer.
   Liquid eye liner is quick drying. It takes a deft hand but is longer-lasting than pencil.

☐ **MASCARA:** Make a choice between the two types.
   Cream mascara is easy to use because it can be applied without water. However, some experts complain because its consistency is not adjustable.
   Cake mascara is mixed with water to apply. It can be made thicker or thinner as you desire. For instance, you may wish to have your eyelashes appear heavier at the outer corners and you can accomplish this by using a thicker mascara.

☐ **LIPSTICK:** You should have a "wardrobe" of lipsticks.
   Regular lipstick has enough oil in it to keep your lips soft. This is quite important, the lips have no oil glands of their own.
   Indelible lipstick is advertised to stay on. It may be kissable, but it's drying so don't wear it all the time.

☐ **LIPSTICK BRUSH**
   Sable hairs are usually used in the better brushes. Don't settle for less than this.

IMPLEMENTS AND MATERIALS

☐ *Eyelash Curler* Use before you start your make-up application.
☐ *Eyebrow Tweezers* The scissor-type with handles are easy to use.
☐ A very *clean skin*.
☐ A *hair net*.
☐ A *cosmetic cape* or *towel* over your shoulders.
☐ *Facial tissues*.
☐ *Cotton balls*.
☐ A *stand-up mirror* with a magnifying side.

COSMETIC APPLICATION AND CORRECTIVE MAKE-UP

THE EYEBROWS

It is interesting to note that movie actresses do more than half of their acting with their eyes. They can portray practically all of the emotions with the position of the eyebrows. Properly done, your brows should give "character" to your face. The "surprised" look should be avoided by all means as should the "vacuous stare" look. And how about the "dark cloud" look caused from having the eyebrows too close together and too thick by the nose?

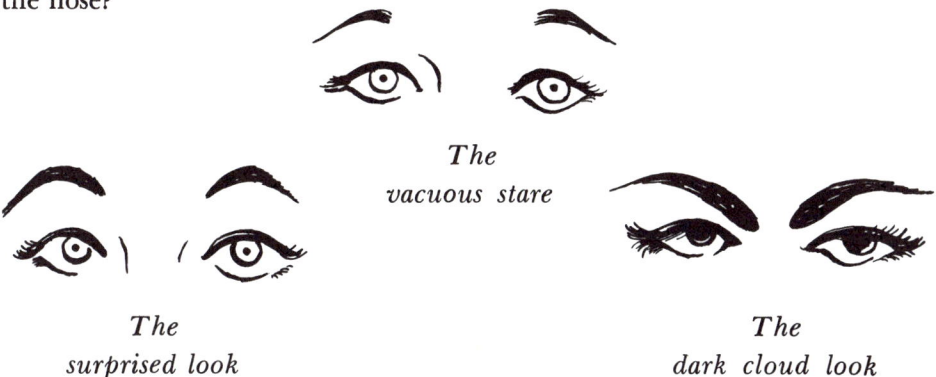

The vacuous stare

The surprised look

The dark cloud look

An eyebrow should be a flattering frame for the eye. It should be in proportion to the other features of the face, and to the size of the face itself. It should not be bizarre nor pencil thin. It should, in fact, be so carefully considered that it lends interest, balance and intrigue to the facial features.

PLUCKING THE BROWS

Before plucking your eyebrows, it will be easier for you to imagine the finished product if you will apply your eyebrow pencil in advance. Now you can see which hairs stay and which ones must go.

Try penciling the inner corner and working outward and upward. The apex of the brows should come just above the outer edge of the iris. The sweep of the brow should be wing-like.

If there is no special effect to be achieved, the eyebrow should start just above the inner corner of the eye and should end far enough out so that if a straight line were drawn from the corner of the nostril past the corner of the eye, it would touch the tip of the eyebrow.

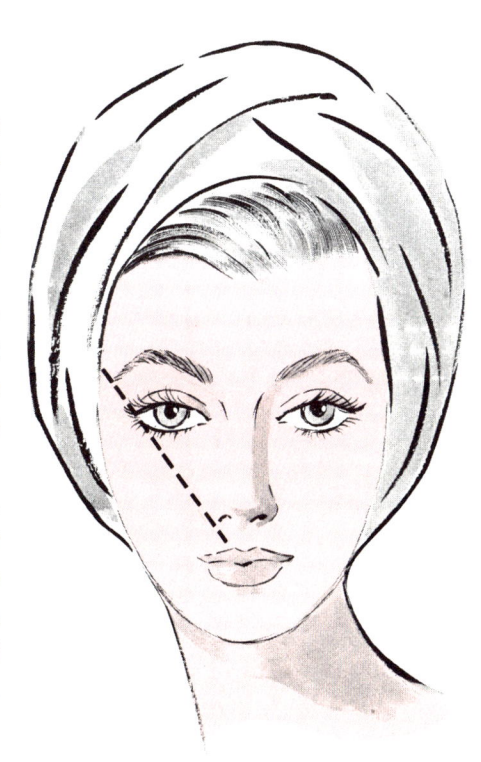

Just a word to the wise on plucking. You will be able to avoid some pain in the process if you will:
1. Oil the skin to first soften it.
2. Pull the skin taut with one hand.
3. Tweeze the hairs in the direction in which they grow.
4. Apply rubbing alcohol immediately after.

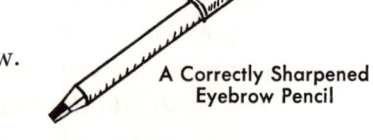

A Correctly Sharpened Eyebrow Pencil

The eyebrow pencil should be sharpened so that you can get either a thin or broad line. This can be done best by sharpening the pencil with a one edged razor. The pencil will then look like a screw driver.

ADDITIONAL HINTS FOR EYEBROWS

You have probably discovered that we are searching for ways and means to look more lovely in a natural way. You probably will want to pluck your eyebrows to achieve this. Just be sure that you stop plucking the moment the strays are gone. Don't make the mistake of plucking until your face is as bare as a plucked Christmas goose. Because the tendency is to pluck too much, rather than too little, you had better decide in advance how you want your eyebrows to look, and then start plucking them from underneath and from the center.

Because the distance between "normally" set eyes is the width of one eye, it may be that you will want to make close-set eyes look farther apart or wide-set eyes closer together. You can do this and make other facial corrections with your eyebrows and eye make-up.

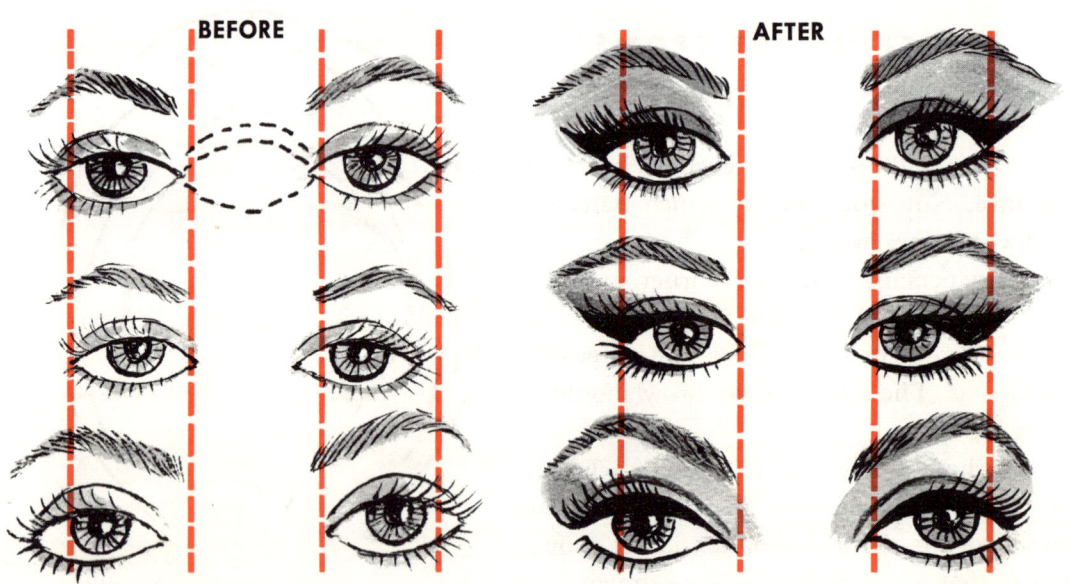

BEFORE **AFTER**

CLOSE-SET EYES Pluck the eyebrows so that the distance between them equals the width of one eye. This may mean that they will start over the tear duct rather than over the corner of the eyes.

WIDE-SET EYES Will seem closer together if the eyebrows are plucked to the distance of one eye span from the other. This may mean that they will start in, beyond the corner of the eyes.

COSMETIC APPLICATION AND CORRECTIVE MAKE-UP

BROW SHAPES FOR CORRECTING OTHER FACIAL FEATURES

An "abnormal" nose may be corrected by eyebrow lines as may a too-high or too-low forehead.

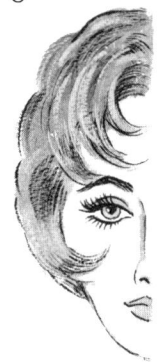

TOO-LONG NOSE If the nose is narrow as well as long, pluck the eyebrows slightly farther apart and keep the inner edges curved rather than squarely perpendicular. Place the arch farther out than the outer edge of the iris. If your nose is long and broad, it is probably large and should be minimized with dark foundation.

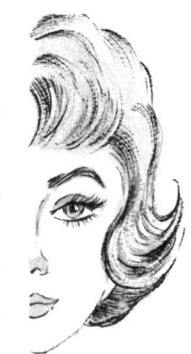

Long Nose

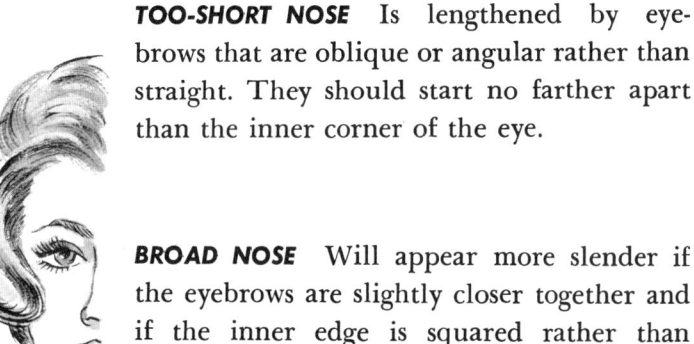

Short Nose

TOO-SHORT NOSE Is lengthened by eyebrows that are oblique or angular rather than straight. They should start no farther apart than the inner corner of the eye.

BROAD NOSE Will appear more slender if the eyebrows are slightly closer together and if the inner edge is squared rather than rounded. The arches should be slightly closer together too.

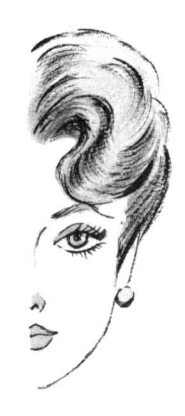

Broad Nose

Narrow Nose

NARROW NOSE Is made to look wider if the eyebrows are plucked out beyond the corners of the eyes and if they are more or less straight rather than highly arched.

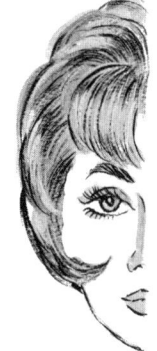

HIGH FOREHEAD The expanse will be broken by an eyebrow that is slightly elevated in the arch.

LOW FOREHEAD Requires normally arched eyebrows, not exaggerated.

High Forehead

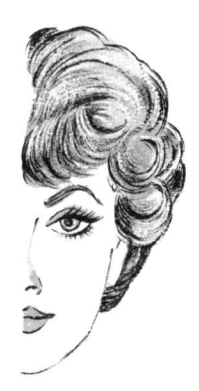

Low Forehead

LIPS

What part does your mouth play in telling people what kind of a person you are? Right away it discloses your disposition and lets others in on the horrible truth. If you are a perpetual pouter, your mouth reflects this attitude. If you are jolly and friendly and approachable, your mouth reveals this fact too. Your mouth is a sort of mirror for your soul. Let it be as inviting as possible.

RULES FOR LIP LINE:

1. It is easier for you to use a brush. You can get a more clean-cut line with a brush in applying your lipstick than you can with either a lipstick tube or your finger.
2. The upper and lower lip should be nearly the same size. If one is much larger than the other, correct this fault. Color over the natural line with foundation and start from scratch—or better yet, start from an objective viewpoint. Maybe the very fault that you wish to disguise is the feature that makes you different. This very difference is an important part of your charm.
3. The highest points on the upper lip should come just below the nostrils. For them to come much farther out declares you an outmoded demoiselle.
4. The lower lip will not drag the mouth down if you use a straight line from the corner to the point just below the nostril.
5. The mouth will have an upward tilt if you will give the upper lip its full value. You might even try building it up at the corners just a little. See the difference!

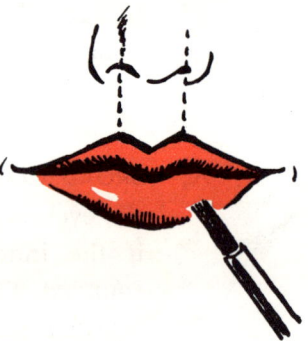

Correct Lipstick Application

SPECIAL TIPS FOR LIPSTICK APPLICATION

What about white lipstick? It may be used to advantage over or under other colors but by itself it creates a ghastly effect. Don't destroy your beauty with cosmetics, enhance it.

Your lipstick will have more "staying" power if you apply it once, powder over it, apply a second time, then blot.

Blot both lips at once with the mouth open as though you are saying "oh." This enables you to get the inner edges, which should be well rouged, as well as the corners.

Don't be guilty of transferring lipstick from your upper to your lower lip by pressing them together. They are not the same shape, or shouldn't be.

COSMETIC APPLICATION AND CORRECTIVE MAKE-UP 39

CORRECTING THE LIP LINE

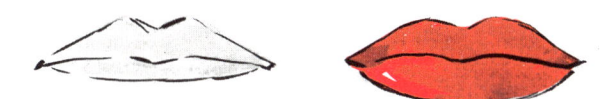

1. **THIN LOWER LIP.** Extend curve of lower lip to balance.

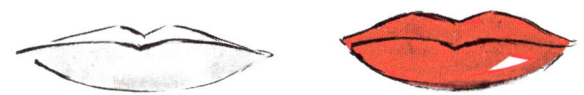

2. **THIN UPPER LIP.** Build up curve of upper lip to balance.

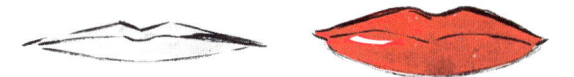

3. **THIN LIPS.** Increase size of both upper and lower lips with a gentle, curving line.

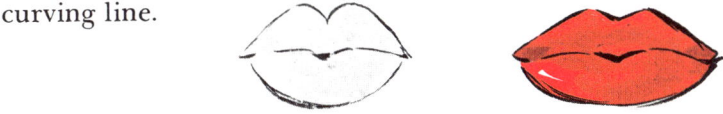

4. **SMALL MOUTH.** Build out sides of upper and lower lips and extend the corners of mouth.

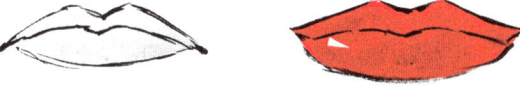

5. **DROOPING CORNERS.** Build up the upper lip at corners of the mouth.

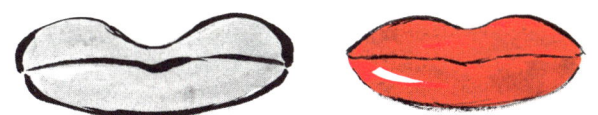

6. **LARGE FULL LIPS.** Keep lipstick coloring inside of the lip line. Shade color off at sides. Keep corners very sharp and clean-cut.

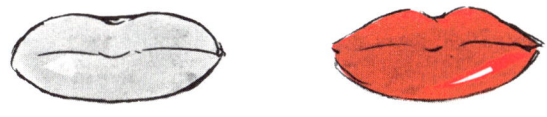

7. **MOUTH TOO OVAL.** Color the center upper lips into a slight Cupid's bow.

8. **SHARP CUPID'S BOW.** Fill in most of the Cupid's bow; widen the sides of upper and lower lips.

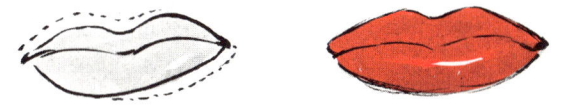

9. **UNEVEN LIPS.** Fill in areas as shown on the illustration.

COSMETIC APPLICATION AND CORRECTIVE MAKE-UP

COMPLETE MAKE-UP APPLICATION

Now you are equipped and ready to start. Just be sure you are in a good light. Diffused daylight is perfect. Here we go!

PROCEDURE

1. **FOUNDATION** is first. It is applied evenly over the entire surface of the face and is blended under the chin onto the neck so that there is no definite line of demarkation. Use too little rather than too much. For liquid or cream foundation, use the five dot method. Place one dot on the chin, one on each cheek, one on the nose, and one on the forehead. Using a sponge, start with the chin and blend up and out to the hairline.

2. **ROUGE** is next. Apply it according to the rules already given. If you are using a cake foundation and dry rouge you will, of course, apply your powder before rouge.

3. **POWDER** is applied in abundance with a piece of cotton or clean powder puff. Pat it on over the entire surface of the face and upper neck. Take a clean piece of cotton and brush off the excess with downward strokes.

4. **EYEBROW PENCIL** is applied to correct an eyebrow line that has already had the benefit of plucking. It may also be used to slightly darken the eyebrow hairs and underlying skin. Start at the inner corner, use short feathery strokes that simulate the hairs. To finish, brush with the eyebrow brush to relieve any harshness.

5. **EYE-SHADOW** is applied as suggested for your shape face. It is applied to the upper lid only, never to the lower.

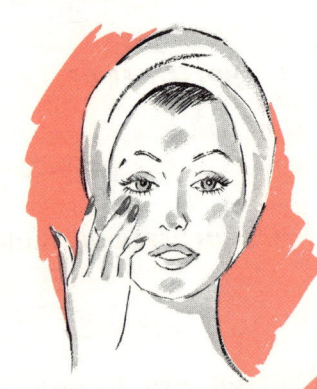

Apply Foundation and Blend

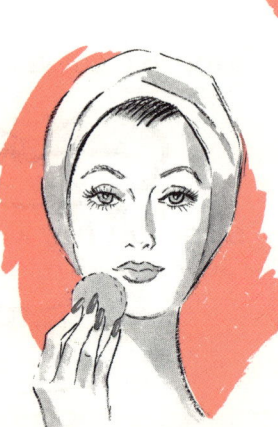

Apply Rouge

Apply Powder and Remove Excess

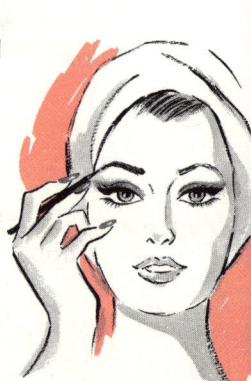

Accent the Brows

COSMETIC APPLICATION AND CORRECTIVE MAKE-UP

6. **EYE LINER** is applied over the eye shadow as close to the lashes as possible. Some girls like to line the entire eye for a more dramatic effect. Save this drama for the stage or evening affairs.

7. **MASCARA** is applied to the upper lashes only unless the lower lashes are so pale they cannot be seen. Avoid the stupid baby doll look that comes from using mascara on both the upper and lower lashes. It is better to give definition to the eye with eye liner.

8. **LIPSTICK** is the last cosmetic to be applied. You may wish to use two shades. Use the lighter shade where you wish to highlight your lips. For instance, if you have a protruding lower lip, you may wish to use the darker lipstick on it. Or you may use the darker to outline your lips and the lighter to fill in. If you think your lips are too full, use a dull color to outline and a more vivid, intense color to fill in.

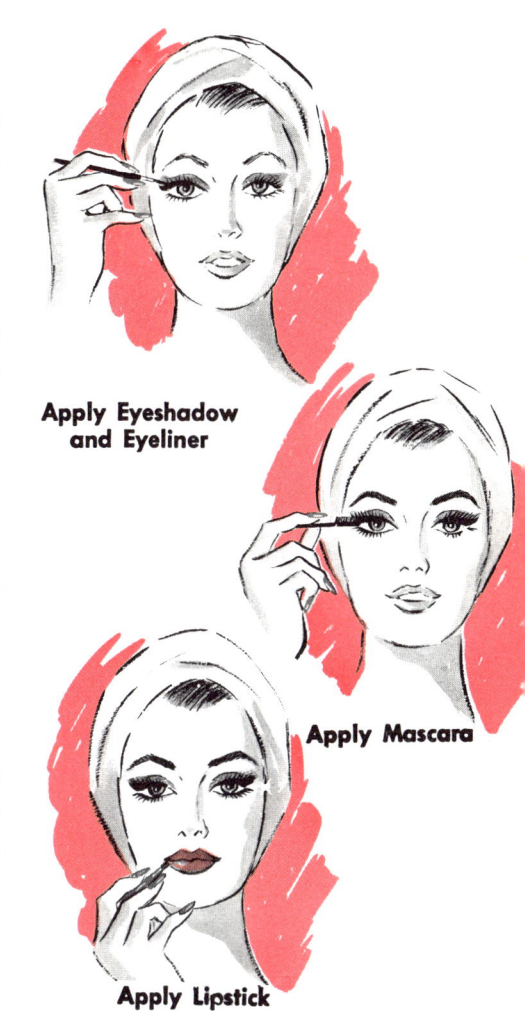

Apply Eyeshadow and Eyeliner

Apply Mascara

Apply Lipstick

HINTS FOR CORRECTIVE MAKE-UP

The objectives of corrective make-up are achieved by playing up the good features and toning down the bad. *Facial features can be accented with proper highlighting and subdued with the correct shadowing or shading.*

CORRECTIVE FOUNDATION

DARKER FOUNDATION will make an area recede, be less noticeable. It is the right answer for large jaws, double chins, protruding foreheads, large noses, heavy-lidded eyes, long chins.

LIGHTER FOUNDATION will make an area advance and is the right answer to the problem of dark circles around the eyes, deep-set eyes, discoloration and lines and wrinkles. It can also be used to create the illusion of width on a long face when it is used across the cheeks and nose. Be sure to extend it to the hairline. It will make a short nose appear longer when it is streaked right down the middle from just above the bridge down to and under the tip. It will make a receding chin seem to come forward and be more prominent.

COSMETIC APPLICATION AND CORRECTIVE MAKE-UP

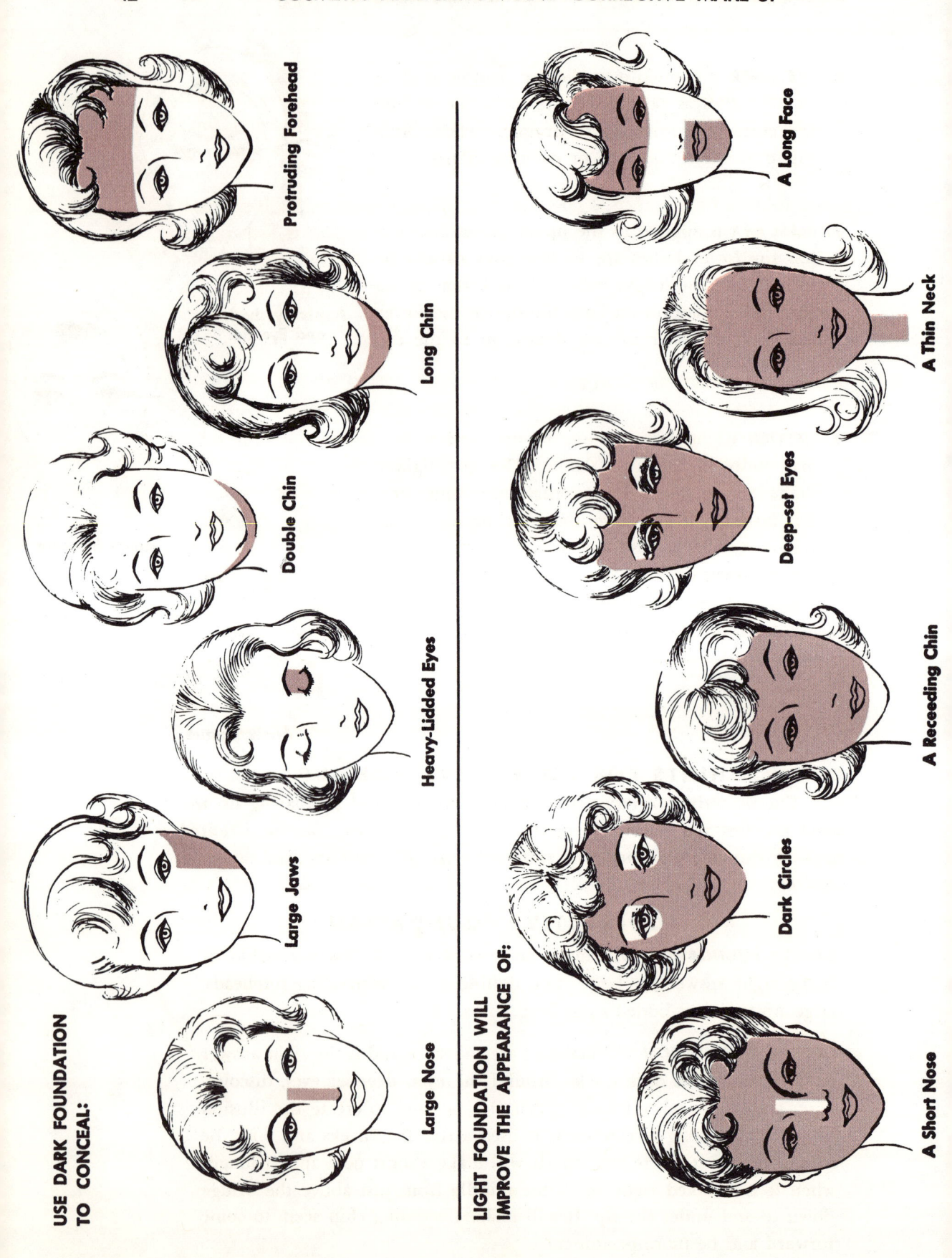

USE DARK FOUNDATION TO CONCEAL:

- Protruding Forehead
- Long Chin
- Double Chin
- Heavy-Lidded Eyes
- Large Jaws
- Large Nose

LIGHT FOUNDATION WILL IMPROVE THE APPEARANCE OF:

- A Long Face
- A Thin Neck
- Deep-set Eyes
- A Receding Chin
- Dark Circles
- A Short Nose

COSMETIC APPLICATION AND CORRECTIVE MAKE-UP

ROUGE

If you have a flawless complexion with good natural coloring, and if you have a face exactly the shape you would like it to be, then you don't need rouge for corrective purposes. That's for sure. However, we will assume that you are the average woman who would like to enhance her natural loveliness as much as possible. You will use rouge not to add a blob of color to your face like a spot of red ink on a white towel, but rather subtly, so that your audience will be unaware of just what the new enchantment is. You should hope for a heightening of your natural color and a recontouring of your features. If you see this effect, you are using rouge with purpose and effect.

RULES FOR ROUGE APPLICATION:
1. Match the rouge color to your lipstick color. If you are wearing a lipstick with yellow undertones, the rouge should have the same underlying tones although it may be a shade lighter in color.
2. Never apply rouge in, beyond the center of the eyeball.
3. Never below the bottom of the nose.
4. Never above the eyebrow.
5. Never in a conspicuous circle.

The foregoing sound like never, never rules. Now let us get a few constructive ideas. There are three types of rouge; dry, cream, and liquid. Because the cream or liquid rouge can be applied under your powder, and because they can be made to look more natural, they get our vote on the beauty ballot. We hope they get yours.

Their application will depend upon the shape of your face and where you wish the accent to be. Almost invariably, however, you will find the three dot method the most desirable. Blend together these three dots until there is only a trace of color with no definite beginning or end. Like an old soldier, let it just fade away.

Please refer to your face shape, and decide what you want the rouge to do for you—*heighten, broaden,* or *erase circles under your eyes.*

A miracle!

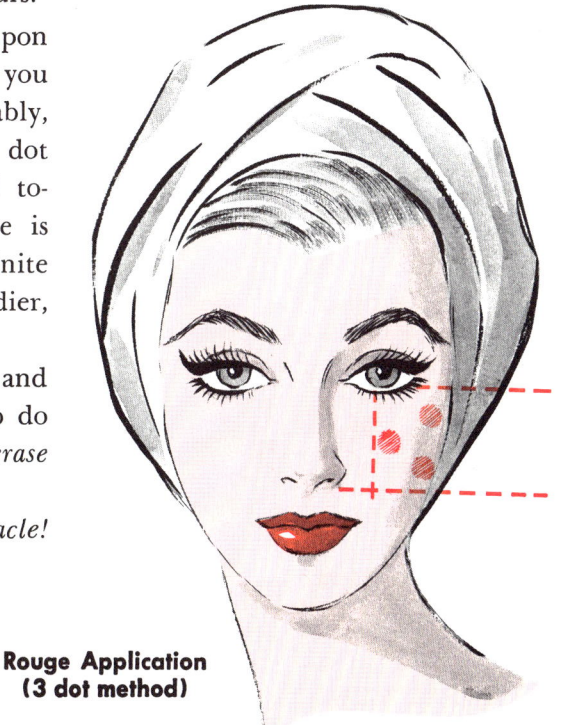

**Rouge Application
(3 dot method)**

COSMETIC APPLICATION AND CORRECTIVE MAKE-UP

USING ROUGE FOR CORRECTION

Rouge is some shade of red; therefore, it is a very advancing and noticeable color. Use it where you want definite emphasis.

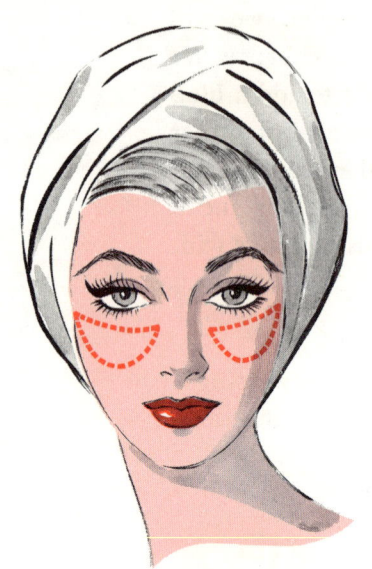

AVERAGE FACE: Dot your rouge wide on height of cheekbones, smooth up and outward evenly.

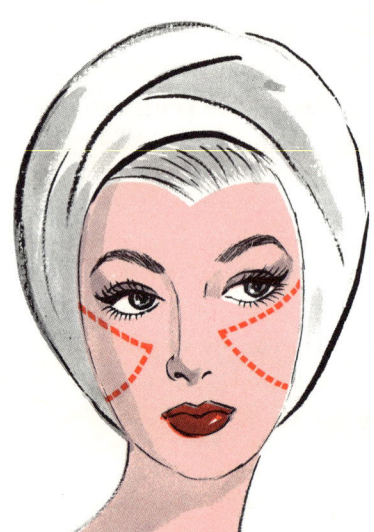

WIDE FACE: Keep rouge closer to nose carry up at an oblique angle for a look of length.

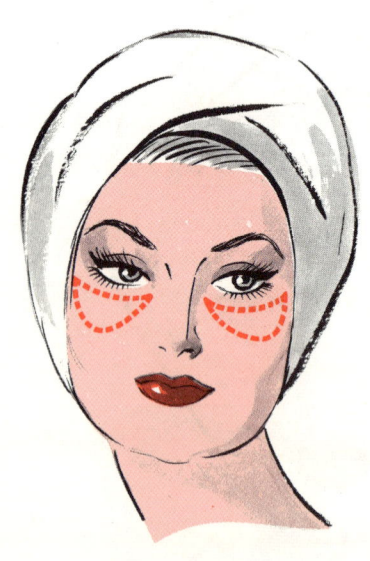

NARROW FACE: Use rouge for illusion of width. Apply from cheekbones back to hairline.

WIDE JAW: Give emphasis to upper part of face by applying rouge on upper cheekbone.

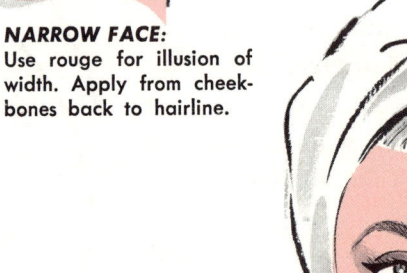

NARROW JAW: Give illusion of width to lower half of face by applying rouge low on the cheekbone.

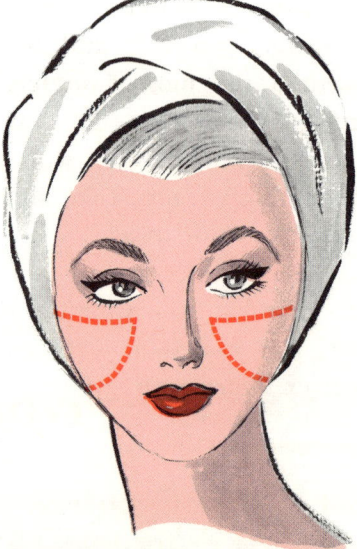

COSMETIC APPLICATION AND CORRECTIVE MAKE-UP

CORRECTIVE MAKE-UP FOR THE EYES

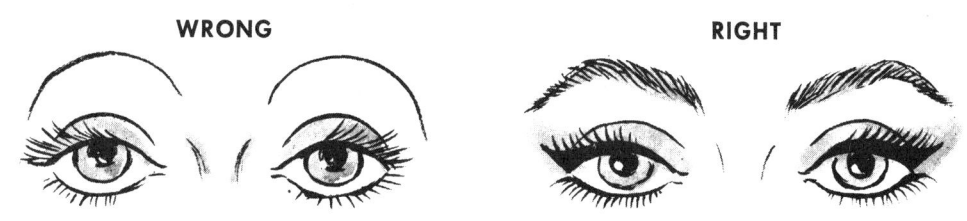

WRONG   **RIGHT**

ROUND EYES can be lengthened by extending the shadow beyond the outer corner of the eyes.

CLOSE-SET EYES. For eyes that are set too close together, apply shadow lightly up from the outer edge of the eyes.

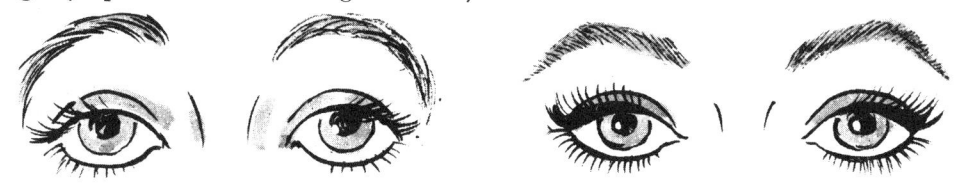

BULGING EYES can be minimized by blending the shadow carefully over the prominent part of the upper lid, carrying it lightly to the line of the brow. Use **dark** shadow as in illustration.

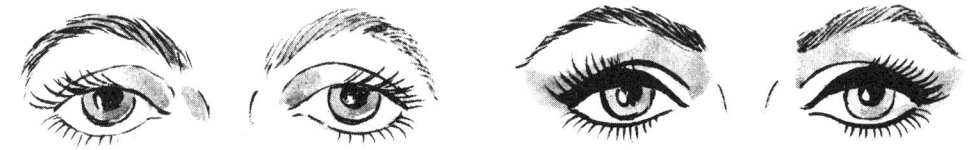

HEAVY-LIDDED EYES. Shadow evenly and lightly across the lid from the edge of the eyelash line to the small crease in the eye socket as in illustration.

SMALL EYES can be made to appear larger by extending the shadow slightly above, beyond and below the eyes.

EYES SET TOO FAR APART. For eyes that are set too far apart, use the shadow on the upper inner side of the eyelid.

DEEP-SUNKEN EYES. Use very little shadow on the lids nearest the temples and leave untouched the part next to the nose and inner corner of the eyes.

DARK CIRCLES UNDER EYES. Apply a **lighter** foundation cream, blending it into the dark area.

EVENING MAKE-UP

Introduction

Dusk throws a new light on your make-up. Light—moonlight, candlelight, all kinds of electric light—has an effect on your make-up. If you want to predict how your make-up will look for a special occasion, try it on under a light similar to the one you will be under for the Big Date.

COSMETIC APPLICATION AND CORRECTIVE MAKE-UP

EFFECTS OF ARTIFICIAL LIGHT

Artificial light drains color so you can wear more make-up and brighter colors. Accent your features with more rouge, thicker mascara, darker eye liner, brighter eye-shadow, darker lip liner.

Evening is the time to really make *up*. Here are ten glamourizing tricks for fun and festivity.

1. An attention-getting beauty mark in dark brown or black.
2. Shining eye shadow of silver or gold.
3. Red spotted at the inner corner of each eye.
4. White used as an undercoat for regular eye shadow.
5. False eye lashes.
6. Eye entirely lined with with black, or
7. Eye liner, eye shadow and mascara all worn in matching bright blue or green.
8. Lip gloss applied for permanent sheen, over lipstick.

FASHION EFFECTS IN EYES AND BROWS MAKE-UP

- Natural
- Oblique Oriental Effect
- Dramatic — Beauty Mark
- Evening
- Daytime
- Exotic

A GLOSSARY OF CLEANSERS

Cleansers today do more than clean. They help treat dry, oily or blemished skin. Some of them sooth, refine, protect or tone up. You'll find an explanation of cleansers here. Note the special properties of each; then choose the kind that suits the condition of your skin.

CLEANSING CREAMS, AND LIQUIDS:

All-purpose
    Has more than the function of cleansing, it may also soften, nourish and act as a make-up base.

Antiseptic
    Is designed to counteract harmful bacteria.

Astringent
    Is formulated to stimulate and contract tissues or pores.

Cold Cream
    Is a non-liquefying emulsion type cleanser designed principally for normal or oily skin.

Deep-pore
    Is a penetrating cleanser for deep-cleaning clogged pores.

Emulsion
    Is a cleanser composed mainly of water and mineral oil, brought together by an emulsifying agent.

COSMETIC APPLICATION AND CORRECTIVE MAKE-UP 47

Estrogenic
> Has hormone content to help retain moisture and revive ageing skin cells.

Hormone
> See estrogenic.

Humectant
> Is a cleanser with a material that moisturizes skin by absorption and retention such as glycerin.

Hypo-allergenic
> Is special cleanser for skin irritated by or sensitive to certain ingredients.

Liquefying cream
> Is a cleanser with oil that melts and glides on smoothly; for normal to dry skin.

Medicated
> Is formulated to treat or heal specific skin disorders; designed for acne and similar eruptions.

Moisturizing
> Cleanser contains humectants designed to benefit dry or ageing skin.

CLEANSING SOAPS:

Baby
> Very mild, often contains olive oil.

Castile
> A very mild soap with vegetable oils. Originally applied only to soaps made with olive oil.

Cream
> Soap in cream form for skins sensitive to ordinary soaps.

Hypo-allergenic
> Soap for skin irritated by or sensitive to certain ingredients contained in most other soaps.

Medicated
> Has ingredients designed to treat skin disorders such as sulphur or tar.

Oatmeal
> Contains oatmeal which acts as a mild abrasive for tougher cleaning action.

Superfatted
> Are soaps to which lanolin, cold cream or other extra fat or oil has been added.

ADDITIONAL CLEANSERS

Granules
> Fine grains that cleanse by abrasive action.

Pads
> Saturated with a liquid cleansing agent.

A GLOSSARY OF CREAMS

Science, not sorcery, has brewed the many creams that do more than cleanse the skin. These are in addition to those already listed.

Acne
> A special cream for the treatment of the inflammatory disease of the sebaceous glands characterized by eruptions.

Blemish
> A medicated cream with antiseptic agents; in tubes, sticks or jars and in neutral tints to blend with complexion tones.

Conditioning
> Cream especially formulated to restore oils, elasticity, tone, texture.

Contour
> Thin, film-like cream which temporarily lifts and firms tissues.

Depilatory
> Cream chemically constituted for hair removal.

Foundation
> An oil base cream used as a base for make-up; may be colorless or variously tinted to blend with specific complexions.

Lanolin
> A purified fat from sheep wool; non-alkaline emulsifer used in creams for dry skin.

Massaging
> Lubricating cream to be used for kneading, rubbing, stroking or patting the skin.

Placental
> Cream containing biological material extracted from the human placenta; used as a healing and restoring treatment for damaged tissue.

Poly-unsaturate
> Fat material found chiefly in grain oils and vegetables; used to offset dry, flaky skin conditions and premature ageing.

Protective
> Sun cream, hand cream or face cream which screens against harmful-to-the-skin factors like dirt, dust, grime, sun, wind and water.

Royal Jelly
> Vitamin-rich substance which comes from the food of the Queen bee; Royal jelly contains nitrogen, proteins, B-complex vitamins; is formulated to nourish, moisturize, lubricate and condition.

Silicone
> Crystalline element which acts as a barrier or screen; silicone creams keep skin moisture in, keep harmful drying detergents, chlorinated water, chemicals out.

Vitamin
> Enriched with various vitamins which penetrate and nourish the skin.

CHAPTER 3

HAND CARE AND MANICURING

Introduction

The care a beauty contestant gives her hands and nails is considered so important to her over-all beauty that, in major contests, she is automatically eliminated for biting her nails. It is taken for granted that you do not indulge in this de-glamourizing habit. Even so, are your hands as well groomed as they might be?

No excuses! You can protect your hands with gloves whenever you do work that will roughen your hands. Or, at the very least, you can use one of the new protective lotions. If you don't, your hands will in all probability, become rough, red and calloused.

HAND CARE

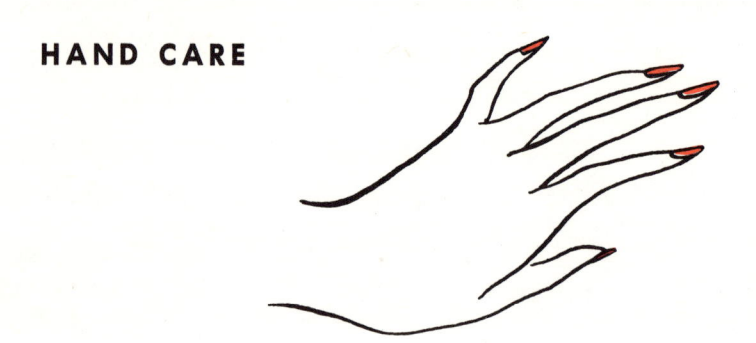

If your hands are not now the "hands you love to hold," then you must spend a little extra time on them each day. The four steps to beauty that were covered in Chapter 1 apply to your hands as well as to your face. Your daily beauty ritual should include time for *cleansing, lubricating, stimulating* and *protecting* your hands. You can keep the cuticle soft by applying cuticle oil, your skin soft by lubricating it with a rich hand lotion. Or perhaps you should try the model's trick of applying a generous amount of dry skin cream at night and then wearing an old pair of white cotton gloves to bed. By morning the skin will be soft enough to respond to a stiff hand brush that will remove old, dead cells.

For the woman whose hands are showing her age, or maybe lying about it to her disadvantage, there are hormone creams on the market to plump up the cells and give the hands a more youthful appearance. There are also creams to lighten the "liver" spots of old age.

You may not believe in palmistry (the science of reading the lines in the palms), but you must admit your hands tell others a story. What can others "read" in your hands? Is it a story of care—or carelessness? If it is anything less than the beauty achieved by daily grooming, it is not good enough.

PROFESSIONAL-LIKE HAND CARE

You must reserve time somewhere along the way for the beauty rituals that will make you a desired employee, a beloved wife, an admired social butterfly.

One of the items on your weekly beauty ritual should be a professional-type manicure.

If you will think of your nails as jewels, decorative accents to your hands, you will give them the care they deserve. They can have a romantic drawing power when they are colorful ovals, glowing like gems. Learn to give yourself a perfect manicure; use nail polish to accent your color scheme as well as make your nails more beautiful.

HAND CARE AND MANICURING

MANICURING

Start out by assembling the equipment and materials necessary:

EQUIPMENT

Emery boards
Orangewood stick
Nail brush and bowl
Cuticle nippers (optional)
Nail buffer (optional)
Towel

MATERIALS

Polish remover
Cuticle remover
Cuticle cream
Absorbent cotton
Base undercoat
Nail polish
Colorless topcoat
Hand lotion

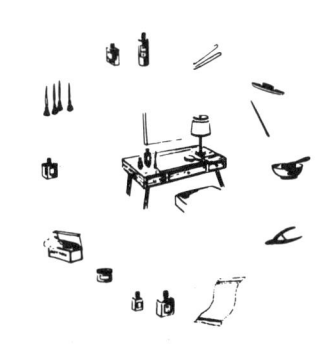

Find a spill-proof table surface that you can use for your manicure, don't try to do it in your lap. You'll need good light too so you can see the details of what you are doing. One more word before you begin: Don't hesitate to remove all the polish and start over again if your nails are not just right. It is patient practice today that makes perfection tomorrow.

PROCEDURE

Here is the procedure to follow for a professional-type manicure.

1. **REMOVE OLD POLISH** It will be easier to remove if you will allow it to soften for a few moments under a cotton pad that has been generously dampened with polish remover. Having moistened a piece of cotton with polish remover, press over old polish on each nail and use a rotary motion to remove old polish. Start with the little finger and work toward the thumb. Repeat with the other hand. If you are right handed, do this hand first, then if you are clumsy and make a boo-boo you can correct it without spoiling the other hand too. If there is any stubborn polish still adhering to the nails, use clean cotton and repeat. This method prevents getting diluted polish on the skin around the nails.

    Remove Old Polish

2. **FILE THE NAILS** An emery board is easier on the nails than a metal file. A long emery board, seven inches long, will do a better job than a short one. File in one direction only, preferably from the side toward the center. Avoid filing down too far, it spoils appearance and weakens the nail. Avoid a too sharp point. Make the curve oval and rather shallow like the curve at the base of the nail.

    File The Nails

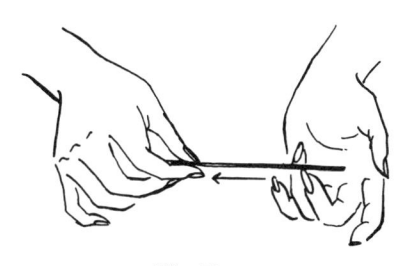

Finger nails should not be more than one-quarter inch beyond the ends of the fingers. All the nails should be approximately the same length. Avoid having one nail much longer than the others, it may look fine on a Chinese mandarin, but not on you.

3. **SOAK NAILS IN WARM SOAPY WATER** Clean your nails thoroughly with the nail brush to remove as much cuticle as you can from the nail surface.

4. **PUSH CUTICLE BACK** This can be done partially with the towel as you dry your hands.

5. **APPLY CUTICLE REMOVER** Use the orangewood stick wrapped in cotton to get the cuticle remover down around the edge of the nails.

6. **LOOSEN AND REMOVE DEAD CUTICLE** with the flat end of the orangewood stick. Use it without cotton. Be sure to get all the cuticle off the surface of the nails; otherwise, you will not get a smooth polish application. Work steadily but lightly; with one circling movement, lift the rim of cuticle free of the nail.

7. **CLEAN UNDER FREE EDGE** Use the cotton-tipped orangewood stick dipped in soapy water or cuticle oil.

8. **TRIM HANG NAILS** Do not make a habit of cutting your cuticle, it will make it tougher. If you are tempted to cut too often or too much, it is better to leave well enough alone.

9. **WHITEN UNDER FREE EDGE** This can be done with nail white in cream or pencil form. If you are going to cover the entire surface of the nail with polish you may feel this step is unnecessary. It might be if you keep your nails scrupulously clean.

10. **APPLY CUTICLE OIL** Get around the sides and the base of each nail. Push cuticle back and gently massage each nail with the thumb of the opposite hand.

11. **REMOVE OIL FROM NAILS** Brush toward the tips of the nails with the hand brush and soapy water.

12. **MASSAGE HANDS AND ARMS** Massage with hand lotion right up to and including your elbows.

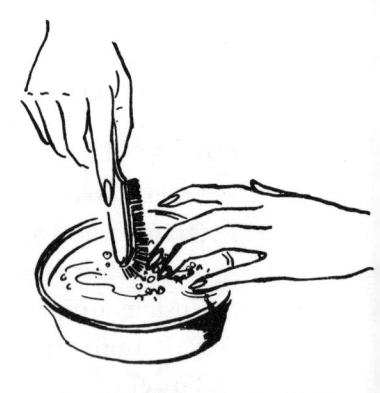

Soak and Brush the Nails

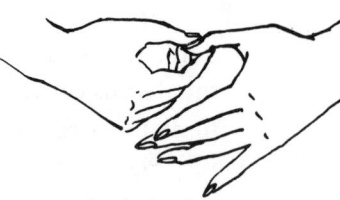

Push Back Cuticle

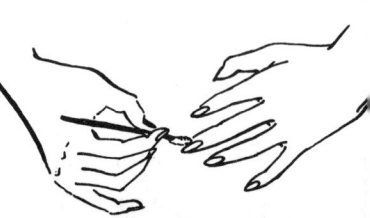

Apply Cuticle Remover and Remove Cuticle

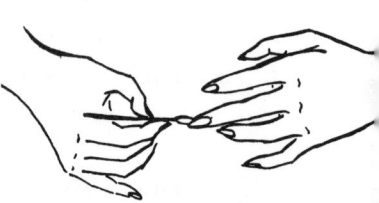

Clean Under Free Edge

Massage Hands and Arms

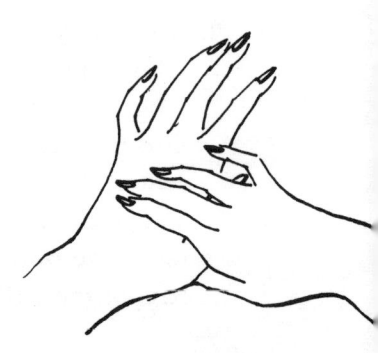

HAND CARE AND MANICURING

13. **GO OVER NAILS LIGHTLY WITH POLISH REMOVER** This will remove all trace of oil from the nails and will assure you a long-lasting polish job. Use cotton-tipped orangewood stick soaked in remover.

14. **APPLY BASE COAT, POLISH COLOR AND SEALER (TOP-COAT)** You will get pleasing results if you will observe these general suggestions:

    ▸ The base coat, polish and sealer should not be so thick that they "string" as the applicator is pulled out of the bottle. If they are, thin them with polish solvent that is sold expressly for this purpose.

    ▸ There should be just enough polish on the applicator to do one nail without redipping. This polish should be applied to the nail with as few strokes as possible. It is suggested that only three strokes be used: one from base to tip in the center of the nail, one on either side of the middle. Avoid brushing over what has already been done.

    ▸ Avoid touching the cuticle with polish. Leave a hair line between polish and cuticle, if possible. Otherwise, use the orangewood stick (without cotton) to remove the excess polish immediately.

    ▸ Removing a hair line from the tip will help to prevent chipping. This must be done with the thumb of the opposite hand as each coat is applied. If the polish is partially dry, it will ripple.

The normal shaped nail may have its entire surface covered with polish.

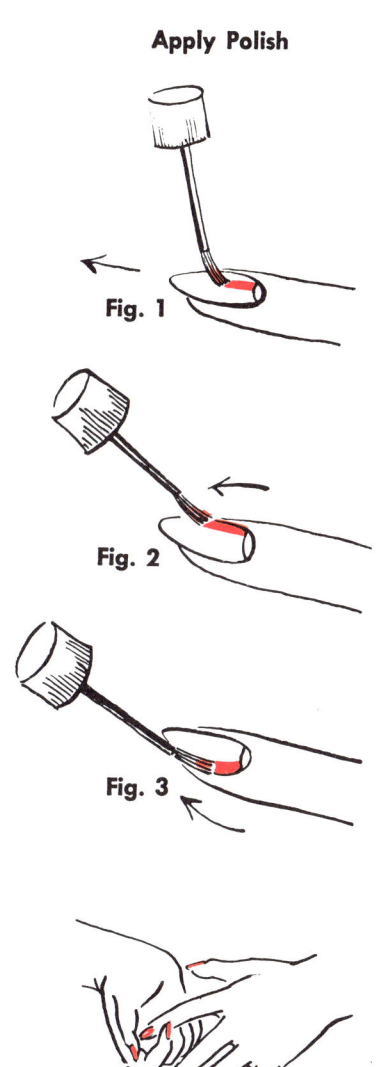

Apply Polish

Fig. 1

Fig. 2

Fig. 3

Remove Hairline Tip

CORRECTIVE USE OF NAIL POLISH

You can use polish to improve the shape of your nails.

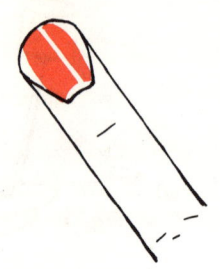

The splay shape of the *Spatulate* nail can be disguised by polishing it to look oval.

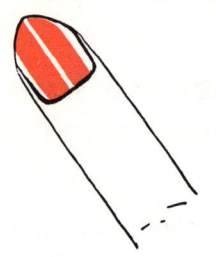

The *Broad* nail will look less so if only the middle section is polished.

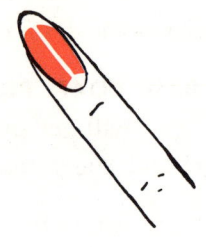

The long, *Narrow* nail will appear more oval if the moon and white section at the tip are left unpainted.

COLOR Dark polish makes the nails look smaller; medium polish larger; light polish, delicate. (Exaggerated dark or weird colors are not recommended.)

CORRECTIVE COLORS FOR THE HANDS

For plump hands: Dark polish covering the entire nail will make them look slimmer.

For bony hands: A medium or light shade is flattering when applied according to the shape of the nail.

For large hands: Medium polish applied according to the shape of the nail.

For small hands: Light polish will make them look delicate.

For reddened hands: A medium to dark shade will avoid accenting the redness.

For white hands: Light polish will make them look delicate. A medium or dark tone will make them look whiter. What do you prefer?

BEAUTY TIPS FOR HANDS AND NAILS

Avoid biting the nails or cuticles.

Avoid letting the cuticle grow up too far on the nail. Loosen it daily.

Avoid nails that look like claws because they are too long.

Avoid wearing chipped polish. Repair it as soon as possible.

Avoid putting new polish over old, chipped polish. It will never look neat.

Avoid wearing each nail a different length. If you break one, cut them all off or buy a false nail to wear over the broken one until it grows out.

Avoid putting one coat of polish on top of another until it is five or six coats deep.

CHAPTER 4

LEG CARE AND PEDICURING

Introduction

Superfluous hair should be removed as regularly from the legs, especially below the knee, as it is from under the arms. How often will depend upon you and how noticeable the hair is. There is nothing more unsightly than a grown girl wearing nylons with long hair poking out like a porcupine. Ugh!

What's that you say? It will grow in longer and blacker? Oh, no it won't, you are never going to let it grow in again. In our society, hairlessness is a sign of femininity; qualifying that statement, hairlessness of the face and extremities is a sign of femininity. For femininity and a dainty appearance, remove hair where and when you must.

LEG CARE

Authorities seem to agree that *the best way to remove hair from large areas is by shaving with a razor*, either safety or electric. If you are going to try a chemical depilatory, give yourself a skin test to determine if you are sensitive to the action. Select a hairless part of the arm, apply a small portion according to the manufacturer's direction; leave on the skin for about seven minutes. If there is no redness or swelling at the end of this time, you may assume it can be used safely.

If your choice is a safety razor, use shaving cream or soap on your legs. Don't shave them dry. Shave downward with the grain of the hairs; then if you want a really close shave go over them the second time upward. Please be careful so that you don't knick over your shin or ankle bone.

You can finish by washing away the soap, drying and applying a creamy hand lotion. This will prevent dry, flaking skin. Try it and see for yourself.

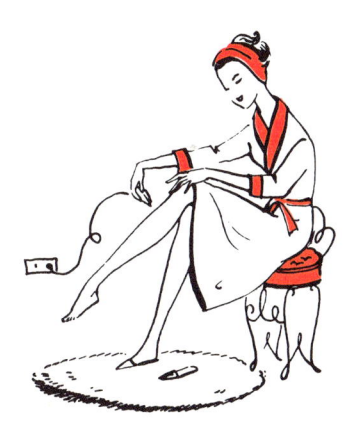

Shaving The Legs

PEDICURING

A number of beauty authorities are against a woman ever exposing her feet to the public view except around a swimming pool or at the beach. Considering the number of malformations and abnormalities due to improper shoes, it's no wonder. But exposed or no, you should take as good care of your feet as you do of your hands. It is your feet that have to, literally, carry you to success.

FOOT CARE

The daily care of your feet should include *bathing* for cleanliness; *creaming* for lubrication; *hot and cold baths or alcohol* for stimulation; *powder* for protection.

The weekly care of your feet should include a complete pedicure that follows the same procedure as manicuring except for a couple of changes. These are:

1. File your nails straight across or cut them with a special toenail clipper.
2. Keep your toenails shorter than your toes but do not cut the corners.
3. Place a small roll of cotton or foam rubber between the toes while you apply the polish. This will facilitate neat polish application.

Spread the Toes With Cotton Rolls

The benefits that will accrue from taking care of yourself are more than just physical. They are mental and emotional as well. What woman can look beautiful and relaxed when her feet are hurting? Besides, you want to have fun dancing and dating and your feet have to be healthy to carry you through a strenuous day and a glamorous night.

FOR BEAUTIFUL FEET:

Avoid corns, bunions and callouses by wearing the proper shoes.

Avoid pump bumps by using a pumice stone after every bath.

Avoid ingrown toenails by cutting the nails straight across.

Avoid wearing hose that are too short.

Avoid snagging your hosiery by keeping your toenails, feet and legs smooth.

Avoid foot fatigue by pampering your feet with the correct shoes and with foot baths and massage.

Avoid foot odor by using foot powder in your shoes.

Avoid fungus growth by keeping your feet as dry as possible.

CHAPTER 5

HAIR CARE, SHAMPOOING AND COIFFURE ARRANGEMENTS

Introduction

You are going to need a good hair brush, a comb with both fine and widely spaced teeth and a hair dressing. That is all in the line of equipment, but you are also going to need a persistence for brushing your hair until it becomes your "crowning glory." Or until it is, as Massey had said, "Soft hair, on which light drops a diadem."

BRUSHING THE HAIR

Once you realize that brushing will not destroy your hair set but will actually make it more manageable, you will enjoy brushing your hair one hundred strokes a day. Lean forward with your head bent low, brush away from the scalp turning the brush slightly as you do so. This position for brushing loosens the scalp, stimulates the circulation, helps correct dandruff problems, distributes the natural scalp oils evenly on the hair and encourages hair growth.

A professional brush like this one is recommended as the best type for women.

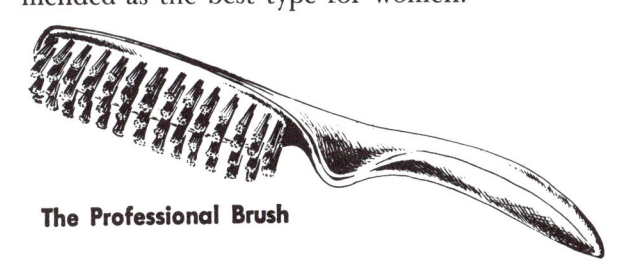

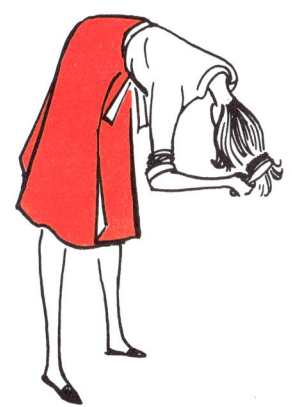

Correct Brushing Technique

The Professional Brush

A hair dressing whether it comes in a spray can, tube or jar will keep unruly wisps in place and will give your hair a professionally-done look.

58   HAIR CARE, SHAMPOOING AND COIFFURE ARRANGEMENTS

If you have scalp or hair troubles that do not respond to simple home remedies, see your physician. However, most dandruff problems will respond to treatments. If you cannot have these in the school or in a salon, do-it-yourself at home.

For an excessively dry scalp, here is a simple treatment that is often effective. Simply heat olive oil in a bowl to body temperature, apply to the scalp with a small pledget of cotton by parting the hair from front to back in one-half inch parts. Roll a towel around your head, leave on overnight, then shampoo.

SHAMPOOING

The first requisite for beautiful hair is, of course, cleanliness. You should decide how often you think you should shampoo your hair and then make it a habit. If your hair is somewhat oily, you will need to shampoo more often than the gal who has normal or dry hair. There is nothing that smells worse than rancid oil, if your hair is the oily type, keep it clean, clean, clean.

One of the best tests for clean hair is the smell test. Ask mom or teacher or someone you can trust to help you decide how often you should shampoo your hair. Then choose a type of shampoo that is formulated for your kind of hair; be sure to follow the directions on the package. Usually they will suggest that you thoroughly wet the hair before applying the shampoo. If so, your procedure will go like this:

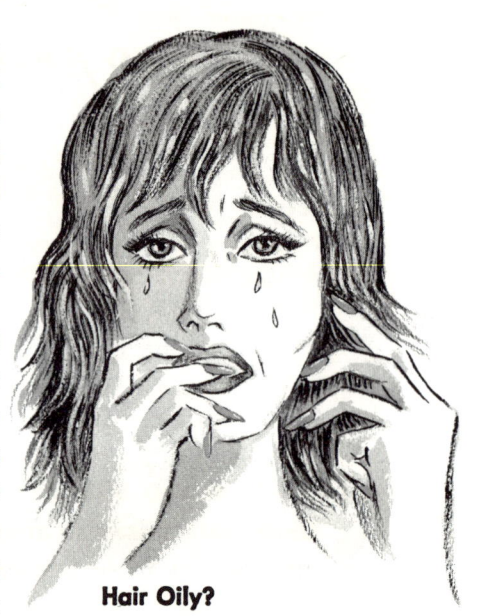

Hair Oily?

1. Wet hair.
2. Apply shampoo and work up to a thick lather by rubbing into scalp and hair.
3. Rinse out.
4. Apply more shampoo and work up to thick lather.
5. Rinse out until hair is "squeaky" clean.
6. Use a rinse.
   For dry hair, a cream rinse.
   For normal or oily hair, lemon (lightens, good for blonds) or vinegar. Both of these cut the soap curds left by hard water.
7. Towel hair until partially dry.
8. Set.

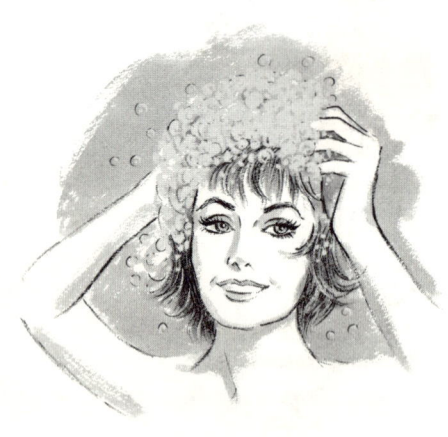

Work Up a Good Lather

HAIR PROTECTION

Your hair and scalp benefit from the four beauty steps: *cleansing* with shampoo; *lubricating* with oil; *stimulating* with brush and massage; *protecting* with hat and scarf.

During the summer especially, your hair needs protection. Don't let the sun and wind and water dry it to a frizzle. These elements all spell d-r-y-n-e-s-s, so you will have to give your hair extra special attention if you are in the habit of swimming or sun bathing. Always cover your hair, with a hat or scarf *out* of the water, and with a bathing cap while *in*. Bleached streaks may be all right for a beach, but how about a ball?

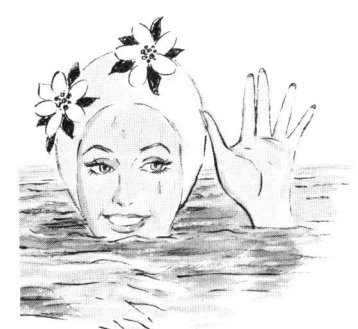

COIFFURE ARRANGEMENTS FOR VARIOUS HAIR COLORING

Speaking of a ball, maybe you would like to have one trying new hair colors. Before you do, consider the amount of time and money it will take to keep it up. Play safe and experiment with temporary tints that are close to your own hair color before you venture far afield. Did you ever stop to think that the color of your hair should make a difference in the way it is arranged?

STYLES FOR BLOND HAIR

Blond hair looks best in soft gentle styles that fit its coloring. This hair has lots of golden highlights that should parade with each other like a halo around the head. If blond hair is tousled, it looks terrible.

STYLES FOR SILVER HAIR

Silver hair needs a glamourized style befitting its dignity. Usually something upswept away from the face.

STYLES FOR PLATINUM HAIR

Platinum hair is for showgirls; it looks wonderful on the stage; it needs impeccable grooming. A sophisticated hairstyle shows it off to best advantage.

STYLES FOR BROWN HAIR

Brown hair doesn't sound very romantic and doesn't look very exotic. It is the outdoor color; keep it free and breezy.

STYLES FOR RED HAIR

Red hair has both highlights and depth of color so select a style that fits the kind of hair you have and your personality.

STYLES FOR BLACK HAIR

Black hair is the siren type. Its silhouette needs emphasis so it can be styled to advantage in everything from the bouffant to the beehive.

HAIR CARE, SHAMPOOING AND COIFFURE ARRANGEMENTS

SELECTING A HAIRSTYLE

Color is one criterion for selecting a hairstyle that is right for you. Here are other factors for you to consider:

1. What kind of hair do I have? Is it coarse or fine, thick or thin?
2. How does my hair grow out of my head? Where are my cowlicks?
3. What kind of hairline do I have around my face? At the nape of my neck?
4. What hairstyle will fit my way of life? Being a school girl, do I have time for an elaborate hairdo?
5. What hairstyle will suit my age?

Note:

(Gray hair hanging down is more witching than bewitching.)

HEIGHT IS AN IMPORTANT FACTOR

How much hair will be in good proportion to my height and build? (A short girl should not have a gob of hair.)

SHORT STATURE

Corrective Hairstyle: One that creates an illusion of height. Hair should be kept short.

TALL STATURE

Corrective Hairstyle: One that offsets a tall appearance. Select a hairstyle which is full. Hair should be medium to long in length.

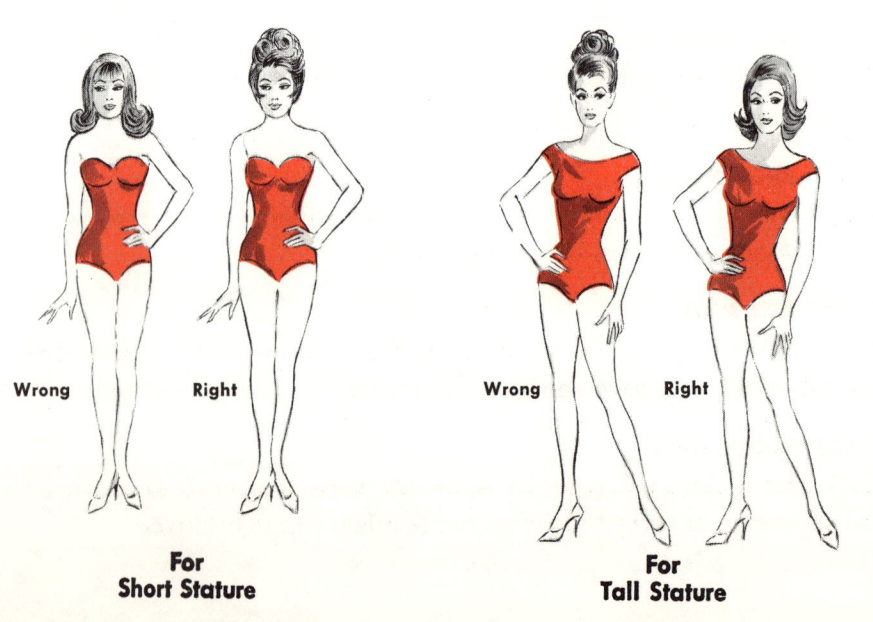

Wrong   Right
For Short Stature

Wrong   Right
For Tall Stature

HAIR CARE, SHAMPOOING AND COIFFURE ARRANGEMENTS   61

NECK LENGTH MUST BE CONSIDERED
What hairstyle will flatter my neck?

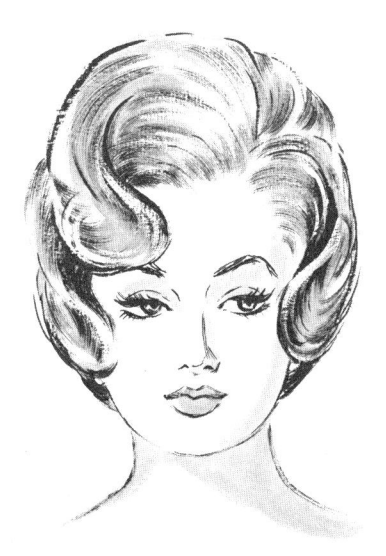

SHORT NECK

Corrective Hairstyle: One that creates an illusion of length by sweeping up, away from the neck. Avoid squareness or fullness at the nape.

LONG, THIN NECK

Corrective Hairstyle: One that minimizes the length of the neck by covering a portion of it. Avoid dressing the hair up from the back of the neck.

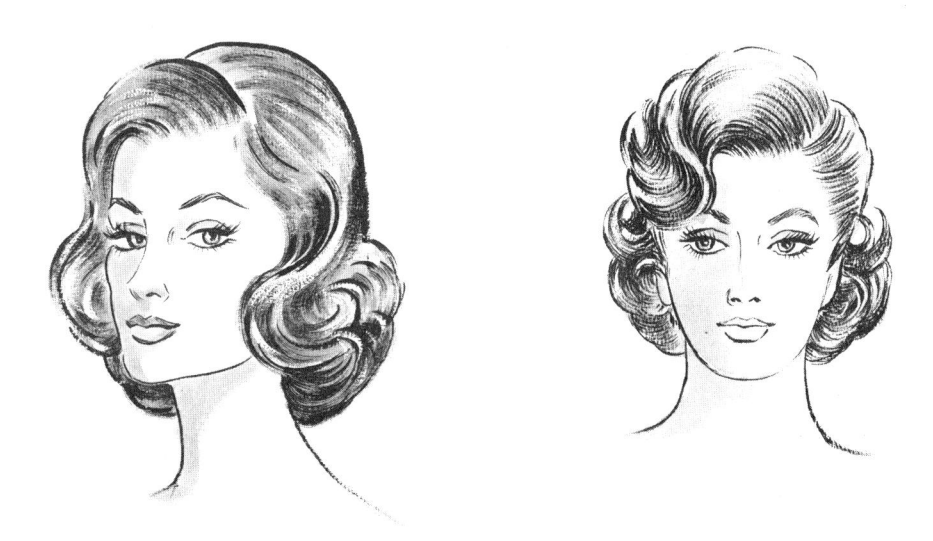

THICK, MUSCULAR NECK WITH BROAD SHOULDERS

Corrective Hairstyle: One that has diagonal waves and a quality of softness. Avoid horizontal lines in the style.

PROFILES

What hairstyle will flatter my profile?

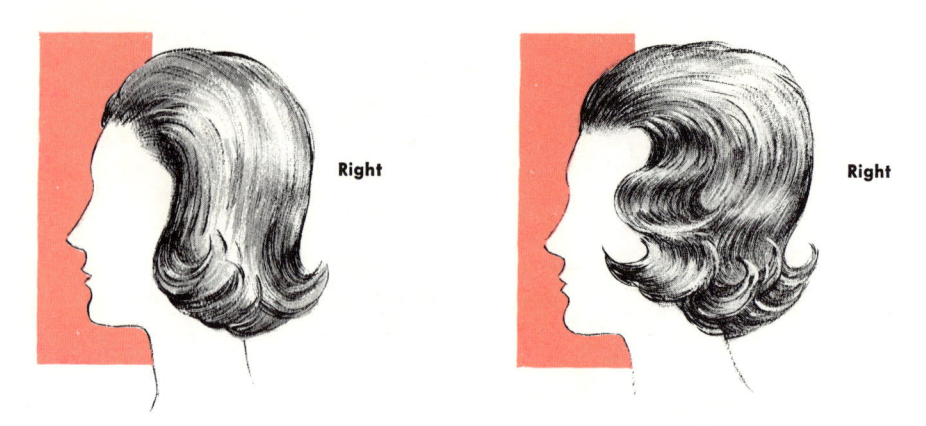

STRAIGHT Usually, all hair styles are becoming to the straight or normal profile.

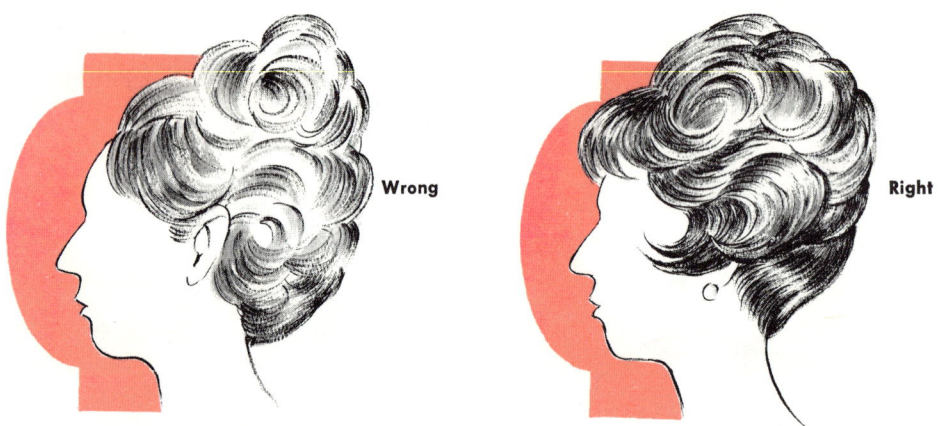

CONVEX Curls or waved bangs should be placed forward on the forehead to conceal receding forehead and irregular hairlines. The hair at the nape of the neck should be dressed close to the head to give it perfect balance.

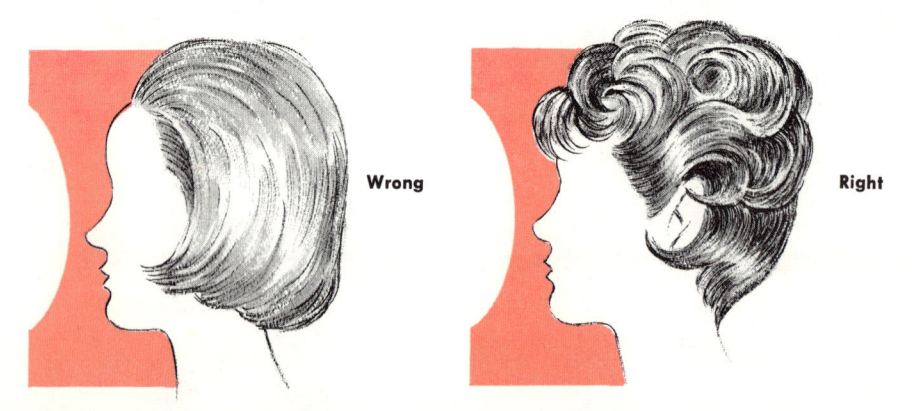

CONCAVE Requires either flat dressing or small curls or waves over the forehead to minimize the bulginess of the forehead. The hair at the nape of the neck should be dressed in small, soft curls to soften the features.

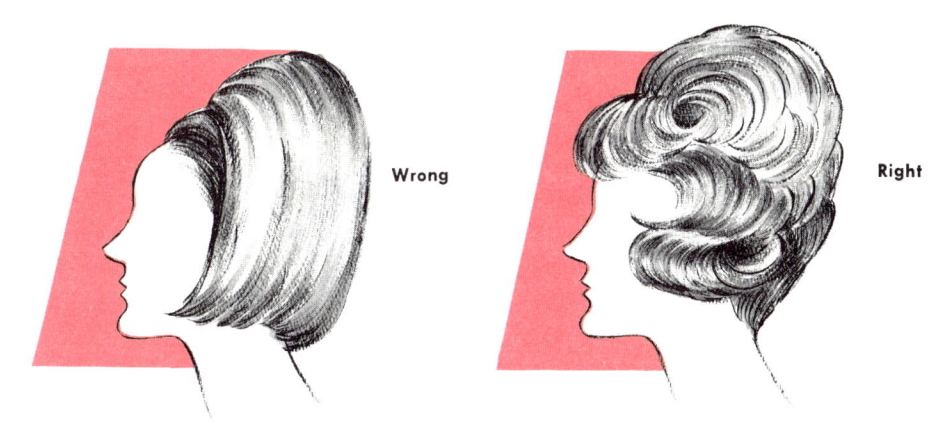

LOW FOREHEAD, SHARP CHIN High pompadour and upsweep movements at the sides will give added length to the face. Soft curls over the jawline will soften the sharpness of the face.

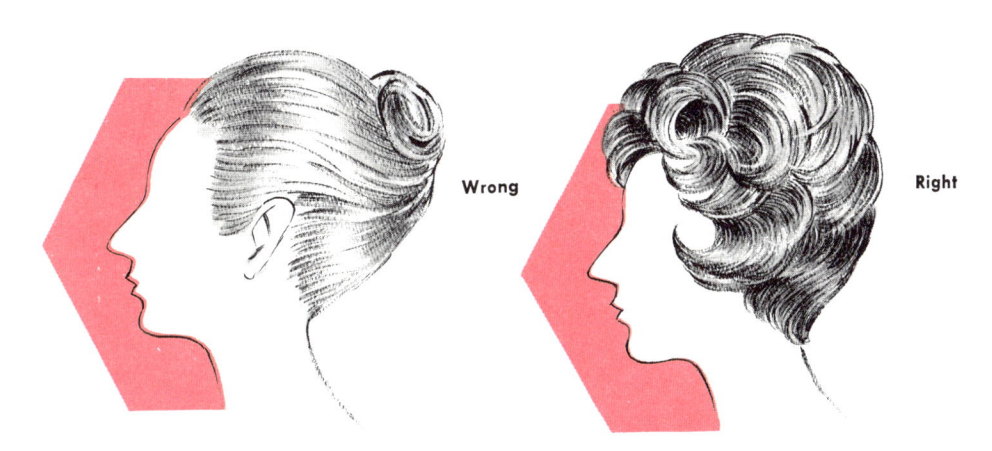

POINTED CONVEX Curls or waved bangs should be placed forward on the forehead to minimize the receding forehead. Dressing the back of the head with soft curls will help to soften the pointed appearance of the face.

FACIAL SHAPE

What hairstyle will flatter the shape of my face?

Your teacher is the one to whom you should turn for professional advice about the hairstyles that will be best suited for you. But one thing you may be able to decide for yourself is the type of silhouette your hair should form around your face.

HAIRSTYLING TO FLATTER FACIAL SHAPE

Just as make-up is used to make your face more oval, so your hairstyle should ovalize your face. Here are the seven *face shapes* and suggestions for coiffures that will make you less (wrong) or more (right) beautiful.

OVAL FACE

This is considered to be the ideal face shape, everything you do with your hair, your make-up and necklines should tend to emphasize the oval.

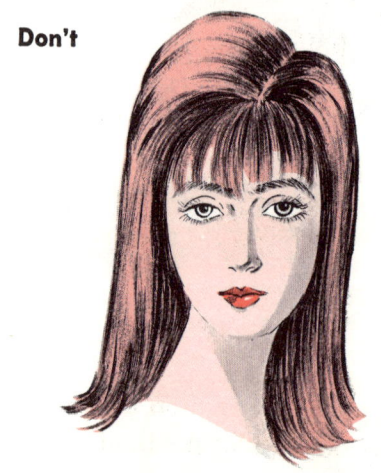

Don't

Do

Don't cover all of your forehead with bangs.

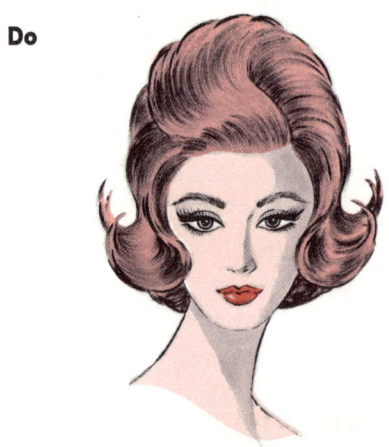

Do retain the oval shape with your hairline.

HAIR CARE, SHAMPOOING AND COIFFURE ARRANGEMENTS

ROUND FACE

This face should be lengthened, or at least not shortened. The coiffure, therefore, should have more height than width. Bangs that form a horizontal line across the forehead will shorten and widen the face.

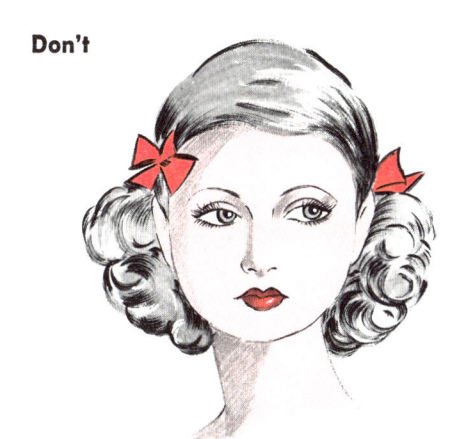

Don't

Do

Don't let it hang like a mop. Don't slick it back where it can't help detract from the roundness.

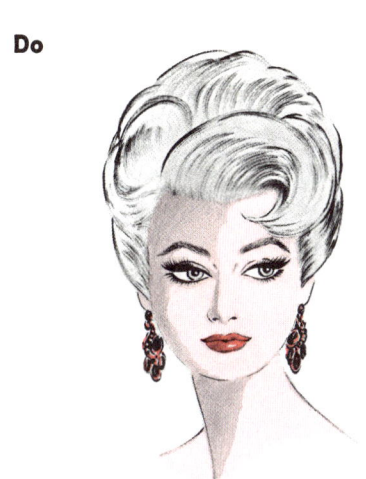

Do lengthen your face by having a built-up hair style above the ears. Do use a side rather than a middle part. Do build your hair higher on one side than on the other.

SQUARE FACE

Coiffures with height arranged unevenly are flattering to square faces, especially so if the silhouette tapers asymmetrically on top. Variety in line and not too much bang on the forehead are best.

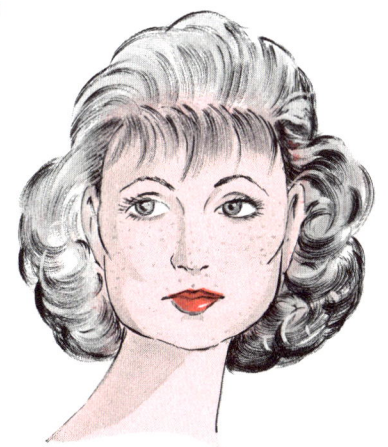

Don't

Do

Don't accent the squareness with a hairstyle that repeats this line. Don't wear your hair slicked back away from your face. Don't wear hair in tiny curls, it just doesn't go with your face.

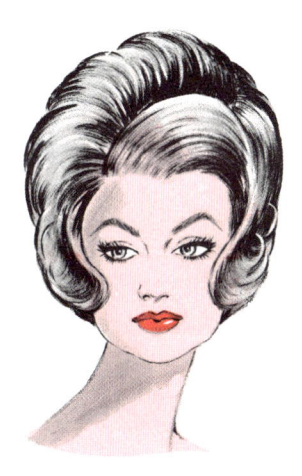

Do counteract the squareness with a hairstyle that has an uneven silhouette. Do wear soft waves around the face to soften the angularity.

OBLONG FACE

A hairstyle that is widest in the middle of the head is best for this face. Usually a symmetrical coiffure without irregularities is most flattering.

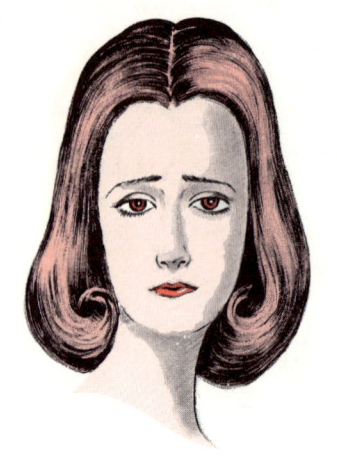

Don't

Do

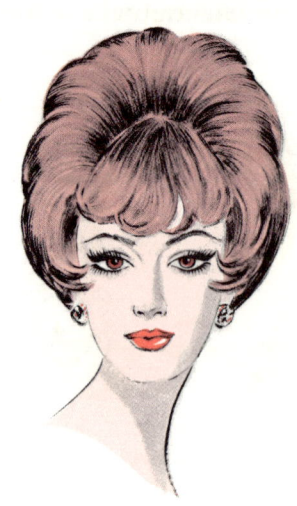

Don't emphasize the long line with hanging hair. Don't wear a middle part.

Do soften the angularity with an asymmetrical bang. Do balance the face; if the lower part of the face is longer than the upper part, achieve balance by building up the silhouette with high bangs.

HEART-SHAPED FACE

Coiffures that are widest below the temples are best for the heart shaped face. Bangs or hair that falls onto the forehead should form oblique lines.

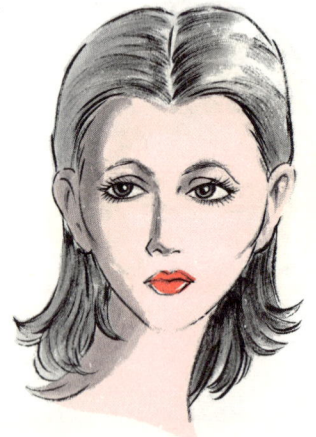

Don't

Do

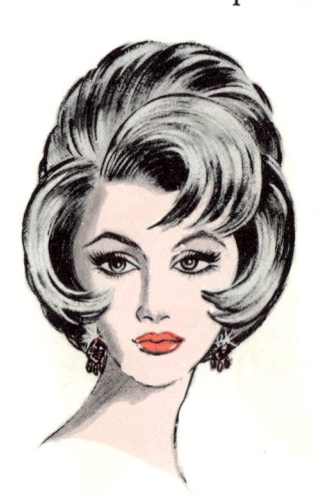

Don't build additional width at the temples with the silhouette of the hairstyle.

Do cover some of the wide expanse of the forehead with a bang. Do flatter the *femininity* of your face with a hairstyle that is soft, not severe.

HAIR CARE, SHAMPOOING AND COIFFURE ARRANGEMENTS

TRIANGULAR FACE

To bring the face into better balance, the silhouette of the hairstyle should create the perfect oval by having fullness that starts at the top of the ears and continues around the top of the head.

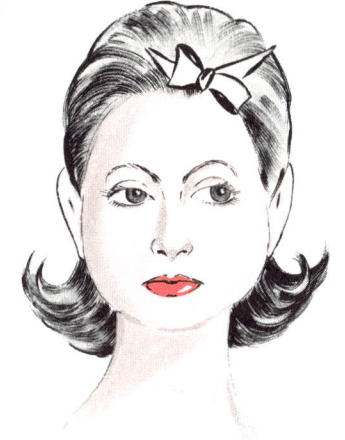

Don't

Do

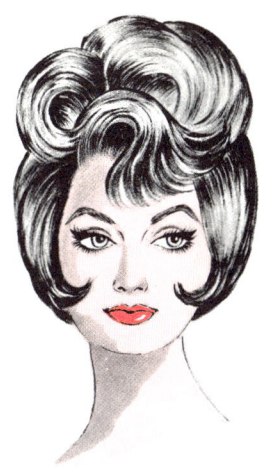

Don't add width to the jaw by having the hair silhouette full below the ears. Don't accent the "pear" shape of your face by slicking your hair flat against your head.

Do ovalize your face by having fullness above the ears and on top of the head. Do bring your face into better balance by having the space from the bridge of the nose to the top of the hairstyle equal to the distance from the bridge of the nose to the bottom of the chin.

DIAMOND-SHAPED FACE

It is plain to see that the hairstyle should broaden the forehead and the narrow chin line.

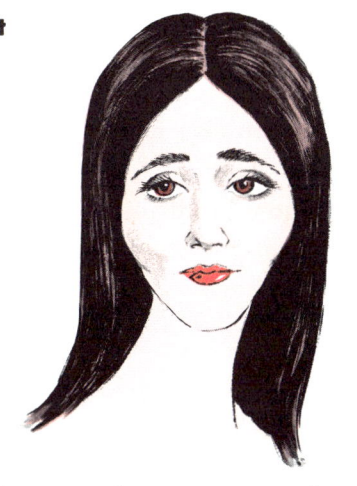

Don't

Do

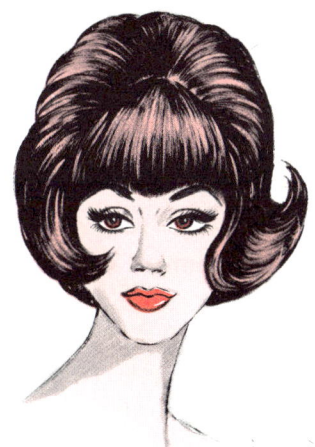

Don't accent the narrowness of your forehead by slicking your hair back at the temples. Don't add length to your face by having your hair too short.

Do wear some sort of bang. Do wear your hair wide across the jaw to "fill in", to give bulk to your narrow chin.

HAIR PIECES

A variety of hairstyles may be created with hair pieces. which can be dressed for either daytime or evening wear.

These hair pieces come in various forms such as:

1. **SWITCHES** — long wefts of hair mounted with a loop at the end. Switches are constructed with one to three stems of hair. The better switches are constructed with three stems in order to provide greater flexibility in styling and braiding. Switches may be worked into the hair or braided to create special styling effects.

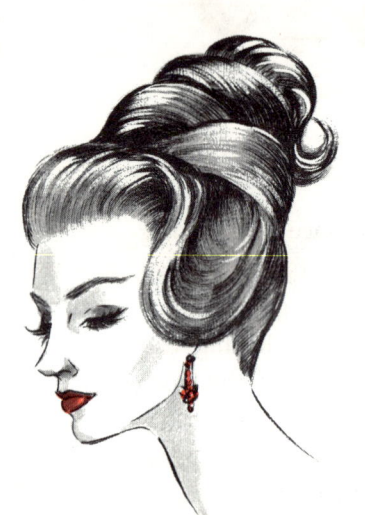

Switch worked into patron's hair

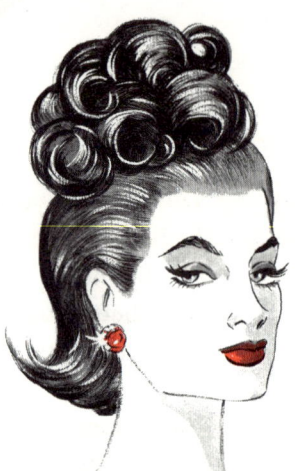

Wiglets attached to patron's hair

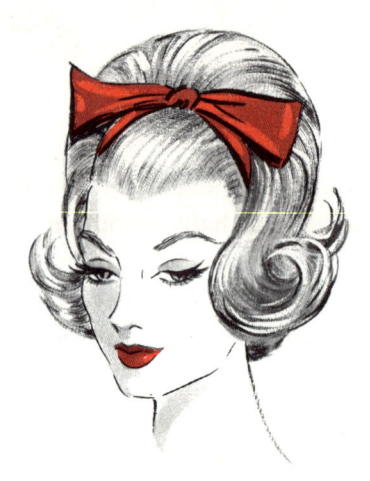

Bandeau type placed back of patron's hairline

2. **WIGLETS** — a hair piece with a flat base which is used in special areas of the head. They are used primarily to blend with your own hair in order to extend the range of the hair. Wiglets can be worked into the top of the hair in curls or under the hair to give it height and body. They are also employed to create special effects.

3. **BANDEAU TYPE** — a hair piece which is sewn to a headband covering the hairline. The headband, which may be replaceable and come in different colors, serves as an excellent disguise for the hairline. The bandeau type hair piece is usually worn over the hair and is dressed in a casual, relaxed manner.

UNIT TWO

VISUAL POISE

Introduction

"Grace is to the body, what good sense is to the mind."

Grace is efficiency of movement. It is the elimination of wasted energy. Movements that are graceful look easy and they are easy because they are right, both from the beauty point of view and from the body mechanics angle. They are coordinated and smooth because the body is being used as Mother Nature intended.

As a student of this Charm Course, you are going to learn how to make your muscles work for you at optimum tension; how to allow one set to take over as another set lets go. You are going to learn how to conserve energy while sitting by learning to sit quietly and at ease. You are going to learn how to increase your self-confidence by removing the causes of your timidity. You are going to know what to do with your hands, so gone will be the embarrassing feeling, "I'm all hands and feet." You are going to know what to do with your body and your belongings, so gone will be the panic of entering into new social situations.

You are going to increase your charm by being sure of your actions and body postures. You will no longer have to be concerned with them. Your mind will be free to concentrate on the people around you and this is the true essence of charm—complete unself-consciousness.

In a sentence, you are going to learn to let your gracefulness be the outward expression of your inner poise. You will have poise because you will know what to do and how to do it. And right now, learn to stand so beautifully in private that you will never have to think about it in public. Here we go!

CHAPTER 6

STANDING

BASIC STANCE

A foot and leg position is called a "stance". There are two for you to learn. One is for a pause or just a second or two, the other is a more stable foot position for those pauses that last any length of time. Both of these positions must be flattering to your legs and must also leave one leg ready for action. Practice the one for long pauses first; it is called the "basic stance". You will need a straight line on the floor and you can make this with a piece of string or with a piece of chalk. As you progress you will often refer to "the line" during exercises in which a positioning of the feet is involved.

Place your left foot across the line pointing outward to the left at a forty-five degree angle. (This is one-eighth of a pie.) The line should run through the instep. Now place your right foot slightly in front of the left foot on the line and slide it back until the heel rests on the instep of the left foot. Very good, you have it. Then you must check on several details:

1. Is your left foot turned out at a forty-five degree angle?
2. Is your right foot on the line and pointing straight ahead?
3. Is your right knee bent over the left knee, *in* not out?
4. Is your left knee also slightly flexed? It should be.

If you have a full length mirror available, go look in it as you repeat the stance. Isn't it pretty? See how it slims your hips and flatters your legs.

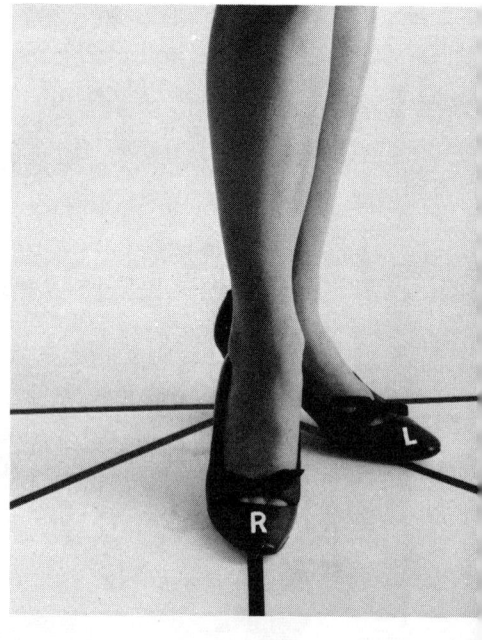

The Basic Stance

STANDING

LEGS CLASSIFIED

If a movie actress doesn't have nicely shaped legs, she must do everything she can to make up for this lack with exercise, diet and correct leg techniques. It is important to her movies and her morale. Not more so for hers than for yours.

Know exactly why your legs are not perfect. Legs are classified as normal, bowed, heavy, thin and knock-kneed.

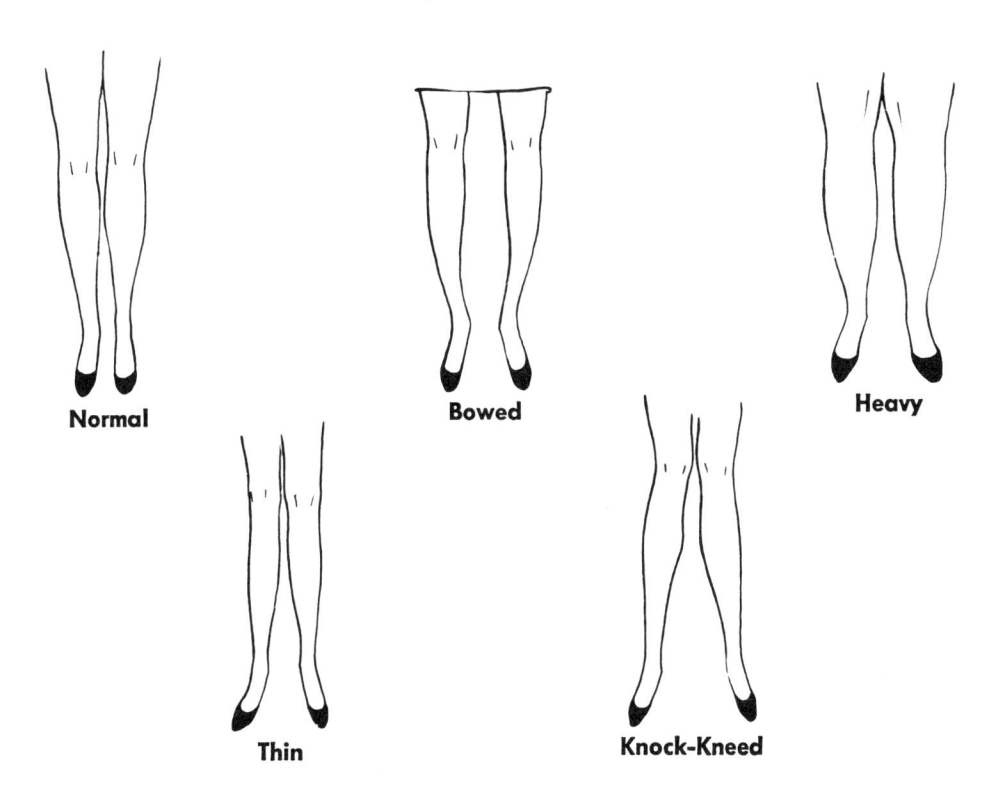

Normal   **Bowed**   **Heavy**

Thin   **Knock-Kneed**

NORMAL LEGS are straight so that when the feet are touching, the calves are touching as are the knees and the thighs.

BOWED LEGS do not meet at the calf, and sometimes do not meet at the knees. Usually this is due to outside leg muscle development rather than bony structure.

HEAVY LEGS have too much bulk. They may be straight or bowed or knock-kneed.

THIN LEGS touch at the knees, but not at the calves. They probably don't touch in the thighs above the knees because they are so slender.

KNOCK-KNEED LEGS are considered normal (because the knees touch) for women, but only if they are neither too thin nor too fat.

STANCE RULES FOR LEG VARIATIONS

No matter what story your mirror tells, there is no need to get discouraged. Keep in mind that beauty is an illusion created by attention to the myriad details that are a part of its composition. Line is one of these and you are going to create pleasing lines for your legs by observing the following rules.

STANCE RULES FOR NORMAL LEGS:
1. Both knees are slightly bent. Neither is held in a "locked" position.
2. The feet should not be farther apart than six inches.
3. One foot is always slightly in front of the other.
4. The heel of the back foot turns slightly in toward the body so that both feet form a forty-five degree angle.
5. The front knee should cover the inside line of the back knee, so bend it. The more beautiful your legs the less bend you will need.
6. Place the major portion of the weight on the back leg.

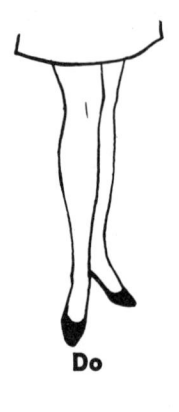

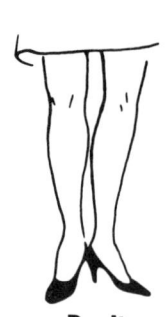

STANCE RULES FOR BOWED LEGS:
1. Bend both knees quite a bit.
2. Put one foot in front of the other enough to hide the back heel. This should hide the back leg inside calf line too.
3. Place the front foot straight ahead.
4. The back foot is placed with the toe pointing out almost far enough to form a ninety degree angle.
5. Put most of the weight on the back foot.
6. Bend the front knee enough so that it covers a part of the back leg.

Often bowed legs are beautiful when seen one in front of the other. Their defect becomes glaringly apparent when placed side by side like two ( ) *parentheses*. So never, never place them in an identical position.

If you will consistently follow the rules for disguising bowed legs, it will be impossible for anyone to discover your secret. Of course you are not going to use it for a conversational topic.

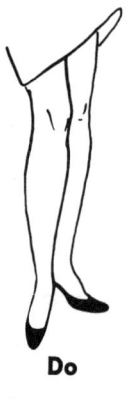

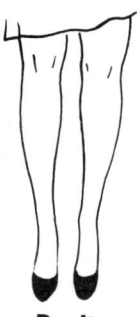

STANDING

STANCE RULES FOR HEAVY LEGS:

1. Strive to create one line instead of two. Do this by hiding the back leg.
2. Balance is achieved by turning the front toe out about an inch.
3. The back foot is also turned out away from the body.
4. There should be about three inches between the heel of the front foot and the toe of the back one. See why the toes are out for balance?
5. Both knees are slightly bent.
6. There is a little more weight on the back foot than on the front.
7. Heels of both feet are in toward the center of the body.

Go look in the mirror. You've subtracted inches from your legs, haven't you? This is a difficult stance but should be used all the time, or at least until such time as you have been able to correct the fault.

STANCE RULES FOR THIN LEGS:

1. Keep them close enough together so that the eye sees both legs as one unit.
2. Stand so that one foot is slightly in front of the other as with normal legs.
3. Back foot is placed at an angle with toe out and heel in.
4. Bend the knee of the front leg so that it barely covers the inside line of the back knee.
5. Put a major portion of your weight on the back leg.
6. The front foot is straight ahead.
7. The front leg covers less than half an inch of the back leg. There should be no space between the two calves when viewed from the front.

Thin legs are usually associated with a slender build. If, however, this is not the case with you and you have an overweight torso, your appearance will be flattered if you will put your feet in the "pedestal stance" as explained in the following paragraph under "Knock-kneed Legs".

STANCE RULES FOR KNOCK-KNEED LEGS:

If your legs are too thin or too fat, you should refer to the rules given for these leg variations. In any case, check the way you stand on your feet in a mirror to see if the arches are pronated. In other words, are you standing on the inside of your feet? You shouldn't, as you will learn in the section on walking.

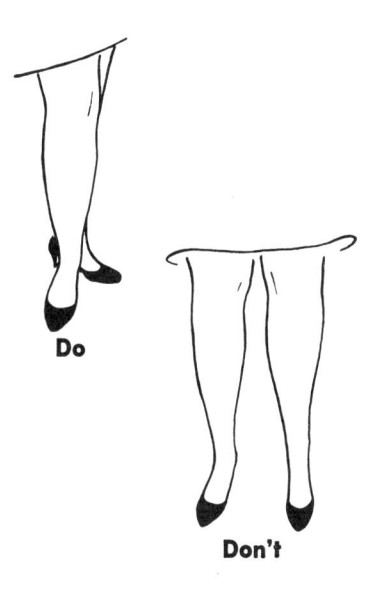

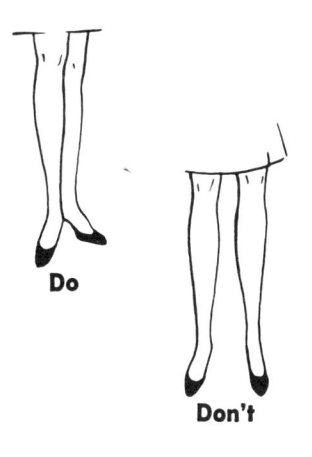

THE PEDESTAL STANCE

Your legs, if they are normal in size, will be flattered by the pedestal stance.

ASSUMING THE STANCE:

1. Place the left foot across the straight line pointing outward at a forty-five degree angle.
2. Place the right foot parallel to the straight line, six inches to the right.
3. Slide the right foot into position with the heel of the right foot even with the ball of the left foot. (It stays six inches to the right.)
4. Bend the right knee toward the left knee. This will rotate the body toward the left.
5. From the waistline up, bring the shoulders around so that they form a right angle to the straight line.
6. Read on to see what you may do with your hands.

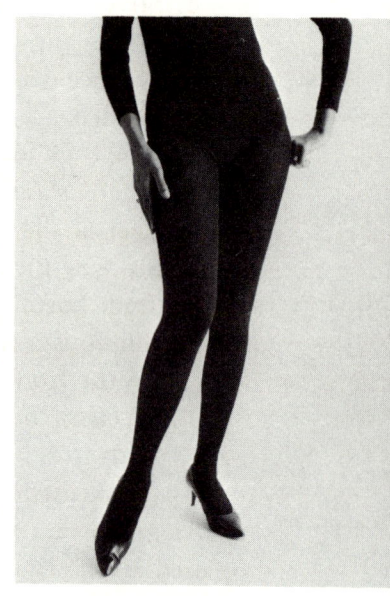

THE BASIC HAND POSITION

Up to this point, what have you been doing with your hands? Have they been hanging like dead fish at your sides? No more.

Do you know that people believe what they see before they believe what they hear? They'll believe in your charm when they see it expressed with your hands. Not that you should over-gesticulate, but your hands do tell a story, let it be one of grace and poise.

It should go without saying that the basic stance with the basic hand position or whatever hand position you may choose to use should incorporate all the rules for good posture and correct body alignment.

The basic hand position that goes with your basic foot position is this: When the right foot is forward, the *right hand* is forward with the little finger edge of the hand resting against the front of the right thigh, the palm facing the center line of the body. The wrist is relaxed backward so that the hand is perpendicular to the floor.

The *left hand* is slightly behind the body with the thumb edge resting against hip.

Both elbows are slightly bent with space between the body and the arms. The elbows are forward rather than back so that the space between the body and the arms can be seen when the figure is viewed from the front.

This hand position is *reversed* when the *left foot* is forward. In short, when the right foot is forward, the right hand is forward; when the left foot is forward, the left hand is forward.

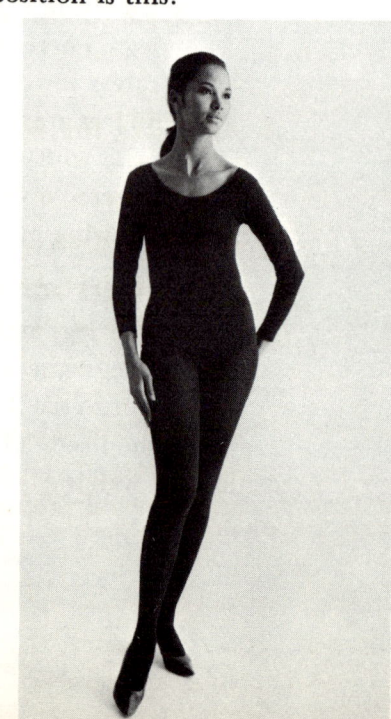

FIVE HAND-HIP POSITIONS

Here are other hand positions that you may use with your basic stance for long pauses. Examine these five and see which ones will be most beautiful and effective for you. Some of them will add width to the hip line, one will reduce the size of the waistline and others are emotionally expressive. Which ones are for you?

1. **ADDS WEIGHT TO THE HIP LINE** The hands are placed on the hips with the fingers forward and the thumb in back. The wrists are bent backward so that the fingers point in a diagonal line upward. The fingers are unevenly spaced from one another. The elbows are held forward so that a definite silhouette of the body is seen from the front.

2. **SLENDERIZES THE HIP LINE** The hands are placed on the hips with the fingers and the thumb together, pointing toward the floor. This hand-hip position is most attractive when one hand is placed somewhat higher on the hip than the other. It will be most slenderizing if the right hand is placed higher than the left when the right foot is forward in the basic stance. Be careful to place your hands on the hips so that the thumb silhouette view is seen from the front. This means that the hands must not be placed too far back nor too far forward.
This hand-hip position will tend to slenderize the hips of a really overweight person if she will place her hands on the thighs rather than on the hips.

3. **MINIMIZES THE WAISTLINE** The hands are placed in the waistline with the thumbs forward, the fingers back. Because the thumbs point downward and toward the center line of the body at a forty-five degree angle, and because the palms tend to press against the waistline, this is the most slenderizing of all the hand-hip positions.
Warning to the overweight: This particular position requires the arms to be akimbo and should, therefore, be avoided. The much overweight figure benefits most in its appearance if the hands as well as the feet are held in asymmetrical positions.

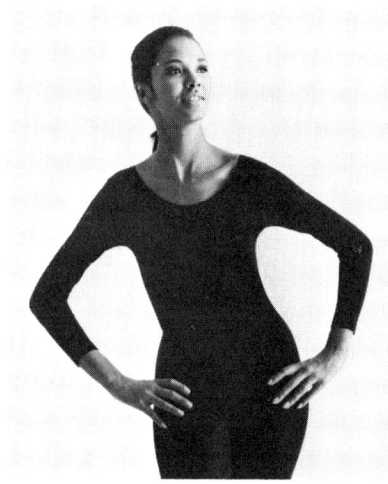

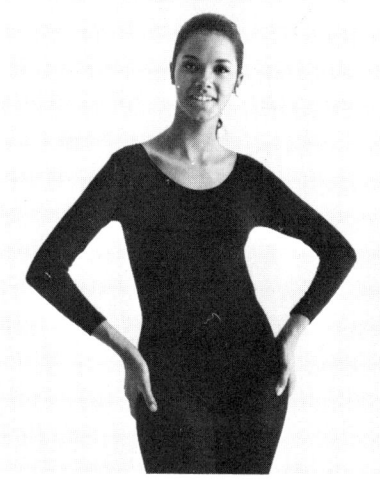

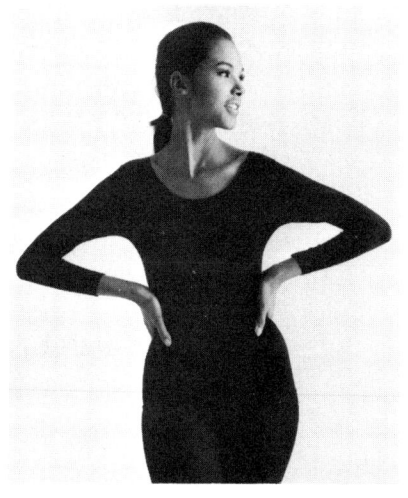

4. DENOTES DETERMINATION The hands are made into light fists and are placed on the hips with the backs of the hands facing forward, the wrists straight. This might be likened to punching yourself on the hips. Don't do it in a lazy or haphazard way. It is a definite, positive position and should be executed with assurance.

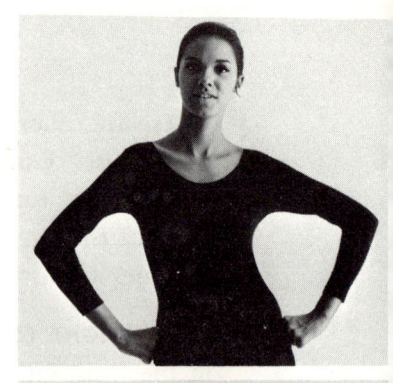

5. EXPRESSES PERTNESS The hands are placed on the hips with the palms facing outward, the fingers relaxed and slightly curled away from the body. This is a sassy position and could be used to advantage in the right situation.

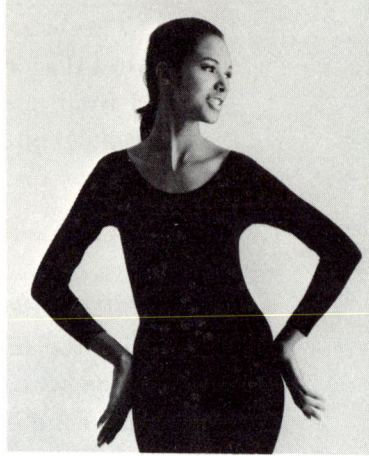

ADDITIONAL HAND POSITIONS FOR EVERYONE

Your main concern about what to do with your hands comes when you have nothing in particular to do with them and when you are not holding anything. Consequently, the hands are empty for the Five Hand-Hip Positions and for these that follow.

SINGER'S HAND POSITION Place one hand on top of the other just below the waistline with both palms up.

THINKER'S HAND POSITION Place the right hand up by the face with the palm facing toward the center line of the body. Extend the forefinger upward along the side of the jaw. Curl the remainder of the fingers and the thumb under the chin.
Place the back of the left hand against the elbow of the right hand. The palm of the left hand is facing toward the floor.

LEANER'S HAND POSITION Place one hand on the hip in whichever one of the Hand-Hip Positions you like best; place the other hand on the top of a table or back of a chair. Don't actually lean your weight on this hand, just look as though you are.

COWBOY'S HAND POSITION Place the thumbs of both hands in the belt; let the wrists relax and the fingers slightly curl.

TALKER'S HAND POSITION Allow the hand by the back foot to rest slightly behind the body with the elbow relaxed. The hand by the front foot is placed just below the waistline with the palm up ready to gesticulate.

STANDING

THREE RULES FOR BEAUTIFUL HANDS

By observing these three rules, your hands will always seem lovely no matter what their size or shape.

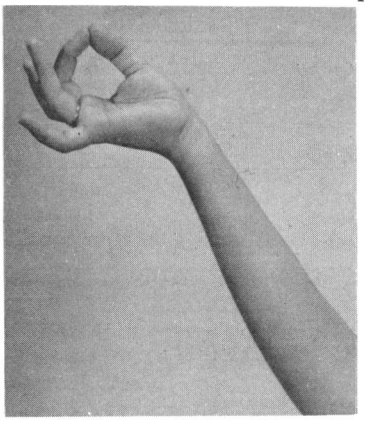

The Hand In Profile

1. The fingers should be relaxed and *unevenly spaced* from one another. This may be achieved by doing as dancers do—place the thumb and the middle or longest finger together and then slowly open the hand keeping the middle finger in toward the palm more than the other fingers.
2. The hand should be at an *angle from the wrist*. This gives the hand a relaxed "at ease" look.
3. The hand should always be *seen in profile*. Either the little finger profile or the thumb profile.

HAND DON'TS

Just as there are certain hand positions that will enhance your appearance and heighten your beauty, so there are things you should avoid doing with your hands, because they detract. Here are five:

1. Do not let the hands hang like dead fish at the sides. This detracts from the silhouette of the figure and looks lifeless.

2. Do not fidget. The more quiet the hands, the more poise there is expressed.

3. Do not squeeze the hands together. This screams of tension.

4. Do not hold both hands interlocked at the waistline. It adds weight to the figure.

5. Do not fold the arms and hide the hands. It drags the bustline down, makes the shoulders sag and adds weight to the waistline.

   Exception: If you are tall and thin, you may fold your arms if you keep your hands exposed and watch your posture.

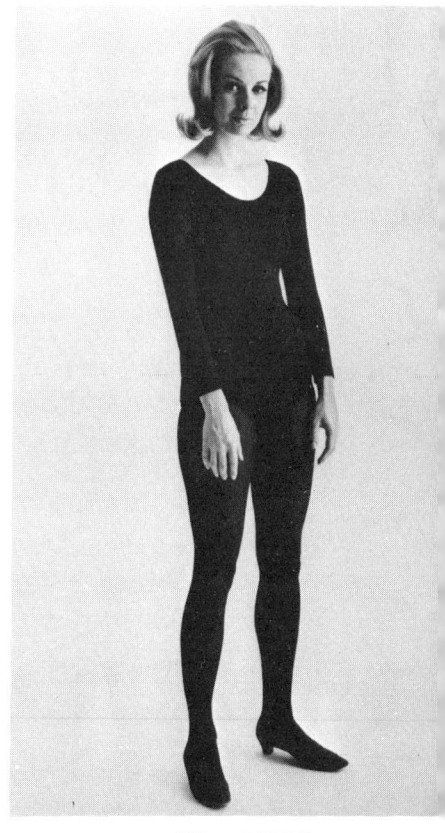

"Dead Fish"

REVIEW ON STANDING

You have now analyzed your legs and you know what position is most flattering to them. You have also discovered a variety of hand positions. You can now look animatedly beautiful even when you do nothing but stand still. Review the rules to make sure the picture you present is the loveliest one possible.

RULES FOR STANDING.
1. The feet are placed with one foot forward.
2. The feet form an angle to one another.
3. The front knee is crossed over the back knee.
4. The major portion of the body weight is on the back leg.
5. The body is correctly aligned with the middle of the shoulders over the middle of the hip bone.
6. The body as a whole presents an asymmetrical or unevenly balanced picture which is pleasing to the eye.
7. The arms form angles to the body.
8. The hands are used for expression.
9. The hands are placed to heighten figure beauty.
10. The hands are shown relaxed and in profile.

CHAPTER 7

WALKING

Introduction

Ethereal qualities are associated with those who walk well. It is said that they "float" or "glide" as though there were no earthly connection between their feet and the ground. Story and song abound with such phrases as "I saw a dream walking." It has been the smooth, elegant and seemingly effortless grace of attractive women who have inspired poets, writers and artists from time immemorial.

A woman who walks beautifully is a delight to behold. Of all the qualities any woman can develop, this is the one which will make her admired even after she is no longer young. It is the one quality by which men universally judge beauty. Men instinctively watch a woman in motion, it is a part of their masculine nature. Let's hope they say of you, "she walks like a queen."

LEARNING TO WALK CORRECTLY

Much has been written about the beauty of a graceful walk, but little about the techniques that make it look fluid and smooth. Where are the feet placed and what do the hands do? These are questions that need to be answered before you, as a student of charm, can learn to walk well.

Just as a ballerina must learn the basic foot and hand positions before she can dance, so you must learn the basic rules before you can walk—in beauty. The following pages are intended to light the path of progress for a more graceful *you*.

Find some area in your house where you can take five steps, that is all, just five. Put a string, chalk mark or something on the floor to indicate a straight line. If you can practice in front of a full length mirror, all the better, for you will be able to see yourself as others see you. What a revelation.

Do practice in shoes with heels. There's nothing more ungainly than a girl who looks as though she is wearing her first pair of high heels. The shoes you wear should be comfortable with a heel that is from two to three inches high. You'll have more luck with the execution of your pivots if the shoes are pumps with closed heels and toes.

Assume your basic stance with the right foot in front. Correctly align your body, balance your pelvis over your feet, your chest over your pelvis and your head over your chest. Place your hands where they will not interfere in front of you with the palms together, the fingers pointing toward the ceiling. Get them out where they are "floating," free from contact with the chest.

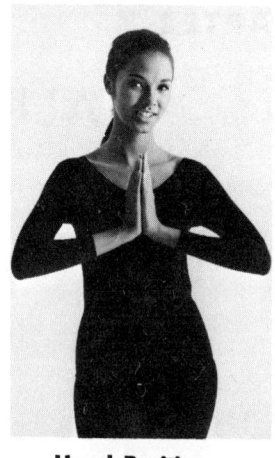

Hand Position For Practice Walk

Even though, in the basic stance, the weight is carried more on one foot (the back one) than on the other, there should never be such an uneven distribution of weight as to cause the hips to slip out of line. *Stand tall.*

As with acquiring any other skill, it will be better for you to practice a little each day rather than devoting several hours one day a week to learning to walk well. Actually, you will have no excuse, for these are techniques that you can put into practice at odd moments and in actual situations.

WALKING

THE FIVE-STEP PRACTICE WALK

Your instructor will tell you whether she prefers to teach a one line or a two line walk. Whichever she chooses, your practice sessions will consist of walking five steps in one direction and five steps back to where you started. For you to do this gracefully and efficiently, you should first learn the *Walking Pivot*. This same pivot will be used later on for leaving a room and for sitting, so learn it well.

PROCEDURE You are in the basic stance with the right foot in front and the back foot at a forty-five degree angle. The major portion of your weight is on the back foot. In order for you to take the first step, you must transfer *all* your weight to the back foot.

Before starting to walk, lift your right foot to make sure it is free.

TWO LINE WALK

The lines on the floor will be approximately two inches apart. The right foot is on the line on the right side and the left foot is crossing the left line at a forty-five degree angle.

ONE LINE WALK

Both feet are on the same line, right foot pointing straight ahead, left at forty-five degree angle.

Further instructions in this paragraph will be given as though you are using two lines.

Step one. When taking this first step, place your right foot on the right line with about the length of one of your own feet separating the heel of the right foot from the toe of the left.

Step two. Place your left foot on the left line with about one foot in between.

Step three. Right foot steps forward on right line.

Step four. Left foot steps forward on left line.

Step five. You are at the completion of your five steps. As soon as your final step contacts the floor, you are ready to execute the walking pivot.

It's difficult to hold your balance with both feet pointing straight ahead, so turn the toes out somewhat while you study:

THE EXECUTION OF THE WALKING PIVOT Come onto the balls of both feet and pivot toward the left until you are turned in the direction from which you just came. Keep your feet "glued" to the floor, don't pick them up.

In order for you to keep your balance during and after the execution of the walking pivot, it will be necessary for you to keep your feet opposed to one another. In other words, they must be at a forty-five degree angle to each other. This means that as you turn, you must arrange to have your right foot stop at an angle to the line. It should be at a forty-five degree angle and your left foot should point straight ahead.

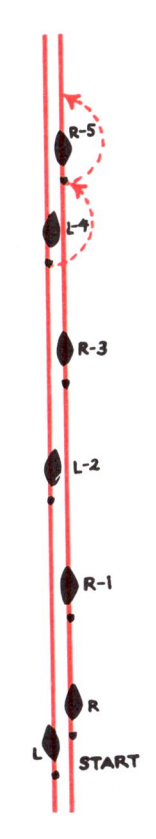

Two Line Walk

One Line Walk

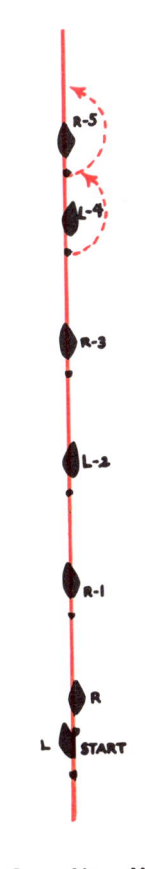

The Walking Pivot

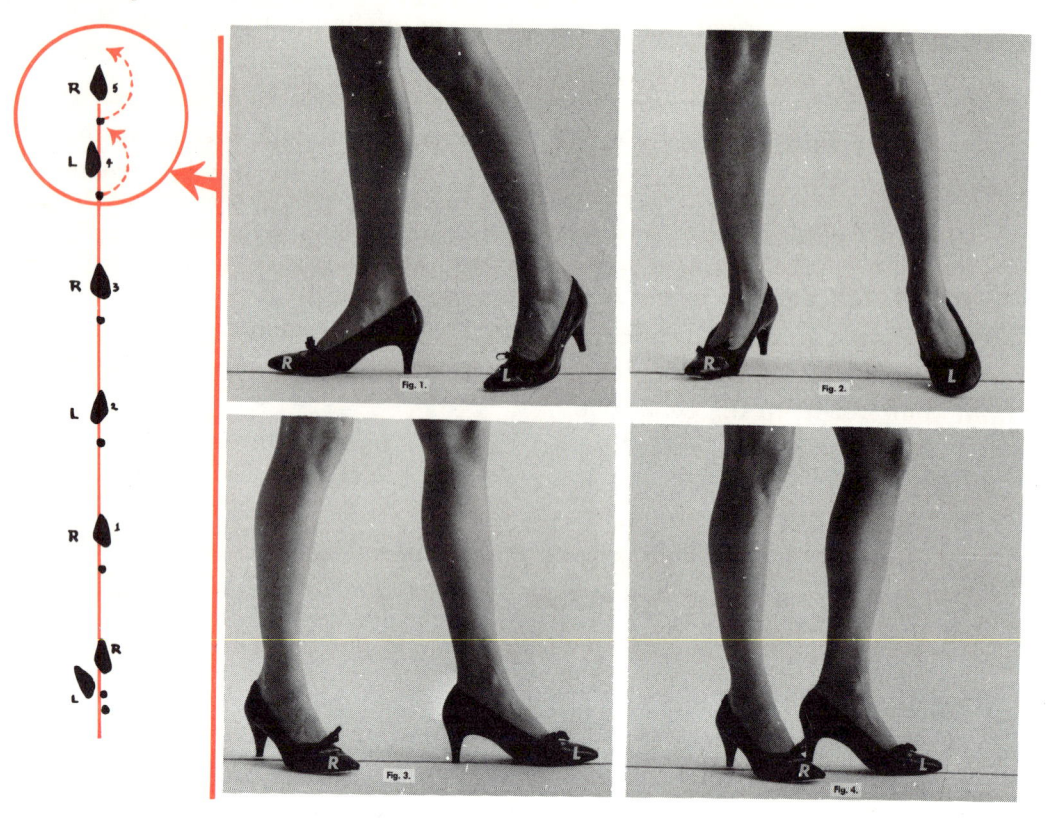

Perhaps it will help you to place the left foot in the instep of the right before starting to walk back. Otherwise, make sure your weight is on the back or right foot, start walking with the front (left) foot. Take five steps.

Upon completing the five steps, your left foot will be in front. Execute the pivot to the right by coming onto the balls of both feet and turning the body toward the right until you are facing in your original position.

As you turn, stop the left foot as soon as it is at a forty-five degree angle to the line. Let the right foot continue to pivot on the ball until its entire length is on the line. Draw the right foot back into the instep of the left.

There you are, you have just completed walking forward five steps, executing a walking pivot to the left, walking to your original position by taking five steps and executing a walking pivot to the right.

Continue to practice walking on the line and executing the Walking Pivot until you can do so with perfect balance. Keep those hands up in front.

TECHNIQUES FOR A GRACEFUL WALK

You are going to say, "For goodness sake, how does all this walking back and forth on a straight line help me acquire a beautiful walk?" Well, let's see.

Poise and balance are synonymous. *If a beautiful walk is anything, it is well balanced.* Walking on a line like a tight rope walker will give you balance; this is the beginning of learning to walk well. It is the beginning, but not the end. Obviously, there is more than this that goes into a beautiful walk.

First of all, a beautiful walk should appear effortless and smooth. This calls for the most efficient movement possible. The muscles must take over and let go at precisely the right moment. They must work at optimum tension. The direction of the walk must be forward, not up and down or from side to side.

You must not "settle" with each step. You must think tall and light. You must keep your weight forward toward the balls of the feet. To check this, stand with your feet side by side, close your eyes and imagine that you are a puppet being pulled up and up by strings attached to the crown of your head and to your ears. Where is your weight? It's definitely not on your heels and never should be as you walk. Carry your weight just in front of the ankle bone. If you sink onto your heels your walk will lack the "heavenly" quality that reaching for the sky will give it.

Keep your chest high. The grace of your arms, neck and head depend upon your chest position. If it is balanced over the feet, the shoulders will act as ballast so that your entire torso from the waistline up will seem like a ship skimming over calm seas.

Keep your chin up. You don't want to lose by a head. There's something queenly about the woman who carries her head held high. What's the saying about it's better to see the stars in the sky than the mud on the ground?

Acquire an evenly spaced momentum. How fast or slow you walk will depend upon your personality. Most of all, you should look for a nice balance between the slouching, idling gait and the "going to a fire" gait that looks harassed. Whatever the speed of the rhythm you choose, let it be a natural rhythm that will vitalize your movements.

Rhythm makes the difference. It will be helpful if you can do your walking practice to music, if not, count aloud to yourself in soft and relaxed tones, "One, two, three, four, five, pivot; one, two, three, four, five, pivot."

Now that you have your legs and torso working, you can begin to coordinate your arm movements with your feet. A moment of observation will convince you that the arms naturally swing at the sides as you walk.

HAND COORDINATION WITH THE FEET

When a step is taken with the right foot, the left hand swings forward in a slight semi-circle around the body. Simultaneously, the right hand swings backward. The more vigorous the walk, the more vigorous the hand swing. We might say that the hands swing forward to the toe and backward to the heel.

The palms of the hands face the body so that when the figure is seen from the front, a profile view of the hands is visible. The elbows are kept relaxed and the hands swing from the shoulders, not from the elbows like a tin soldier.

It is surprising the number of women who lose all semblance of serenity by allowing their arms to become uncontrolled when they are self-conscious. Some are so at a loss as to what to do that they fold them tightly over the chest. This might be all right for a prize fighter, but hardly for a lady. Practice now with your arms at your sides until you are sure of them and know that they will behave under any amount of social pressure.

PRACTICE HAND COORDINATION Assume the basic stance for the feet with the right foot in front. Assume the basic hand position. Remember, your right hand will be in front on the thigh and the left hand will be slightly behind. As you take your first step with the right foot, the left hand must swing out around the body in a slight semi-circle until it is forward with the right toe, the right hand simultaneously swings back to the heel of the left foot.

If you have difficulty getting your hand forward to the opposite toe on each step, try holding a pencil in each hand and say, "Point, point, point, point, point, pivot."

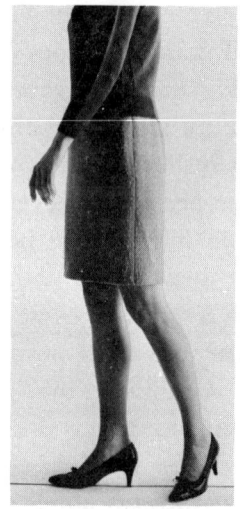

Foot and Hand Coordination

REVIEW ON WALKING

Question: If you have started walking the five steps with your right foot in front and you are ready to pivot after the five steps with the right foot in front, which hand is forward?

Answer: The left hand is forward slightly in front of the body and even with the right toe, the right hand is back toward the heel of the left foot.

As you execute the Walking Pivot toward the left, the left hand remains in front. Upon completion of the pivot the left hand rests in front on the left thigh and the right hand is slightly in back. Now you are ready to start walking with the left foot.

You will encounter a great deal of difficulty if you fail to keep your weight on the back foot or insist on turning in the wrong direction. In this case, slow down to a "slow motion" gait so that you may analyze each action separately.

Get off your heels, get that chin level, back straight, pelvis under, chest up, tummy in, and walk with the fluid grace of a native woman who carries a basket on her head and who wears no shoes on her feet. In high heels, this is no mean trick.

In just a moment, you are going to read the Ten Rules for a Beautiful Walk. As you do so, read just one rule at a time and practice it on your line until you are sure of the "feel" of it. There is a word for this, it is "Kinesthetic sense." It may take a week or more before you get your knees to stay flexed or your hips to come forward, but don't get discouraged. You really only have two legs, a right and left; not three, a right, a left, and a wrong.

Have fun!

TEN RULES FOR A BEAUTIFUL WALK

1. **THE BODY MUST BE CORRECTLY ALIGNED** with the back as straight as possible. To start, the knee bone should be over the ankle bone, the hip bone over the knee bone, the shoulder bone over the hip bone and the head over all. Maintain this torso alignment while the legs are in motion.

2. **THE STEP SHOULD BE NO LONGER THAN YOUR OWN FOOT** so that the distance between the heel of the forward foot and the toe of the back foot does not exceed the length of the foot. Do not reach for your steps and do not mince along.

3. **THE TOES SHOULD POINT STRAIGHT AHEAD** or be turned slightly outward as models and dancers walk.

4. **THERE SHOULD BE NO PERCEPTIBLE CHANGE OF WEIGHT** from one foot to the other. This can best be achieved by keeping the weight on the balls of the feet and by "pushing off" with the ball of the back foot.

5. **THE KNEES ARE KEPT FLEXED** so that they may act as the "spring" for the body to give a smooth, glide appearance.

6. **ONE FOOT IS PLACED DIRECTLY IN FRONT OF THE OTHER** on one line. This method gives a feminine look and when done with balance and grace might be called a "show girl's walk."

7. **THE LEGS SWING FORWARD FROM THE WAISTLINE** so that the hips also move forward and forward. They do not move from side to side, nor do they undulate. This avoids hosiery rub. When the right leg comes forward, the right hip comes forward.

8. *THE ARMS MOVE IN OPPOSITION TO THE FEET* for balance so that when the right foot is forward, the left arm swings forward and vice versa. The hand should swing forward to the toe and backward to the heel. The more vigorous the walk, the more vigorous the hand swing.

9. *THE ARMS SHOULD SWING RELAXED FROM THE SHOULDERS* with the elbows held fairly close to the body but not tight. They should remain relaxed and should not bend as the arm comes forward.

10. *FLOAT FROM THE WAISTLINE UP, WALK FROM THE WAISTLINE DOWN.* The head, shoulders and upper torso move forward smoothly as though disconnected from the rest of the body. The control of the walk comes from the midriff, and the leg moves forward from the waistline.

YOU MUST PRACTICE

From here on out, your success will depend upon practicing the foregoing techniques until you have a "naturally" beautiful walk. Because it is difficult to analyze ourselves objectively, let others comment on your progress.

Your walk tells a great deal about you. It reveals carelessness, timidity, shyness, aggressiveness; or it can bespeak the loveliness of you. *It is worthwhile to learn "to walk in beauty."*

CHAPTER 8

SITTING

Introduction

Airplane pilots say the most difficult thing about learning to fly is landing the plane. It is well done only when the landing is so smooth that the passengers are not jolted when the plane touches down. There's an analogy here. You, as a student of charm, will have perfected your sitting on a chair only when you sit so gently that your audience will not be able to detect the instant of your "landing."

You will be able to "land" smoothly, no matter what the height of the chair, bench, stool or whatever, if you keep control of your body weight by keeping it over your feet. *This means that as you sit you lower your body into a sitting position with the back held straight, the hips under and the large muscles of the thighs and buttocks doing all the work.*

It's when you "fanny reach" that you fall into a chair like a ton of bricks. Don't do it, you're out of control and will undoubtedly "crash land."

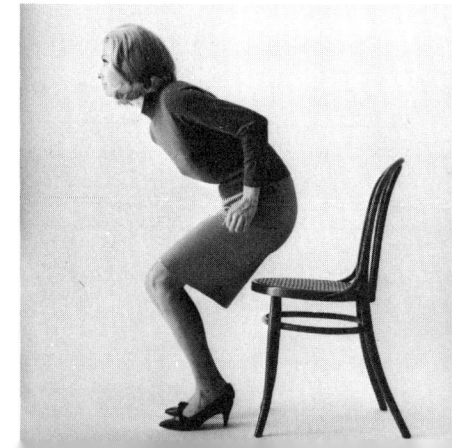

"Fanny Reaching"

LEARNING TO SIT CORRECTLY

Preserve your energy, be efficient, eliminate all unnecessary squirming and wriggling after you are seated. To do this, you sit in a particular position that is the logical result of the direction from which you approach a chair. Also, you adjust your skirt, if it is essential, as you sit, not after you are seated.

APPROACHING THE CHAIR

There are two different ways to approach a chair; one is straight on, the other is from an angle. The first requires that you sit in a "T" position and the latter requires that you sit in an "S" position. You will practice your approach for each "landing" in just a minute or two, but first, learn what to do with your clothes so that you won't have to adjust them once you are seated.

CLOTHES ARRANGING

Your back is to the chair, your body is just beginning to be lowered, the large muscles of the thighs are doing the work, the coccyx (tail bone) is under and the back is only slightly curved as both hands arrange your clothing for comfortable sitting.

STRAIGHT SKIRT Place the right hand on the right thigh just below the hip joint and the left hand on the left side in the same position. Raise the skirt slightly by giving a firm pull upward with both hands. This will keep your skirts from getting "rump sprung."

FULL SKIRT Place both hands slightly behind and below the buttocks. The palms are facing the body as the hands gently pull the skirt outward and upward so that it will wrinkle as little as possible.

PANTS Men raise their pants as they sit by grasping the pant legs just above the knee. The feminine gender will do likewise. (Men do a lot of things right, instinctively, as you'll see when we come to coats.)

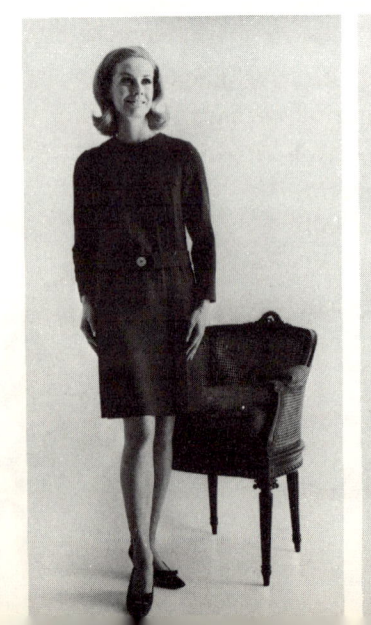

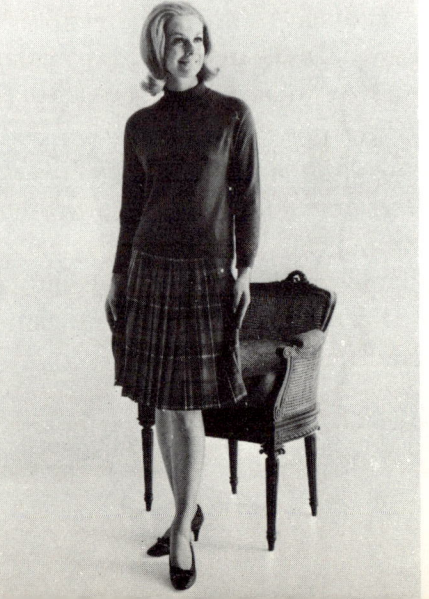

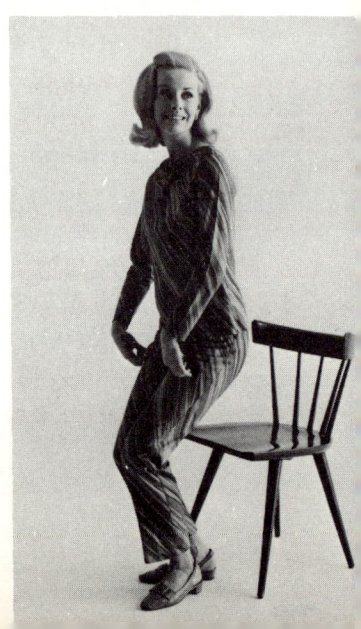

SITTING

THE "T" SITTING POSITION

When you approach a chair from directly in front, your body will form a "T" in the sitting position. Your feet will be perpendicular to your knees, your hips even on the chair, your spine straight. It's your shoulders that form the cross bar. Look in the mirror, you'll be able to see for yourself.

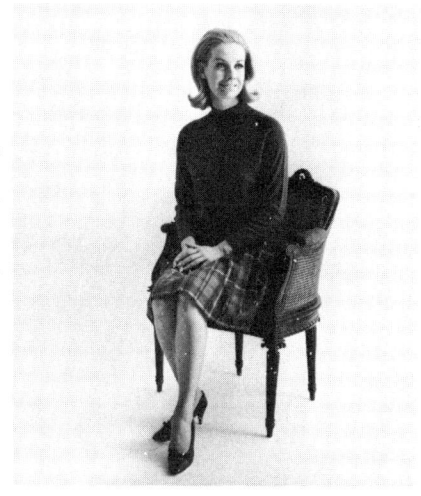

Place a chair at the far end of your straight line. Have the line long enough for you to take three steps that will bring the forward foot about twelve inches away from the chair. Test the distance a couple of times. Are you ready?

APPROACH PROCEDURE FOR THE "T" POSITION Start with your right foot forward, approach the chair by taking three steps, starting with the right foot. Now with the right foot in front, do the walking pivot to the left. *If you have judged your distance correctly, the right calf will be touching the forward edge of the chair after the pivot.*

Walk back to starting position beginning with the left foot which is in front. Pivot. You are now where you started. Repeat until you can judge the distance to the chair so precisely that the calf just touches after you have done the pivot. When you are judging correctly, you will neither push the chair backward with your calf nor miss the chair entirely.

To graduate with high honors from this approach "landing." You should be able to walk from any distance across a room and turn in exactly the right place for easy sitting. Your calf will tell you the chair is there so there is no need for you to look over your shoulder to check. This is the elimination of another unnecessary movement.

As soon as you feel confident of your "approach," you may "land."

PRACTICE PROCEDURE
1. Approach three steps.
2. Pivot, calf touches chair.
3. Arrange skirt.
4. Sit, with the body weight forward in the chair.

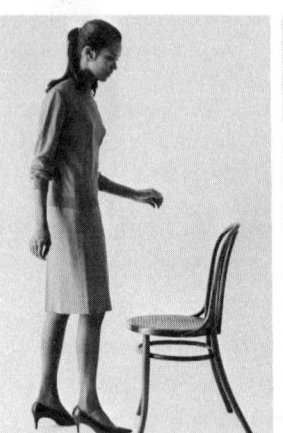

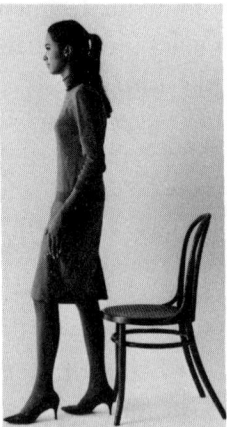

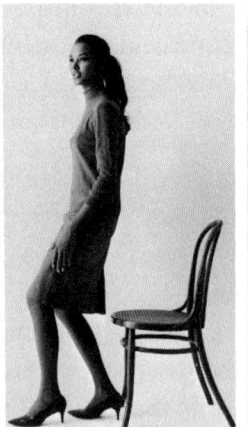

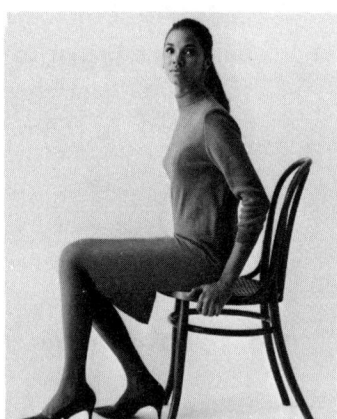

In order to lower the body gracefully without "fanny reaching" and not *fall* into a chair, it is necessary for us to sit down in the front portion.

According to a book on charm written around the turn of the century, "a lady always sits with her hips touching the back of the chair." You may not want to be so straight-laced, there's no rule that says you must sit all the way back. But if you want to be a "lady" by nineteenth century standards, slide back in this fashion:

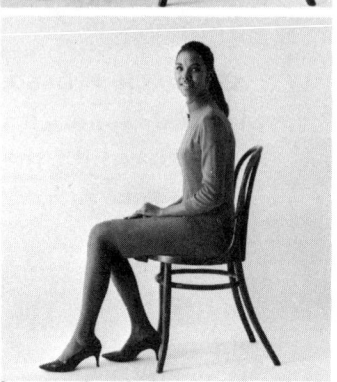

SLIDING TO THE BACK OF CHAIR Place both hands on the forward edge of the chair at either side of the hips. Raise the body slightly, resting the weight on the hands. Slide back. Don't wiggle back.

ARISING FROM CHAIR

Before arising. The torso must again be brought forward so the weight is over the feet. The same technique of raising the body to slide forward is used.

This idea of lifting the body from the chair with the hands to adjust a position is particularly useful when:
1. Sitting in a deep, soft chair or sofa.
2. Sliding over on a bench.
3. Arranging a comfortable position in a car.

There's one important difference between the graceful landing of a plane and your sitting. It is this. A plane makes a three point landing, you make a two—the sits bones. Sit down now and place both your hands under your hips. Feel those two bones? Those are the *sits* bones and are intended

SITTING

to be sat upon. The lower back is a part of the wall of your body, not the basement floor. If you insist on sitting on your spine, you will add four inches to your waistline and subtract four skillion from your charm. Sit and look tall.

While you are sitting, read the basic rules for sitting. If you have a full length mirror handy, look at yourself while you follow the rules, you'll be pleasantly surprised at the difference these rules make in your appearance.

BASIC RULES FOR THE "T" SITTING POSITION

For the feet.
1. Keep the feet close together.
2. Keep the knees together.
3. Keep the feet out slightly farther than the knees. This gives a longer line than having your feet directly under your knees.
4. Never push your feet under the chair. This is a negative position that makes you look subdued and timid.
5. Keep the soles of your shoes on the floor. It might be restful to have only your heels touching the floor, but it doesn't make a good impression.
6. Keep your feet in the basic stance position (they are if you did your pivot correctly). It was a good position for flattering your legs while standing and will continue to do so while you are sitting. If your legs are heavy, hide as much of the back leg as possible.

For the hands.
1. Keep the hands quiet.
2. Keep the fingers relaxed.
3. Strive for length rather than width in your hand positions. This means that your hands will be in your lap, not folded across the chest and not on the arms of a chair.
4. Grace is enhanced by placing your hands to one side of the lap rather than smack dab in the middle.

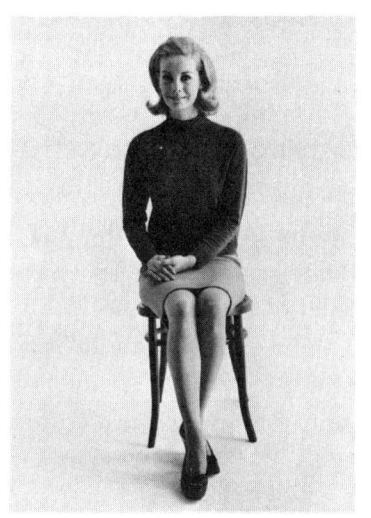

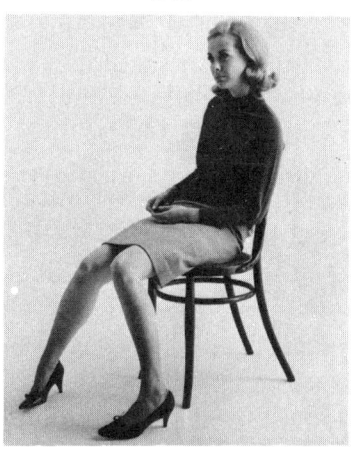

THE "S" SITTING POSITION

The "S" position can be smoothly assumed as a direct result of an angle approach to the object upon which you are going to sit. It is an asymmetrical position. That is, the feet are not under the knees and the hips are at an angle on the sitting surface.

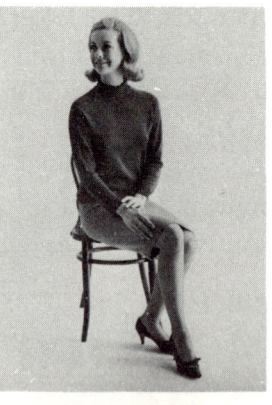

APPROACH PROCEDURE FOR THE "S" POSITION

When a chair, divan or hassock is approached from the side, the foot closer to the furniture is behind. For instance, if you approach your chair from the side, and the chair in which you are going to sit is on your left hand side, you will pause just before sitting with your left foot slightly behind the right. The right foot should be just beyond the center of the front of the seat of the chair. Swivel your hips slightly to the left and sit. Please note that when this is done as directed, the feet are crossed at the ankle.

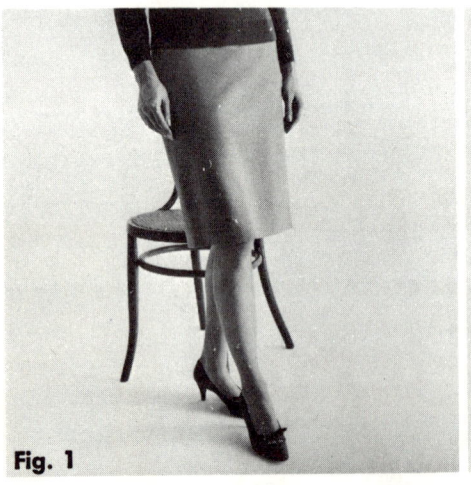

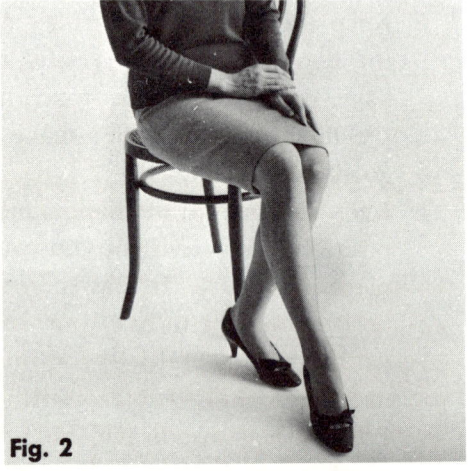

Fig. 1

Fig. 2

SITTING IN THE "S" POSITION

The "S" position is the answer to those sitting situations where the knees would be higher than the hips if they were directly below the knees, such as when sitting on a *low* bench or stool.

SITTING ON A LOW BENCH OR STOOL The technique you use to go down, down, down, is precisely the same except that you use one hand to pilot you. The arm is held straight so that the hand will reach the low sitting surface before you do. It tells you how far down you must go. **Happy landing!**

SITTING

SITTING-PRETTY PRINCIPLES

FOR THE FEET AND LEGS

Crossing the Ankles. Crossing the feet at the ankles is lovely, if you allow no dropping of the arches. The ankles must be controlled so that the entire length, from toe to knee, forms a straight line. Place the left foot behind and to the right of the right foot. Slide both feet to the right side. See that the right leg is making a straight line from the toe to the knee. This is a lovely asymmetrical position and is one of the best for the being-looked-at feeling.

Crossing Legs Above Knee. Shall you cross your legs above the knee? This is not considered good form when applying for a job, sitting on a platform, or when riding a public conveyance. Otherwise, it depends upon the shape of your legs and how gracefully you can cross them. Those of you who are overweight can discard this position without even giving it a try. The rest of you can try it by placing your right hand on your right knee to hold your skirt and smoothly crossing your right leg over the left. Place both feet slightly to the left. The right foot will rest by the left ankle. Remember to keep a straight line on both legs.

Sitting on a Low Chair or Stool. Whenever it is necessary for you to sit in a chair that is so low your knees come under your chin, it will be more flattering for you to put both feet to one side and thereby get your knees down. If you put your feet to the right, the right foot is just slightly in front of the left.

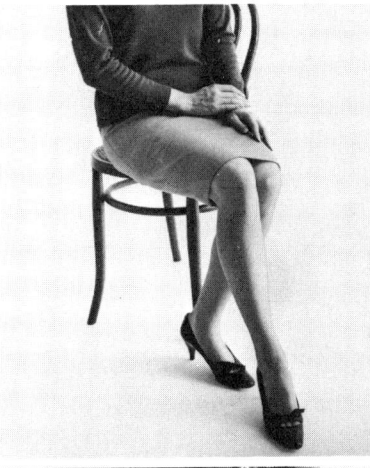

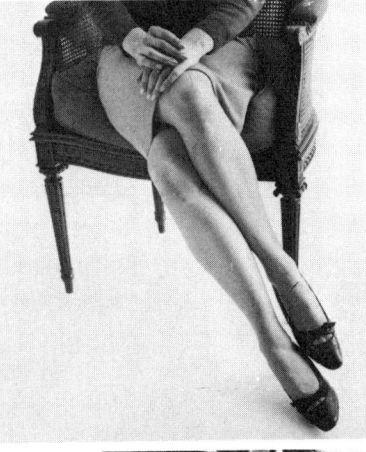

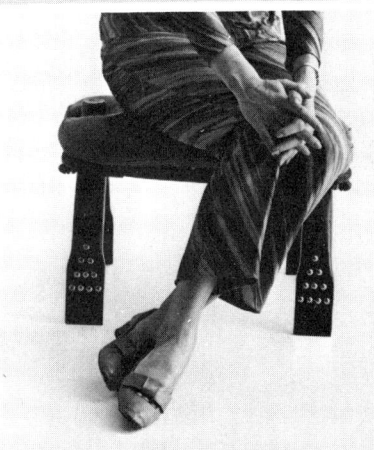

FOR THE HANDS

1. *Palms "Upward" Position.* Turn your hands so that the palms face upward. The fingers are neither too curled nor too straight. Place the thumb of one hand in the palm of the other. This position is one of the best because it is easy to assume, looks natural and gives you something to hold.

2. *Right Thigh Hand Position.* Cross your left arm to the right thigh and join hands. Intertwine the forefinger of the right hand between the forefinger and longest finger of the left hand and alternate fingers as shown in illustration 2. The ring finger and little finger of the left hand are on the bottom to support the weight of both. This may sound difficult, but it isn't. It's one of the most graceful positions.

3. *Encircle Finger Position.* Place one hand in the other, palms facing up. Encircle the index and middle fingers of the upper hand with the thumb of the lower hand. Whether you have square fingers, short fingers or whatever, they will be flattered by this position.

4. *Arm Chair Hand Position.* If your chair has arms, it will be relaxing for you to place one hand on the arm and the other hand, palm up, on the lap. This will give the body a wider line, but this can be counteracted by being sure the legs point in the opposite direction. For instance, if you are resting the right hand on the arm of the chair, then the legs should extend to the left.

SUMMARY OF DON'TS FOR SITTING

1. Don't rearrange your skirt after you are seated.
2. Don't allow your underclothes to show.
3. Don't let your feet be pigeon toed.
4. Don't let your ankles turn outward.
5. Don't let pressure distort the contour of your legs.
6. Don't let your knees separate.
7. Don't sit on the end of your spine.
8. Don't add weight to your figure by "sprawling" your arms or legs.
9. Don't tightly fold your arms or hands.
10. Don't fidget and fuss.

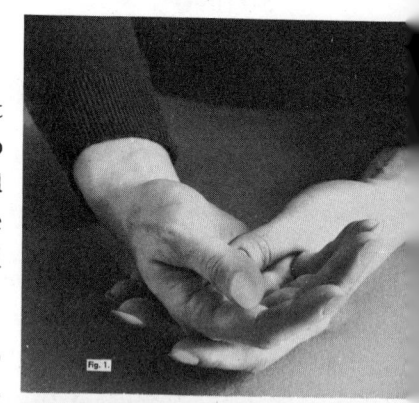

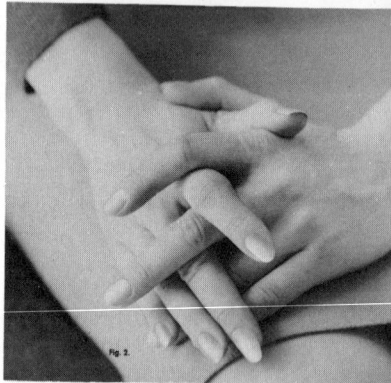

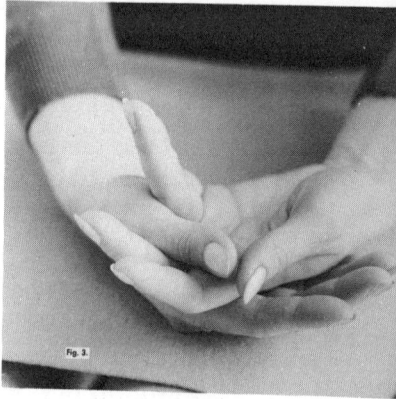

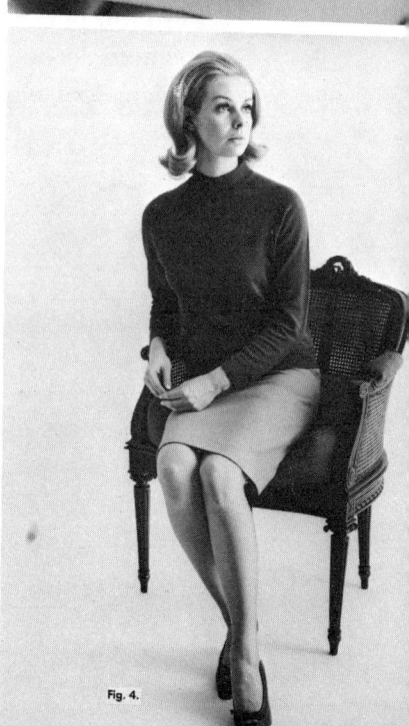

SITTING

GETTING IN AND OUT OF CARS

Introduction

How nice it would be if we could always look graceful when getting into and out of a car. However, some cars are so small and compact that it is necessary to fold up like an accordion. Oh, well, there is a *best* method for everything and that is what we are after.

GETTING INTO A CAR

STANDARD MAKE Let's get into the right front seat. Open the door on the right side, stand facing the front of the car, the left leg almost touching the car by the seat, the feet close together, then:
1. Place the left foot on the floor boards.
2. Turn the hips slightly to position the buttocks correctly and sit down.
3. Bring the right foot into the car immediately.

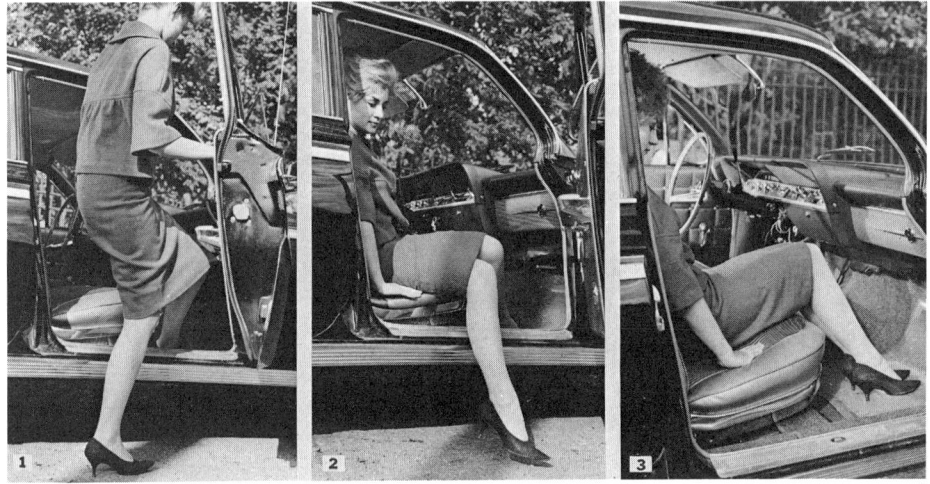

Another version that might be more convenient is to stand as above and then:
1. Turn the hips over the car seat and sit, using the left hand on the seat for balance.
2. Lift both legs and swing them into the car.

In any case, the hands are used on the seat at each side of the hips to lift the body over into a position that is comfortable.

TWO-DOOR CAR Now let's get into the back seat of a two-door. The only solution is to stoop, bending the knees, not the back, and walk in. Keep the buttocks tucked under as much as possible. Again use the hands on the seat to adjust your position.

COMPACT CAR You're on your own. See the Do's and Don'ts which follow right after Getting Out of a Car.

A couple of tidbits of advice. Don't hesitate to use your escort's hand for balance or to give him your belongings so your hands will be free to assist yourself. Have a good trip!

GETTING OUT OF A CAR

STANDARD MAKE Getting out of the right front seat.
1. Slide over as close to the door as possible.
2. Place the right foot on the ground.
3. Lift the body out of the car with the weight on the left foot which is still in the car.

The variation of this would be:
1. Place both feet on the ground.
2. Use your left hand as a lever to lift yourself out of the car.

It is permissible, even advisable, to accept your escort's hand for assistance.

TWO-DOOR CAR To get out of the back seat of a two-door car, slide as close to the door as possible and get out head first. Do not back out with your buttocks leading the way.

COMPACT CAR Again you are on your own. Just follow as closely as you can the following:

DO'S AND DON'TS FOR GETTING IN AND OUT OF A CAR

1. Do keep your hips tucked under.
2. Don't let your skirt hike up around your hips.
3. Do keep your knees together.
4. Don't attempt to ride in a sports car without appropriate clothing. On the other hand, go along for the fun, not the beauty of it.
5. Don't lose your balance. Use your hands for assistance.
6. Don't hesitate to ask for assistance.
7. Do be a good sport about your boy friend's car, no matter what make it is.

CHAPTER 9

SOCIAL POSTURES

Introduction

You've seen women who destroyed any illusion of beauty by being as awkward and jerky as the first model "T." Efficiency as well as beauty depends upon your ability to get into action with the least effort. This is the reason that the body weight is invariably placed more on one foot than on the other. You are poised for action.

You can learn to anticipate your movements and manage your feet with the same precision you manage your car (unless you are the typical female driver, they say). At any rate, it is going to take concentration to learn to approach a chair, come through a door, greet people and handle your personal effects. But just as you concentrated to learn to write so that you could do so without thinking about the mechanics of writing, so you are going to practice all the social postures so that when the time arrives to actually use them, you will not have to think about them. Your mind will be free to be charming and scintillating.

The first social posture you are going to learn is "The Arch" which is a foot position similar to the basic stance except that it is used for momentary pauses such as the one encountered when shaking hands.

THE ARCH

In the arch position, the body is prepared to "arch" from standing to walking, or from repose to action. No matter how heavy you may be, you will appear light and graceful if your weight is smoothly transferred as you go from a stationary position to a walk. Here's how you smooth out the weight shifting transition. Up on your feet!

ASSUMING THE ARCH POSITION
1. Stand in your "stance" position with the right foot in front.
2. The weight is mostly on the back leg.
3. Shift your weight so that most of it is on the front or right foot.
4. Lift the heel of the left foot so that only the ball of the foot is touching the floor.
5. Turn the left toe out so that the heel turns in toward the center of the body and is about an inch off the floor.
6. The left knee touches the right knee.

THE ARCH

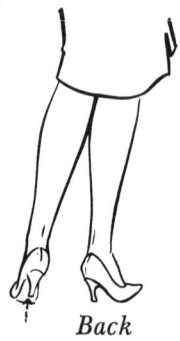

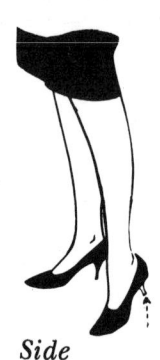

Back   *Side*

PRACTICE THE ARCH Now practice this around the room with a count of "step, arch; step, arch; step, arch." This will look much like a wedding march. If you walk from the position given in number six, your weight is on the right foot and you are ready to step out with the left. Step, now bring the right leg up into the "arch" position. It is free of weight so step. Arch with the left foot again and so on.

This arch position can be used for going forward, backward, or to either side. You arch with the foot in the direction in which you are going. If you are going to the right, arch with the right foot.

Pick out a chair to your right and pretend that there is someone sitting in it with whom you would like to speak. Start out with your right foot and end up in an arch with your right foot. (It's behind). See, the right foot is free for you to continue to the right to greet another guest. Reverse this and go to the left.

Under no circumstance are you to start walking to the right with your left foot. Try it, see how clumsy it is. Hazardous! If there is a time when you find yourself with weight on the right foot when you must go to the right, simply shift your weight to the left leg and proceed with the right.

SOCIAL POSTURES

GREETING PEOPLE

The Arch is the social posture your feet assume when you meet someone. It is gracious in that your weight is forward and you look interested and enthusiastic. You should transfer your weight to the forward foot whenever you meet a new person whether or not you shake hands.

You can add to your charm by practicing your greeting in front of a full length mirror. Inasmuch as all of the following actually happen simultaneously, read them over carefully, lay the book down and try them all together.

THE GREETING

1. Come forward into the "Arch."
2. Bring both hands up toward the waistline.
3. Nod your head with the chin pointing toward the right shoulder.
4. Say, "How do you do."

The only correct thing to say when you meet someone is, "How do you do." But if you are young and the introduction is informal, you **might say,** "Hi." You'll find more on this in the chapter on Social Graces—Introductions.

Pay particular attention to nodding your head. Make sure you tilt it only once. Don't bob up and down like a chicken eating breakfast.

THE HAND SHAKE

A woman has the prerogative of shaking hands with whomever she wishes. However, she would usually accord an older woman the privilege of extending her hand first. Naturally, she would accept the hand of **anyone** who wanted to shake hands.

1. The right hand is brought from the side of the body to the waistline with the inner wrist leading in a semi-circular motion and is placed firmly in the palm of the other person's hand for one or two visible hand shakes.
2. The left hand may be allowed to remain at the side or may be brought toward the waistline. It also may be necessary to use the left hand to hold one's purse and gloves while shaking hands.

Please don't hand someone a "wet dishrag" hand to shake. Be vital, be alive. Let the other person know and feel that you are genuinely glad to make his acquaintance.

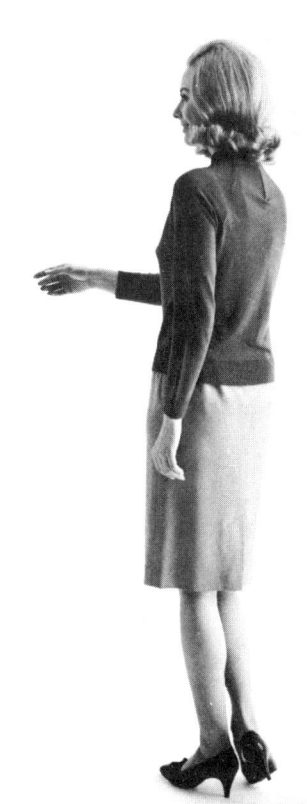

Note Arch Position of the Feet

THE OPEN DOORWAY

ENTERING THROUGH AN OPEN DOORWAY When a poised woman comes into a room through an open doorway, she pauses for a moment to orient herself. You are now going to learn the "Picture Pose." This may seem dramatic to you at first, but its primary purpose is not glamour but courtesy. It allows others a moment to become aware of your presence.

The self-conscious woman has a tendency to "sneak" into a room as though she had no right to be there. She furtively glances around, selects the first chair in sight and then rushes pell-mell, half seated in the process, to become as obscure as possible. Her first impulse is to sit immediately.

A gracious woman, on the other hand, will take advantage of the moment in the doorway to become aware of those present and to appraise the situation. She will mentally make notes, first of all, on the people in the room. They will be the focal point of her interest. Then she will look for a chair that will flatter her height and build. A large woman will look ridiculous on a small stool. A small girl, five foot two with eyes of blue, will be buried, quite literally, in a large wing-back chair.

You cannot assume that the stage has been set just for you, but the moment you spend in the doorway will give you an opportunity to decide whether to sit immediately or wander around a bit. When you do decide to sit, you will do so gracefully, won't you? But of course.

THE PICTURE POSE

You are going to practice with a particular hand and foot position and then you can improvise from this to fit the situation. In any event, you will use the basic stance for your foot position. OK, up you go to the doorway and try it.

ASSUMING THE PICTURE POSE
1. Place your left foot forward as in the basic stance.
2. Place your left hand on your hip in a loose fist as already described in Standing—Hand-Hip Position No. 4.
3. Place your right hand on the door frame shoulder high. Your fingers will point upward toward the ceiling.

There you are in a beautiful asymmetrical position that will look intriguing to your entire "audience."

Just a minute now, check the fine points. Be sure that your left knee is in front of the right; your knees are flexed; your right foot is at a forty-five degree angle. Have it? Then dissolve the pose. Back up about four steps out of the doorway. Approach it

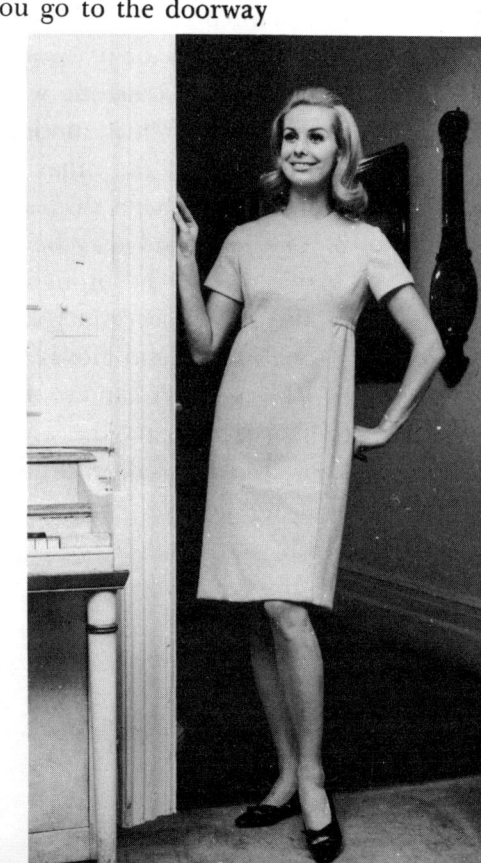

SOCIAL POSTURES

and assume the pose just inside the door. You must judge your steps so that the left foot is the last to come forward. In other words, you literally walk into the position. With some practice, you will be able to judge the distance and gauge your steps accordingly.

LEAVING THROUGH AN OPEN DOORWAY

As soon as you have perfected your Picture Pose, come into the room, walk around to greet imaginary people (or real ones), shake hands, practice your arch and leave the room.

Just for fun, imagine that someone speaks to you just as you are about to go out the doorway, what do you do? You will execute your walking pivot, respond, pivot, and leave the room.

Do not ooze out of the door, nor back out. When you are ready to leave, leave. Practice by turning at the doorway to say, "Goodbye."

Check the fine points. Are you remembering to go to the right with the right foot and to the left with the left foot? Are you remembering to *Arch* for each greeting? Are you nodding just your head and not bowing? Good girl. One last thought, are you leaving the room after your pivot with your forward foot? You must. You don't want to trip over your own foot.

THE CLOSED DOORWAY

ENTERING A CLOSED DOORWAY When going through a closed door it is more graceful and uncomplicated if the door is opened with the hand on the side of the hinges. For instance, if the door opens to your right, you use the right hand. Otherwise, your arm will block your path; you'll be behind the door no matter how far you open it.

Pick up your purse and a pair of gloves and practice going through the nearest closed door. You'll notice that you must transfer your purse and gloves from one hand to the other. If you use your right hand to go out of the room, you must use your left to come back in.

A refined person on her best behavior would not allow a door to slam open or shut. She would control it all the time. You do this by transferring your hand (the same hand) from one knob to the opposite one. You gently close the door as you take a step backward. You do not turn your back on the room, nor do you back out of the doorway.

Now you have the basic technique, go out of the room and enter. The door is closed so you knock, of course, out of politeness. You have anticipated which hand you must use to open the door and have already transferred your purse and gloves to the hand you will not be using. If the door opens to your left, you will have your belongings in your right. Open the door with your hand on the outside knob. Come through the doorway; transfer your hand (same hand) to the inside knob, step inside, close the door as you take a step backward. Keep facing the inside of the room, "feel" for the door to close.

SOCIAL POSTURES

LEAVING THROUGH A CLOSED DOORWAY Greet your imaginary friends, shake hands with about three of them. (Your bag and gloves must be in your left hand for this.) Turn to leave the room. Open the door, look over your shoulder away from door itself to say, "Goodbye." When halfway through the doorway, transfer your hand to the outside knob, walk through the doorway gently closing the door as you do so.

CROSSING IN FRONT OF AND STANDING BEFORE A GROUP

Whenever you are called upon to be in front of a group, you will especially want to present yourself in the best possible light. You can do so if you will remember the following rule:

When crossing in front of a group, stop with the foot by the audience (group) forward. This means that if you cross in front of them with the audience on your right, the right foot will be forward. If you cross with them on your left, the left foot will be forward.

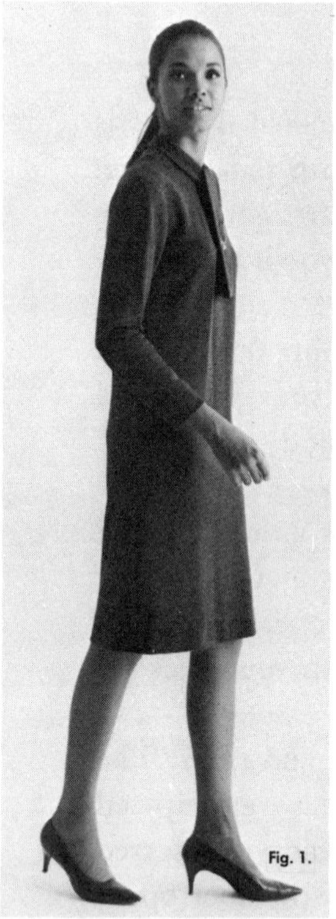

Fig. 1.

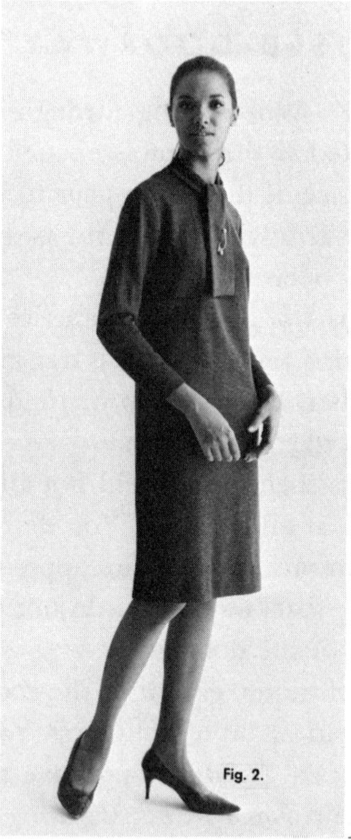

Fig. 2.

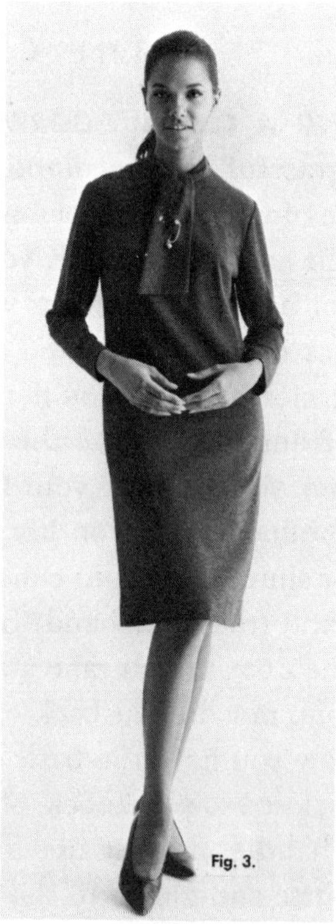

Fig. 3.

Your body will appear more slender and more graceful because your hips will be turned slightly away from the group and because your leg line will be unbroken from the tip of your toe to the hip.

Practice in front of your full length mirror or in front of your friends. You will be pleased with the result.

SOCIAL POSTURES 103

STAIR TECHNIQUES

If you thought the Picture Pose was dramatic, envision yourself poised at the top of a flight of stairs ready to "float" down to your admiring audience. The perspective a stair case gives is so entrancing that it is often used in the theater for emotional impact.

STAIR RULES

It is not suggested here that you attempt to duplicate the performance of great actresses, only that you learn to negotiate steps with grace and confidence. The following rules will help you attain aplomb on the stairway.

DO:

1. Pause before ascending or descending so that you may see the stairs. Look with your eyes, not your head.
2. Hold your body erect. You will get there only when your rear most part arrives.
3. Keep your knees flexed all the time. Don't bend and straighten them. Let the large muscles of the thigh do the work.
4. Place the entire foot on each step. If the steps are too narrow to have the feet pointing straight ahead, turn both feet in one direction.
5. Always come down on the step with the toe first and then the heel.
6. One hand may be placed lightly on a bannister for balance but not for support.
7. Place one foot directly in front of the other.

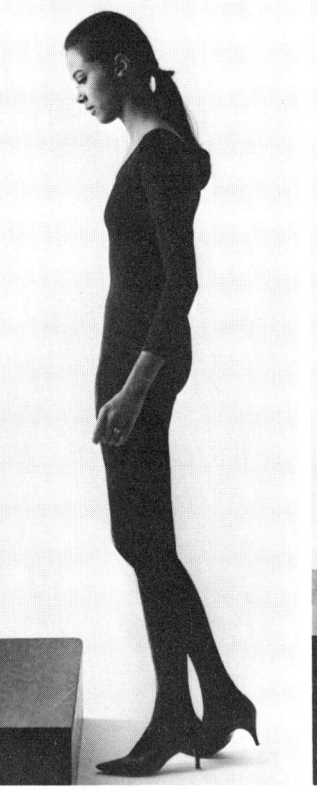

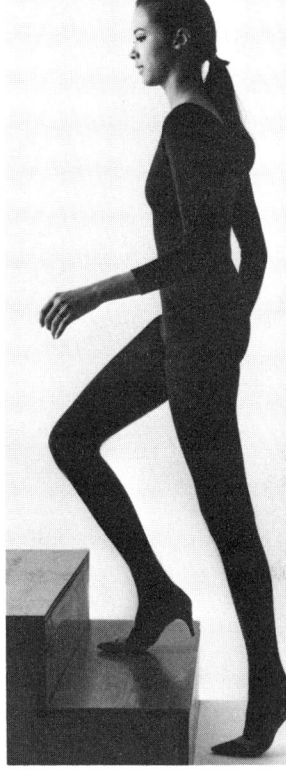

AVOID:

1. Having your heels hang over the edge of the step.
2. Having the body lean forward.
3. Having the knees turn outward.
4. Having the knees straighten with each step.

CHAPTER 10

HANDLING PERSONAL BELONGINGS

Introduction

This section is intended to answer many of the little nagging questions that annoy women who are not quite sure how to handle their personal belongings: their coat, stole, cigarette, handbag and gloves. By answering these questions in your own mind, you will be able to cope with the larger social problems of conversation and graciousness.

There have probably been times when you felt like a juggler in a circus but not half so skillful. If "dropitis" is an ailment that plagues you in the most inopportune circumstances, read on. You'll discover there is a method for handling your personal effects that simplifies the entire performance.

You have probably sat spellbound watching the grace and ease of professional models on the runway. Which only goes to show that it is the *know-how* that makes the operation look easy.

Get the show on the road by gathering the "Props" that you will need. These will include:

    Coat
    Stole
    Handbag
    Gloves
    Cigarettes and a light (if you smoke)

WRAPS

Every wrap, no matter what its name, is worn with sleeves or is thrown over the shoulders. These two techniques, one for a coat and the other for a stole, will cover virtually every kind of over-garment from a cape to a sweater.

Sooner or later we all discover that it is practically impossible to put a wrap on or take it off with paraphernalia in our hands. It is much more convenient to put everything else down somewhere before attempting to handle a wrap.

HANDLING PERSONAL BELONGINGS

COATS

It is not only important to know *when* to put your coat on or take it off, it is also important to know *how*. And up to this point, everything has been very ladylike. Now, however, we are going to borrow from the masculine gender and put on and take off our coats like a gentleman. But don't worry, it will still be graceful, quick and efficient. Besides, it will make you look like a lady.

ARE YOU READY TO PUT ON YOUR COAT?

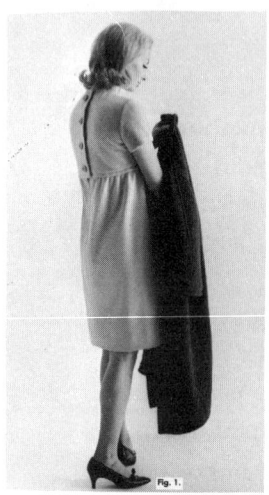

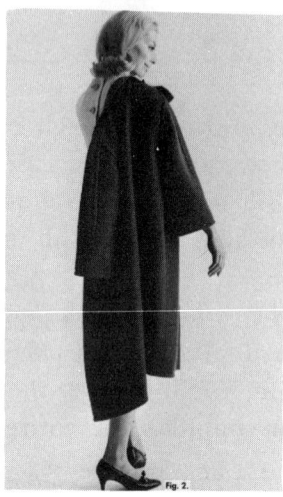

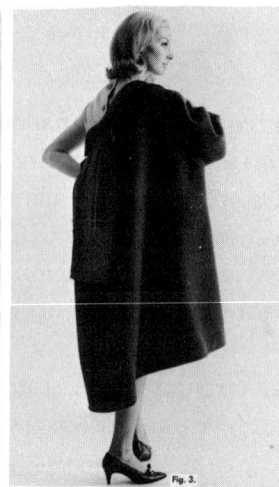

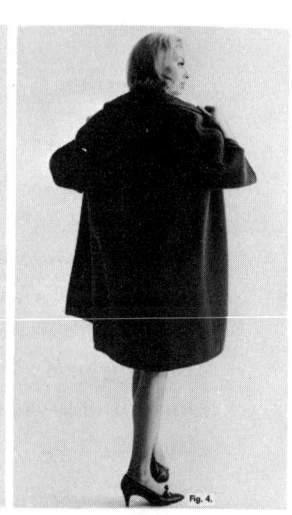

Fig. 1. Fig. 2. Fig. 3. Fig. 4.

PROCEDURE:

1. Grasp the middle of the collar with the left hand.
2. Place the right arm in the armhole that is by your left side.
3. With the left hand, pull the right sleeve all the way up on the right arm until the right shoulder rests on your right shoulder.
4. Take hold of the right lapel with the right hand and push the coat backward.
5. With the left hand, reach around in back, underneath the armpit, until you find the other sleeve.
6. With the assistance of the right hand pulling the coat onto the shoulder, place the left arm all the way into the sleeve and reach up with the left hand to the left lapel to adjust the shoulder line.

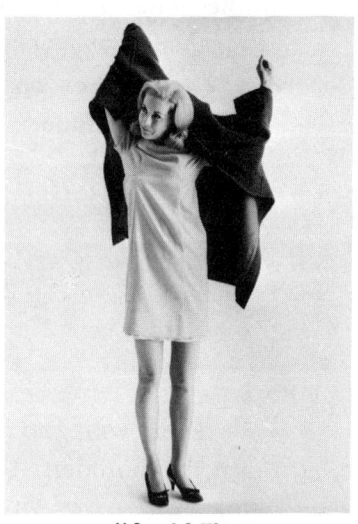

"Avoid This"

Avoid throwing your coat over your head and putting your arms up in the air like a big bird about to take flight.

HANDLING PERSONAL BELONGINGS

Are You Ready To Take Your Coat Off?

COAT "OFF"

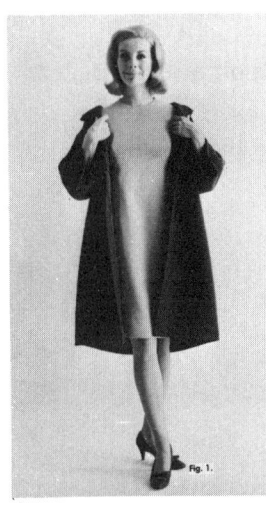

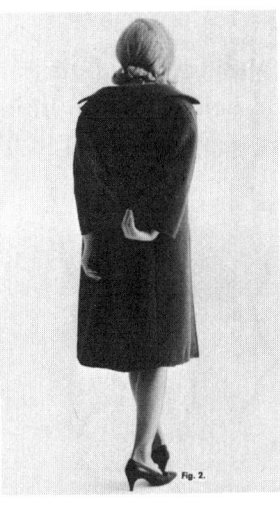

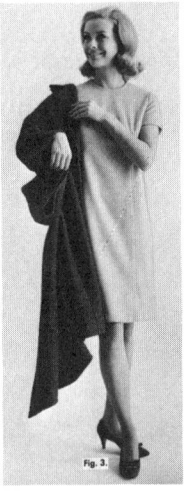

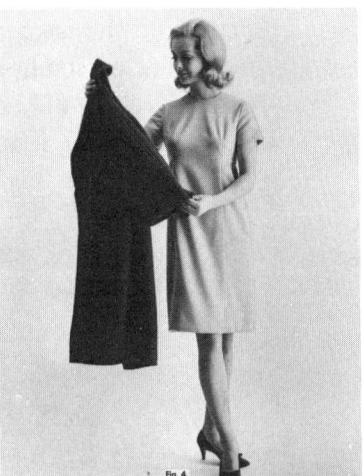

1. Drop both shoulders down your back by grasping the lapels on either side. Don't allow the entire top of the coat to drop all the way to the elbows.
2. Reach around in back with both hands and grasp both cuffs in one hand. Let's make it the right.
3. Bring both cuffs to the front of the body. This will be on the right side.
4. Take both cuffs with the left hand and remove the right arm from the sleeve.
5. & 6. Grasp the middle of the collar with the right hand, and, keeping hold of both cuffs with the left, place the coat over the outside of the left forearm.

If this entire procedure has been followed correctly, the coat will be one smooth bundle of material over the left forearm. No matter what you have heard about this, do not turn the lining out. The only exception to this would be when the lining is a definite part of the costume and, perhaps, matches the dress.

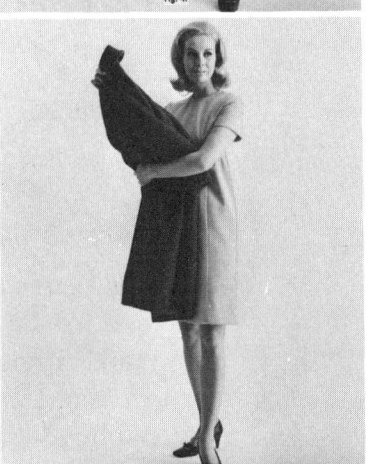

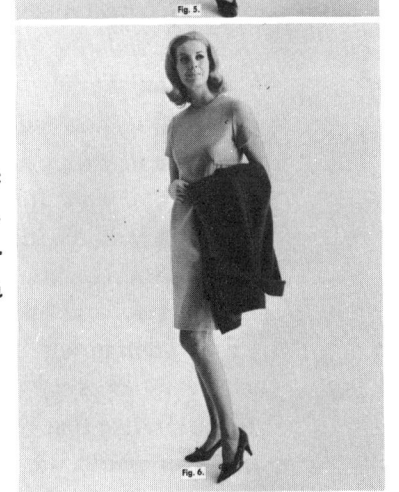

HANDLING PERSONAL BELONGINGS

WHEN YOUR ESCORT ASSISTS YOU

COAT "ON" WITH ASSISTANCE Because it will be easier for your escort to handle only one coat at a time, it it perfectly proper for you to hold your own coat until he has put his on.

The person holding the coat will hold it with both hands on either side of the center of the collar. It will be held with the lining away from the person holding it and toward the person approaching it. The hands will be about shoulder high.

PROCEDURE:

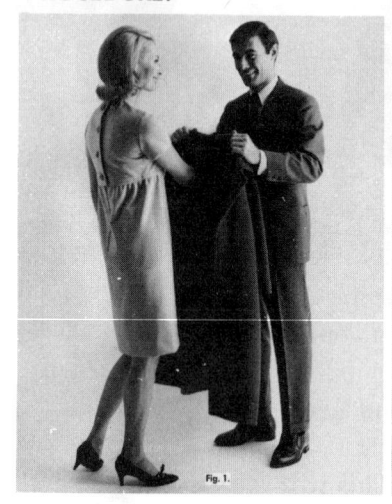

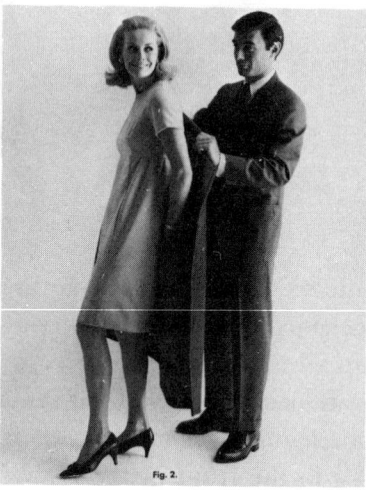

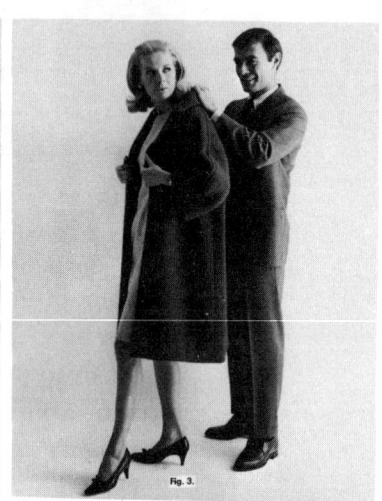

Fig. 1. Fig. 2. Fig. 3.

1. The person approaching will walk up to within about one foot of the coat. She will have her feet in a walking position because she must be prepared to execute a walking turn.
2. While still facing the coat, she places the arm in the correct sleeve. For instance, if the right foot is forward, she places her right arm in the sleeve that is on the left side as shown in Fig. 1.
3. She now pivots to the left without moving her feet and drops her left hand behind her.
4. She waits for the individual holding the coat to place her hand in the sleeve.
5. She reaches up with both hands to the collar of the coat and adjusts the shoulder line.

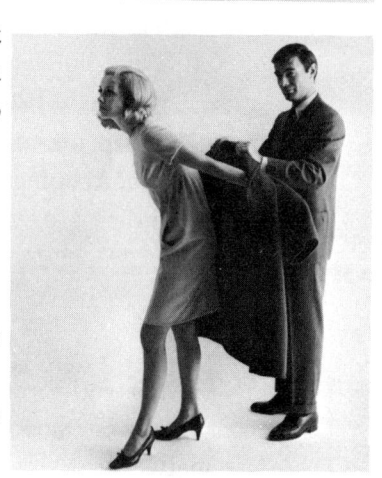

"Avoid This"

Under no circumstance does she turn around to try to see the second sleeve nor does she try to find the armhole by feeling for it. She can relax in the assurance that the person helping her can see both the coat and her arm and can guide them together. The person assisting should pull the coat upward onto the shoulders so that all there is left to do is the adjusting of the shoulder line.

HANDLING PERSONAL BELONGINGS

COAT "OFF" WITH ASSISTANCE Whoever is helping you on and off with your coat should be instructed to stand perfectly still so that you can walk up to him rather than having him approach you. This will give you additional practice with your Walking Pivot and with judging distance.

PROCEDURE:

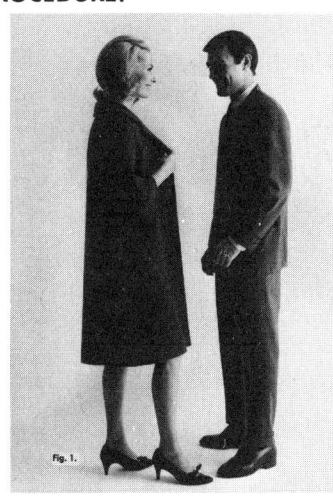

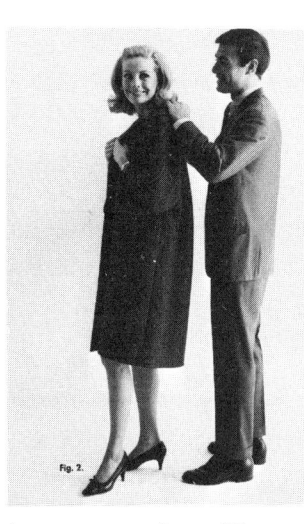

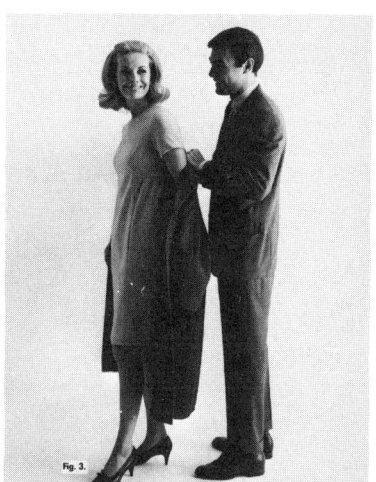

1. Take three steps toward the person who will remove the coat. You should not be closer than one foot nor farther than one and a half feet.
2. The feet are in the walking turn position. If the right foot is forward the turn or pivot will be executed toward the left-hand side.
3. Pivot so that your back is now to the assistant.
4. If the cuffs of the coat are tight, remove the hands from them before placing the hands behind.
5. Drop the coat off both shoulders. The assistant will now take hold of the collar of the coat on each side.
6. Immediately after removing the shoulders of the coat, drop the arms straight down and slightly back at the sides.
7. As the assistant slides the coat off the arms, the elbows may be bent and the hands brought to the front of the body.
8. Your escort will carry your coat over his forearm just as you do.

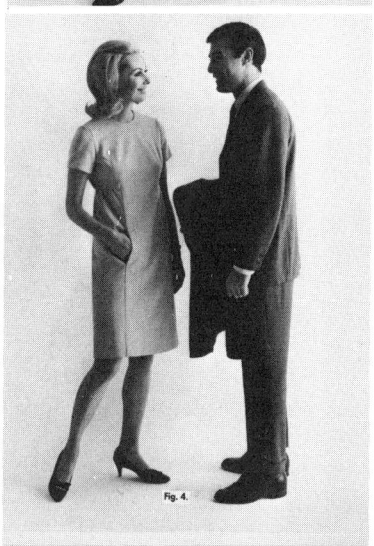

STOLES

Introduction to the wearing of stoles

Many authorities on dress agree that a woman is seen by more people in her coat or other wrap than she is in any other way. If this is true, it is doubly important that she look her very best when dressed to go out on the street. Stoles appear from time to time on the fashion horizon as though they had never made a previous appearance; however, they are so flattering and in such good taste with so many costumes, they will undoubtedly not actually go out of style, ever.

A stole can add a dramatic touch with color, line, texture and movement. It can be used in countless ways too numerous to mention here. Maybe you have some innovations that are not included, if so, use them.

STOLE "ON" By the way, stole is not synonymous with "fur." There are many types and kinds of stoles. Some stoles are reversible, but for now, assume that you have a simple, unfitted length of fabric that is lined. Also assume that you are not in the right circumstance to fling your stole dramatically over your head. The following method is safe and sane.

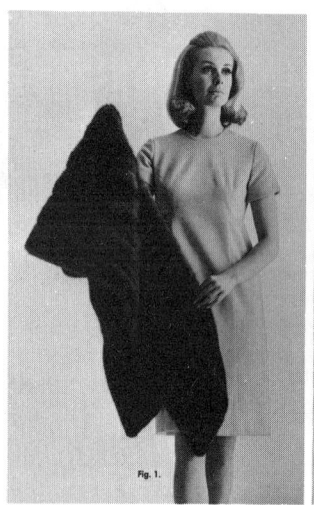

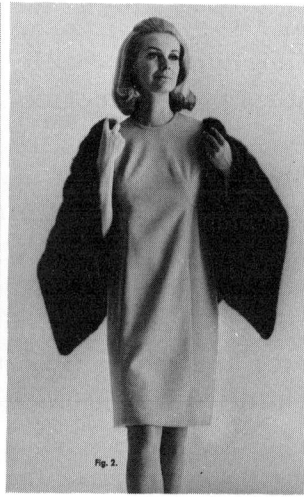

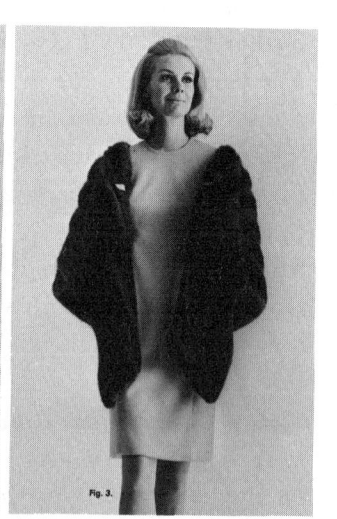

PROCEDURE:

1. With the left hand, place the stole on the right hand where the right side of the collar would be. The right elbow is bent and the right hand is relaxed backward on the wrist with the palm facing the ceiling. It is close to the right shoulder.
2. Now with the free left hand, reach around in back of the neck on the left-hand side. As you do so, bring the right hand over to meet the left hand behind the neck.
3. Sliding the left hand along the stole, bring it over the left shoulder and down the left front.

HANDLING PERSONAL BELONGINGS 111

STOLE "OFF" Reverse the procedure for putting the stole on. Do not take it over the top of the head or duck from under it. Gracefully and simply take it off.

PROCEDURE:

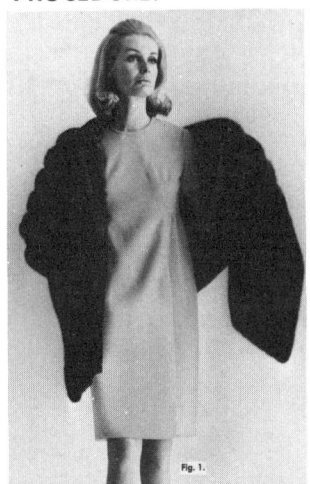

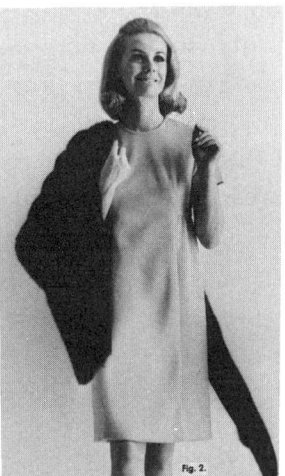

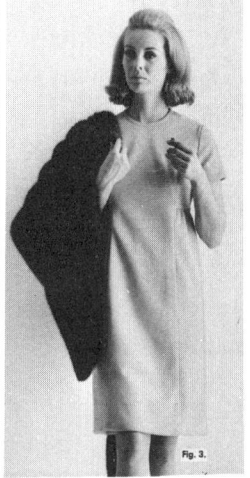

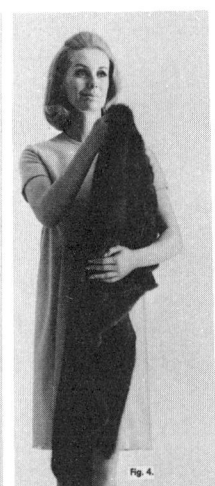

1. With the left hand by the left shoulder, drop the stole to the back.
2. With the right hand bring the stole to the front of the body on the right side.
3. The right hand will be holding the stole approximately in the middle.
4. & 5. Place the stole over the left forearm.

STOLE ARRANGEMENTS:

1. Place the left side of the stole under the right side. Now place the right forearm under the left side of the stole and over the right side. This will hold the stole firmly in one place to the right side of the body. This is an asymmetrical position and is most flattering. Do you understand that once the left side of the stole is crossed under the right that it will be to the right of right side? It is still called the left side of the stole.

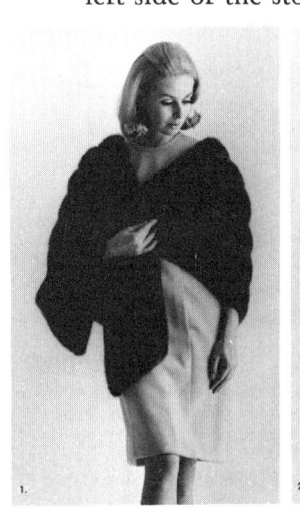

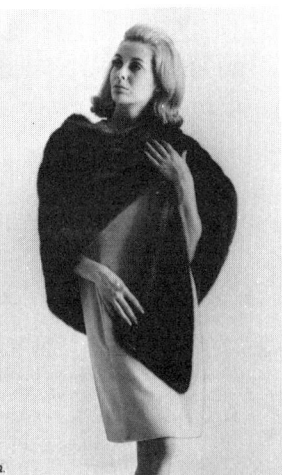

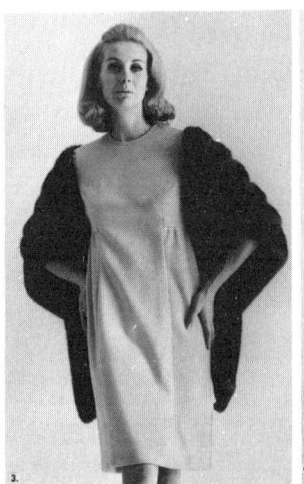

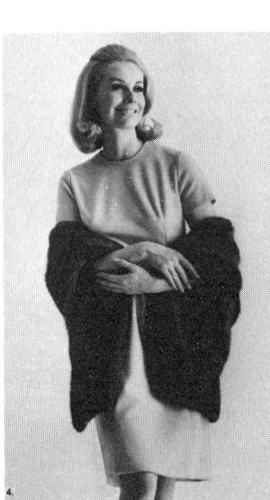

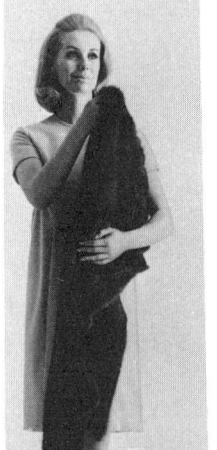

2. With the left side hanging loose, place the right side around the throat and let the end hang over the left shoulder in back.
3. Hold both sides back with the hands on the hips.
4. Drop the stole off the shoulders and catch either side with the elbows. The back of the stole is now down around the waistline.
5. Turn the stole entirely around so that both ends hang down the back. A half knot may be made to keep the stole from falling off the shoulders in back.
6. Pin one side of the stole at the shoulder and allow the other side to drape gracefully over the forearm. This loose side may also be placed under a belt.

In addition to these six arrangements, copy the ones you have seen and admired. Invent some of your own. It's imagination and ingenuity that changes the commonplace into the sublime.

STOLE DON'TS

1. DON'T allow the stole to hug the neckline. It should hang over the tips of the shoulders.
2. DON'T allow the stole to hang loosely over the bustline.
3. DON'T allow the stole to look uncontrolled. Pin it, place it, keep it where you want it.

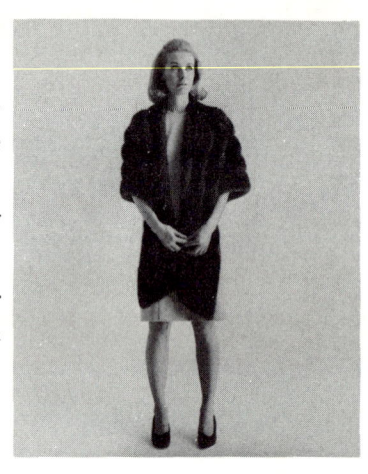

CIGARETTES

Every person who smokes should respect the rights and feelings of others concerning his habit and this is where *smoking etiquette* enters the picture. Your consideration and good breeding show when you:

1. *Do not* light a cigarette when being interviewed for a job.
2. *Do not* light a cigarette in someone's home without asking permission to do so.
3. *Do not* light a cigarette at the dinner table until dessert has been served and then only with permission of those at the table.
4. *Do not* smoke on the street.
5. *Do not* smoke on an elevator.
6. *Do not* smoke where to do so would seem to show lack of respect or reverence.
7. *Do not* smoke when it will be an annoyance to others.

NOTE: *Cigarette smoking is popular and widespread. It is also damaging and deadly. The full seriousness of the cigarette threat was made clear in the report, "Smoking and Health," addressed to the Surgeon General of the United States Public Health Service. Accepted as impartial by both the tobacco industry and health agencies, this report was made by ten eminent scientists, half of them smokers and half abstainers. It officially confirmed fears regarding cigarette smoking which began to arise among scientists more than a quarter of a century ago.*

HANDLING PERSONAL BELONGINGS

CIGARETTE "TECHNIQUES"

The smoking habit was originally strictly a man's habit and although today many women smoke, they should certainly guard against looking masculine or uncouth. Here are a number of suggestions to keep the smoking habit as feminine as possible.

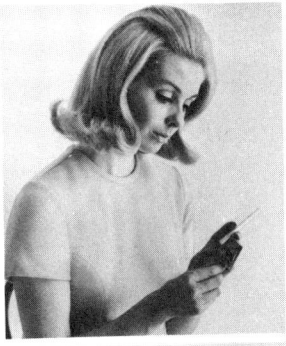

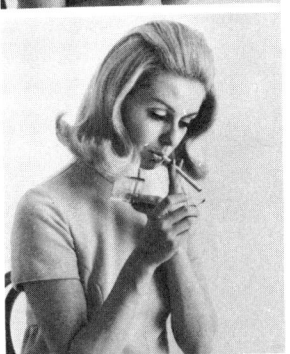

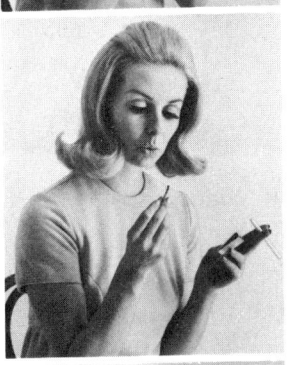

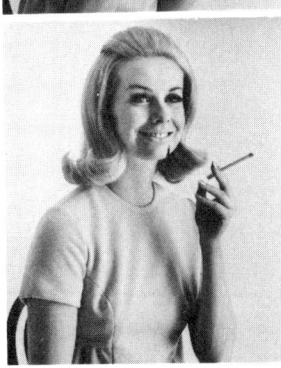

RIGHT **WRONG**

1. Never hold a cigarette in the mouth without the fingers assisting. In other words, no dangling cigarettes.
2. Hold the cigarette in the hand as you strike the match and then place it between the lips for lighting. The fingers must stay in contact with the cigarette.
3. If assistance is offered for lighting the cigarette, graciously lean toward the light.
4. Hold the cigarette as close to the ends of the fingers as possible.
5. Hold the lighted end of the cigarette toward the ceiling so that smoke does not curl through the fingers.
6. Never blow smoke through the nostrils.
7. Do not flick the ashes from the cigarette, roll them off.
8. To put the cigarette out, gently roll it in the ash tray until there is no longer any smoke.

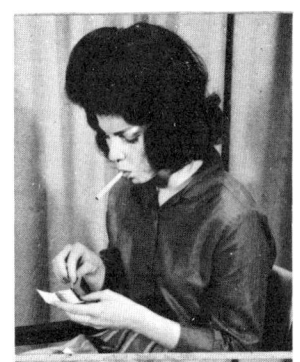

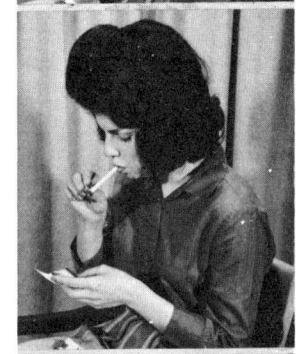

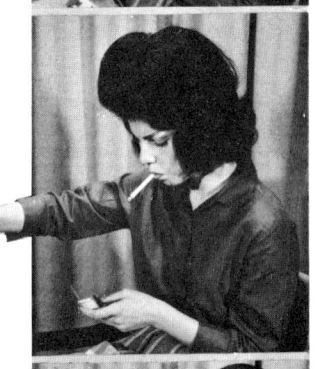

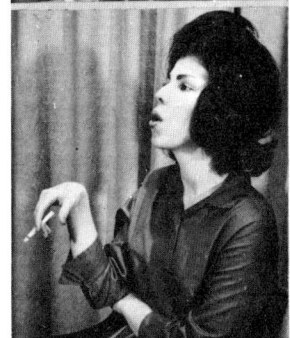

GLOVES

GLOVES "ON" A glove is placed on the hand in much the same way a nylon stocking is put on the foot except that it is slightly more complicated. If the hands have a tendency to perspire, a little talcum powder will help.

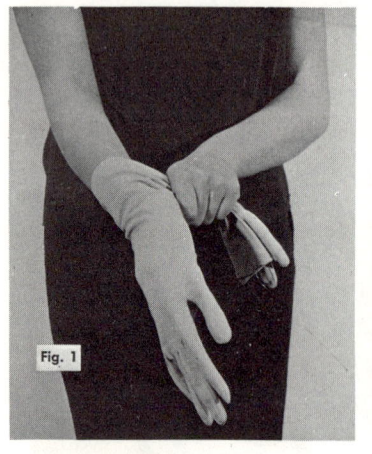

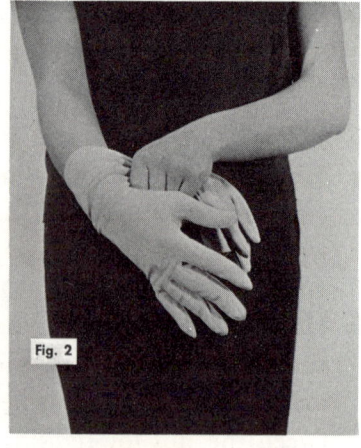

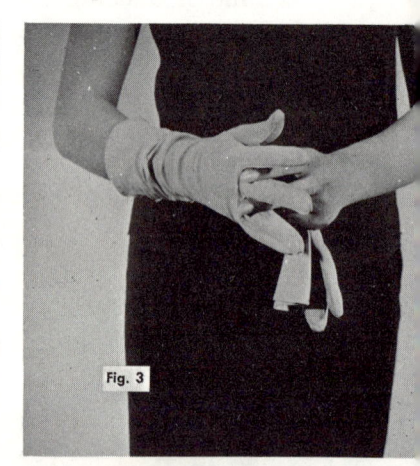

1. Place the hand in the glove and gather the arm length of the glove down to the wrist.
2. Gently pull the fingers of the glove onto each finger of the hand.
3. Gently massage each of the fingers of the glove toward the hand, with the fingers of the other hand.
4. When all the fingers and the thumb are in the glove as far as they will go, gently unroll the arm of the glove.
5. Repeat with the other glove.

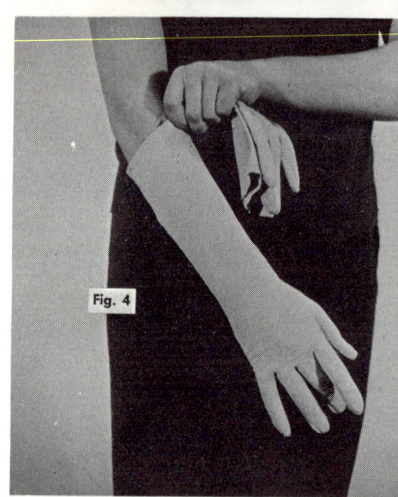

GLOVE "ETIQUETTE"

1. Gloves are always removed for smoking, drinking, eating and dancing. Formal means that the hand of the glove is removed even though the arm of the glove is left on. Buttons at the wrist of a formal glove are placed so that the hand of the glove may be tucked away at the wrist.
2. Gloves are removed when you come indoors. This applies in most churches. However, when it is proper to do otherwise, let the rule apply to you.
3. Gloves need not be removed for hand shaking unless they are garden gloves. A woman does not ask to have her glove excused, she just shakes hands.
4. A woman, to be appropriately dressed, wears gloves on the street even though she may not be wearing a hat.
5. Gloves should always be scrupulously clean.

HANDLING PERSONAL BELONGINGS 115

6. Gloves should never be placed on the dinner table. Only exception is for a dinner-dance. In this instance, the small, evening clutch bag and gloves may be placed on the table after everyone has finished eating and is dancing.
7. Either both gloves should be worn or both removed. The only exception would be on a shopping trip where the right glove is removed to handle change.

GLOVES "OFF" Reverse the procedure in this manner.

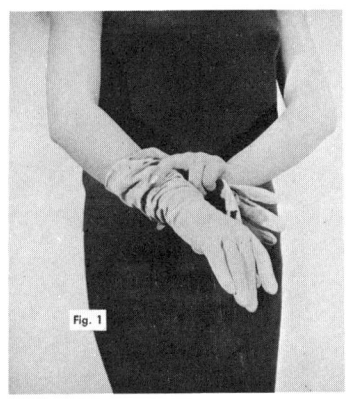

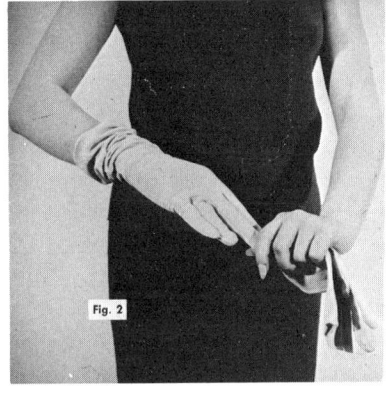

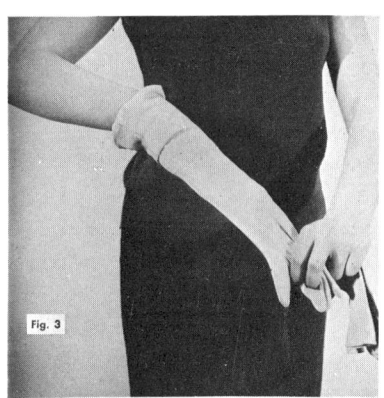

1. Slide or gather the arm of the glove down to the wrist.
2. Gently pull each finger out of the glove, one at a time.
3. Remove the entire hand from the glove, smoothing the arm of the glove by spreading the fingers of the hand from which the glove is being removed.
4. Repeat with the other glove.
5. Place the thumb of the glove over the palm of the glove and smooth. Smooth all fingers until they are straight. Smooth out the arm of the glove. Repeat with the other glove.
6. Place both gloves together with the palm facing one another, the fingers together and the cuffs together.

CARRYING GLOVES

Your appearance will have taken on a high fashion look if you carry your gloves with the cuff over the back of the hand and the fingers of the glove toward the body over the palm. Avoid having the gloves look like a wilted bouquet of flowers with the fingers of the gloves drooping up, out and down.

If the glove is eight button or more, it is advisable to fold the arm of the glove over the palm of the glove, in half, and then to place them together as instructed. This will prevent a long length of fabric from just hanging.

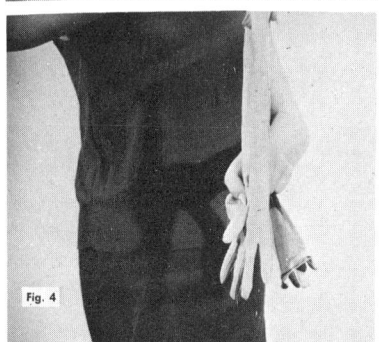

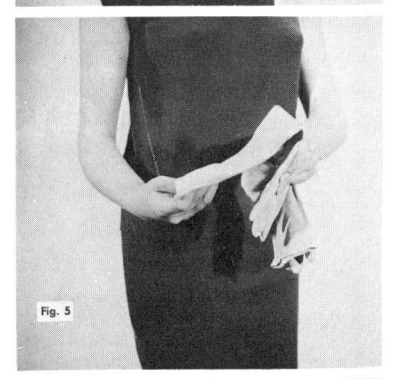

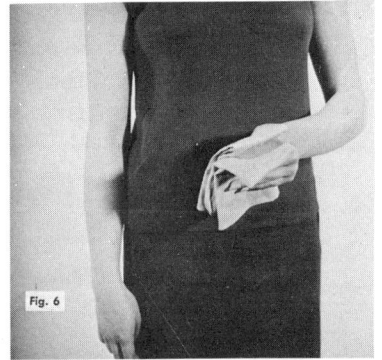

HANDBAGS

Throughout the textbook the aim has been to make you more poised and more beautiful. Learning how to carry all types of handbags will enhance this picture of loveliness. Each bag, because of its own particular size and shape, needs to be handled in its own unique way.

HANDBAGS "HOW CARRIED"

THE CLUTCH BAG The most flattering line to the human figure is the diagonal. Therefore, a "clutch" bag should be carried at the top with the arm straight and slightly in front of the thigh. The bag will slant down and in toward the center line of the body.

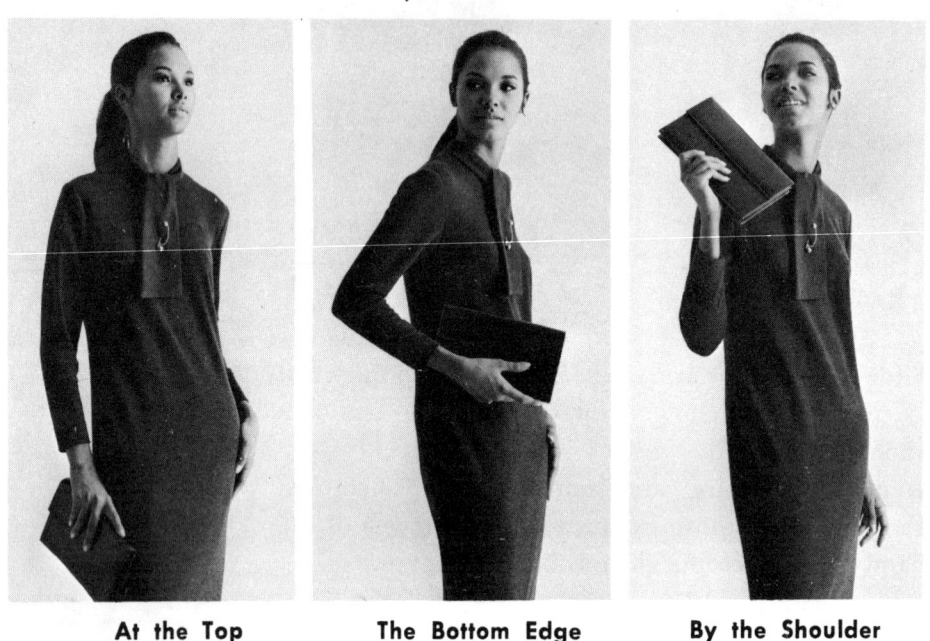

At the Top   **The Bottom Edge**   **By the Shoulder**

A "clutch" bag may also be carried *on the bottom edge* with the bag resting on the palm, the elbow bent and the hand held in front slightly below the waistline. The wrist is relaxed.

This type bag may also be casually placed up *by the shoulder* with the palm up and the fingers pointing away from the body. In this position, the bag will slant upward away from the body.

We usually think of a "clutch" bag for evening and, indeed, it can be a veritable conversation piece. Let it be beautiful and let its contents be a delight to behold—jewelled comb, compact, perfume vial. Incidentally, this is the bag from which you may have a corner of your favorite lace hanky show.

HANDLING PERSONAL BELONGINGS 117

THE "MEDIUM" BAG WITH A HANDLE This type of bag is usually used for *daytime* street wear. It should be carried with the strap or handle over the forearm.

The bag rests against the flat front of the hip bone. The elbow of the arm is bent so that the forearm is just below the waistline.

If you wish to secure the bag when walking through a crowd, you may do so in the following fashion:

Twist the handle forward that is on the outside of the forearm until you can take hold of the upper edge of the purse. If you try this you will see that the side of the bag that was against the body is now facing out. The purse is under control and will be impervious to pickpockets or purse snatchers.

THE "ENVELOPE" BAG This is a *larger* version of the *clutch* bag. It must be carried over the forearm and should not be smashed against the body with the upper arm.

Let the lower edge of the bag rest against the upward palm and the forearm. The forearm is slightly below the waistline.

A little practice will ensure you that the bag is being carried on a slightly diagonal line, pointing down and in.

There are no variations for carrying this type of bag.

THE "TOTE" BAG This is a large, carry-all type of bag resembling a suitcase. Consequently, it is carried at arms length in much the same way.

This is the only bag that should be allowed to hang at the side of the body adding width and weight.

It is to be assumed that it is carried for utilitarian purposes and not for beauty.

Avoid it whenever possible.

Smart travelers often carry a *smaller* bag within the "tote" bag so that they do not have to carry it everywhere with them.

THE SHOULDER STRAP BAG Here in America we have no divisions into royal and peasant classes. Try to avoid looking like a serf. During the Second World War officers were not allowed to carry packages, even for their wives. Do you have a good reason to tote a tote bag?

A "shoulder strap" bag is in the same class and should be avoided. But if you must carry one, place it *behind* the hip and hold it in place with the forearm.

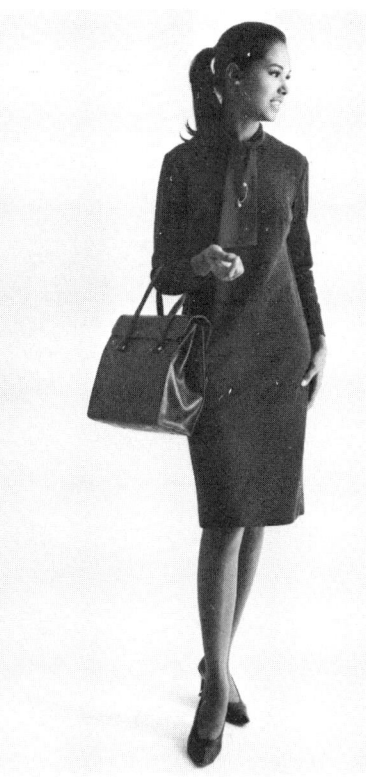

The Medium Bag

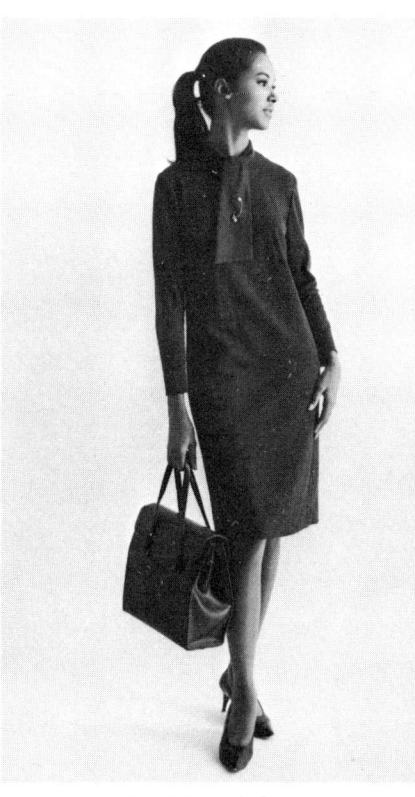

The "Tote" Bag

CHAPTER 11

VISUAL POISE FOR SOCIAL AFFAIRS

Introduction

Social usage, etiquette, is a set of rules that has been devised to lessen friction and make social relationships pleasant. It is not something reserved for the very rich or the very educated, but is a part of every person's everyday life. Etiquette is a part of our contemporary culture and as such is important to every individual no matter what his economic, social, or educational level. Our customs may not be the very best customs because of the outmoded traditions that have come to us from a day gone by, but it is encouraging to note that as the stress is felt, social usage is modified to fit new conditions.

OUR CHANGING CUSTOMS

In our present-day society, social usage is a dynamic, changing cog in the wheel of social progress. It is interesting to refer to "The Ladies' Guide to True Politeness and Correct Manners" by Miss Leslie. In 1864, a lady did not go out by herself after dark. She sent her male caller home by ten o'clock and never called him by his first name. She would not think of corresponding with any man except her husband or a member of her family. Nowadays the telephone, radio and television, to mention just a few inventions, have changed our way of living and our social usages as well. In large cities, it is even considered proper now for a young woman to go to a man's apartment for dinner, because it is his home. Certainly apartment houses with their limited space have affected the type of hospitality most families can offer, and the buffet dinner has become more popular than the formal dinner.

Customs do not change by edict but a gradual breaking away from those usages that are no longer useful. Common sense dictates that customs be changed when they become so extreme as to be a handicap to comfortable living. We see professional women getting away from the high heel during working hours and men giving up a stiff collar, tie, and a coat during hot weather. These changes are good and indicate that we are living in a dynamic, not a static, society. Undoubtedly our customs of today will seem foolish and amusing to a young modern of the twenty-first century, just as the customs of 1864 seem outmoded to us. The social usages of today are, however, an integral part of our daily life, and as such, are important.

You may view social regulations as fetters which are irksome to bear or, on the other hand, you may regard them as essential to the smooth conduct of social intercourse. If you take this position, you will learn the rules of the game so that your attention can be focused on the more interesting aspects of social contact. Just as you have more self-assurance when you know you are dressed properly, so you will have more poise and a feeling of personal security when you are certain of what is expected of you in specific situations.

It's rather safe to say that if the majority in your community of good taste do it, this is the way it should be done. Don't be a stickler for detail. If it doesn't go against your sensibilities you may apply the old saying, *"When in Rome do as the Romans do."*

Get on the magic carpet . . . Take a ride to your favorite social spots. Go to the theater, a party and your favorite restaurant for dinner. All by way of practice for the real thing.

LET'S GO TO THE THEATER

Two couples, you, your escort and two friends arrive at the theater. There is a waiting line. Do you and the other girl go into the foyer and leave the fellows by themselves to buy the tickets. No, not unless the weather is inclement. Otherwise, you *stay by your date's side.* If you are a really charming girl, you talk to your date and not to the other girl.

WHEN TO REMOVE YOUR WRAP Once inside, when do you remove your wrap? In the foyer before going down the theater aisle. The fellows will check their hats and coats, if possible. The girls may decide whether to check theirs or take them to their seats. In any event, it is easier to *remove a wrap in the lobby* than in the aisle blocking someone's view or in a seat.

GOING DOWN THE AISLE How do you proceed down the aisle? If there is an usher it will be girl, boy, girl, boy. Otherwise, one of the fellows will want to lead the way to find the seats. Then it will be boy, girl, girl, boy. It is polite to consider those around you and create as little confusion as possible. For this reason, *proceed down the aisle in the same order you will sit* next to one another.

VISUAL POISE FOR SOCIAL AFFAIRS

GETTING TO YOUR SEAT As you *pass in front of someone who is already seated,* you face directly forward, excuse yourself and "slide" over to your seat like this. If you are going to the left, move the left foot to the left, bring the right foot to it, move the left foot again. There is little danger of stepping on toes this way because the broad side of your left foot acts as a sort of shovel to get the other feet out of the way.

If, in spite of all precaution, *someone is touched or jolted* it is proper to say immediately, "I beg your pardon" or "I'm sorry."

Men who are seated will stand as others pass in front of them. *Women will simply turn their knees sideways* and make as much room as possible.

BEHAVIOR IN THE THEATER Needless to add that talking, noise making, wearing large hats and otherwise *annoying others is taboo* in the theater.

When it's "smoking in the outer lobby only, please," a girl should accompany her date even if it's only to go to the powder room. *Don't stay alone in your seat* and let him fend for himself.

Go over the foregoing material until you are sure. Then your actions will be automatically gracious without the watch-dog of your conscious personality. You will be able to concentrate on being the charming person you are—or want to be.

LET'S GO TO A PARTY

It is considered rude to arrive late when a specific hour is mentioned. True. Especially if the smoothness of the entire event is dependent upon a particular number of people. This would include a card party, a dinner, a shower, etc. In fact, it is good manners to arrive about ten minutes early. Better early than late.

If the affair is an open house or a cocktail party and the invitation states from "six to seven-thirty," you may arrive during this time and *stay not more than one hour.*

REFRESHMENTS

You accept the refreshments offered even though you do not eat or drink them. You mingle with the other guests and you keep in mind that the success of the party is as much your responsibility as it is your hostess's. When it is necessary for you to balance your refreshments on your lap, you do so as carefully as possible. You may assume that anything *served without flatwear* is a finger food. For instance, wedding cake is an item that you eat with your fingers. Be sure to *help yourself to a napkin* or ask for one. It is wise to keep one hand free to balance your plate so you may have to *find some flat surface for a glass.* This could be a table or the floor. *Be sure that you have a coaster under your glass.* Use a napkin or ask for permission to put your glass on your hostess's mahogany. It may be that she has moisture-proof furniture and therefore doesn't serve coasters.

If iced tea is served, the spoon will be removed and placed on the coaster provided. If there is no coaster, hold the spoon in your hand until you have asked for one.

Be considerate about using a linen napkin to wipe your mouth. Lipstick stain is hard to remove. Of course, if you have followed all the hints given in the make-up section, you will have no problem with lipstick on napkins, glasses, cups, spoons and what-not.

A guest's responsibility is to her hostess. It is not necessary to say goodbye to others present unless for some reason or other you must leave early and thereby inconvenience them in some way.

Don't ooze out the doorway, go. Do this immediately *after saying some nice thing to your hostess* about the food, the music, the company or whatever single thing you have enjoyed more than any other. Don't leave it unsaid just because you are shy. Even if you must force yourself the first few times, get the habit of complimenting. *Do it sincerely.*

NEW CONTACTS

With more and more women working after marriage, with more and more companies interviewing the wife as well as the husband, with more and more people in the world with whom we will have social contact, the more important it is for us to be "hip" and in the know.

MEETING NEW PEOPLE

We could stay in our own small world, associate with the same people, do the same things year in and year out, and probably never make any faux pas. But life will be fuller and more interesting if we expand our horizons, make new friends, and acquire new skills. In doing so, we will make mistakes, but then, we can take heart in the fact that no one is so well traveled or so well informed that he always knows what to do.

In addition to meeting people and learning to introduce them with confidence, we should learn to eat graciously and within the bounds of social usage. It might be fun for us to go to an imaginary dinner at a very swank restaurant. Choose your favorite!

VISUAL POISE FOR SOCIAL AFFAIRS 123

GOING TO DINNER

CHECKING COATS First of all, there is the matter of checking coats. Your escort will be required to leave his at the check stand, but you can either leave yours or take it to the table with you. (This must have been designed for the wearers of mink.)

ESCORTING TO THE TABLE You will be met at the dining room entrance by a head waiter, captain or *maitre d'* who will ask whether or not you have a reservation and how many are in your party. If there are just the two of you, you will precede your escort to the table indicated by the head waiter who leads the way.

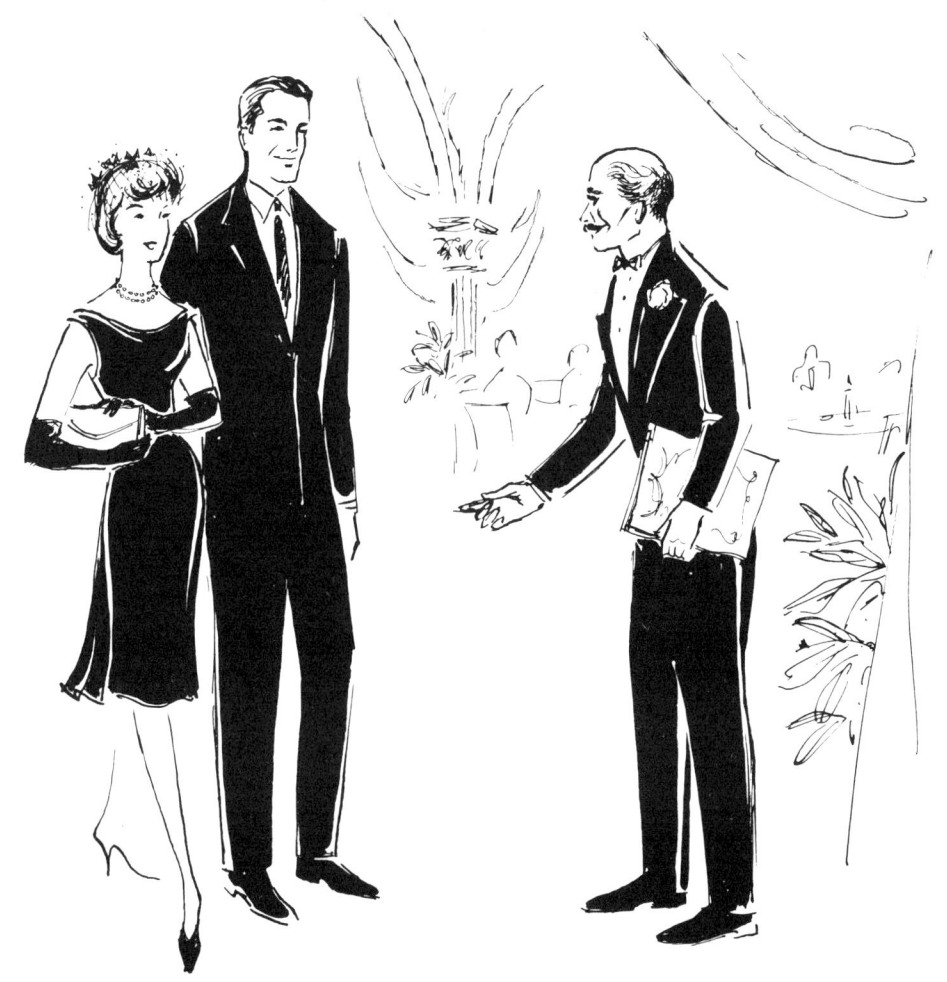

If there are more than two in your party (*and who would invite more than yourself and your love to an imaginary dinner?*) then women will precede the men to the table so that they can be seated wherever it is most comfortable.

If you have dreamed up a very large and formal dinner then the guests will come to the table in pairs (*not with your own husband*). Escorting arrangements are so designed as to separate husbands from their wives during formal dinners.

SITTING AT THE TABLE You will take the seat held out for you by the head waiter, or if he is busy seating one of the other lovelies, you will just lightly touch the back of the chair you have selected. You will make no attempt to pull the chair out (*this injures the male ego and idea of the frail woman*). Incidentally, while we are on the subject: When out with a man, play your femininity to the hilt. Let him open the doors, help you up the stairs, take off your coat, move your chair, order your dinner. It's fun to be helpless, and the man will be helpful, if you'll let him.

PLACING YOUR HANDBAG AND GLOVES Now let's see, where were we? Oh, yes, we have now just been seated. We will put our bag and gloves either on our laps, a spare chair, or on the floor, never on the table. If there is a hostess, we will wait for her lead in placing our napkin on our lap. Otherwise, we can do so now or later when the first course arrives. We want to look as though we came here just to enjoy the company and we must not look hungry even though we are ravenous. This means that we will take time out to scan the menu, to ask questions, to seek advice (*after all, a little ol me can't make up her mind on this important matter of what to order and will let the man assist*).

ORDERING FOOD If we've come this far on our Magic Carpet, we may as well go all out and spend the guy's money. No sense in thinking about the cents, not tonight, but sometimes we may have to think about them (*especially if we are paying the bill ourselves*) so, is it a la carte or table d'hote? If it's the former, the price listed is the price you'll pay for just the item, i.e., "Lobster a la Newburg—4.75." If it's the latter then you will undoubtedly get a choice of appetizer, soup, salad, entree, beverage and dessert. It will not be confusing to your escort or the waiter if you will mention what you want in the order they are listed on the menu. However, because you can't anticipate whether or not you will want dessert (*Who's counting calories? Eat, drink, and be merry, for tomorrow you diet.*), you will not give your order for dessert now, but will wait until you are finished with the main course. You may want your beverage, or you may say, "I will have coffee later."

To clarify any questions you might have about menus, turn to the next page. Don't start eating until everyone has been served unless you ask permission. At a large banquet you would start eating hot food as soon as those around you have been served.

VISUAL POISE FOR SOCIAL AFFAIRS

TIME TO EAT

Our seafood cocktail arrives. We will eat it with a cocktail fork—the little fellow who breaks all the rules and prefers to be an outcast among the spoons. Maybe you didn't order a seafood cocktail and you really don't know what silverware to use. *There are rules to help you.*

1. Use the silverware farthest from your plate first.
2. A fork is preferable to a spoon.
3. Ask.
4. Dry foods not served with silverware are finger foods.

celery	breads	cookies
carrot sticks	pickles	green onions
olives	shrimp (with a tail)	radishes
cheese	sandwiches	potato chips
crackers	some cake	canapes (open-faced sandwiches)

TABLE SETTING

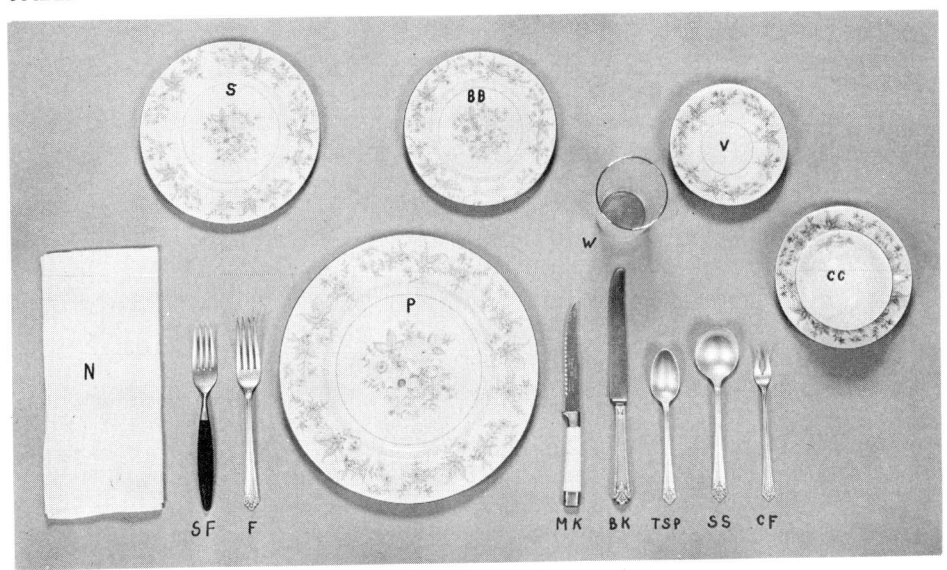

KEY:

N: napkin
SF: salad fork
F: fork
S: salad plate
P: dinner plate
B&B: bread and butter plate
W: water glass
MK: meat knife
BK: bread knife
V: vegetable plate
TSP: teaspoon
SS: soup spoon
CF: cocktail fork
CC: coffee cup

MENU

DINNER

COCKTAILS & APPETIZERS

Crab	Shrimp	Fruit
Sour Cream Herring	Smoked Salmon	Onion Rings
Deviled Eggs	Chopped Chicken Livers	Stuffed Celery

JUICES

Grape, Carrot, Sauerkraut or Clam Nectar
Tomato, Orange, Grapefruit, Pineapple, Prune, V-8 Juice

SALAD

Small Chef's Salad

SOUPS

| Consomme Alphabet | Davenport Clam Chowder |
| Davenport Onion Soup | Bowl Du Jour |

DINNER ENTREES

Poached Filet of Puget Sound Salmon, Egg Sauce	3.75
Dinner Potatoes, Buttered Green Vegetable	
Creamed Crab & Mushroom Omelette	3.60
Long Branch Potatoes, Buttered Broccoli	
Deep Fried Gulf Shrimp, Hot Sauce	3.75
Long Branch Potatoes, Buttered Spinach	
Avocado Stuffed with Seafood Salad, Sliced Tomato	3.45
Veal Cutlet Saute, Talleyrand (a tangy English gravy)	3.85
Baked Potato, Fresh Broccoli	
Roast Prime Ribs of Choice Steer Beef Au Jus	4.25
Baked Potato, Fresh Garden Vegetable	
Pear & Cottage Cheese Salad with Orange & Pineapple Slices	3.25
Grapes, Toasted Almonds	
Roast Young Tom Turkey, Giblet Dressing, Cranberry Sauce	3.85
Whipped Potatoes, Dinner Vegetable	
Broiled Pork Chops, Pineapple Rings, Baked Potato, Spinach	3.85

Dinner Salad, Beverage, Roll & Butter with above Entrees

> **DESSERTS**
> Old Fashioned Brown Betty, Lemon Sauce
> Cocoanut Cream Pie   Peach Pie
> Peppermint Snowball, Chocolate Sauce
> Baked Apple with Cream
> Cup Custard   Peaches in Heavy Syrup   Pumpkin Pie
> Rice or Bread Pudding with Cream   Choice of Sherbet
> Apple Pie   Hot Mince Pie   French Pastry
> French Vanilla, Strawberry or Chocolate ice cream

SILVERWARE AND NAPKINS The place setting will vary with the type of food to be served. The silverware to be used first will be placed on the outside, as mentioned before. The napkin will be found on the left, or, sometimes, it will be placed in the center of the place setting. It is opened only half way when placed on the lap. Luncheon napkins are opened fully.

HOW FOOD IS SERVED AND REMOVED Food is served on the left, except for beverages, and empty plates are removed from the right. Let us hope your plate is empty! Since World War II it is proper to eat everything placed before you. In fact, it is rather poor taste for you not to try each food, even if just a little.

SOUP AND CRACKERS Soup is eaten with the soup spoon and crackers are eaten with the fingers. If you want the very last drop, you will tip the plate away from you, although the less you move your dishes, the better. There's a little poem that will help you to remember.

> *"As a ship goes out to sea,
> So I scoop my soup away from me."*

You might want to launch just a ship or two in the way of croutons or oyster crackers, but no crunching or dunking, please.

BREAD AND BUTTER Shall we insert here that bread is to be buttered with a knife, and that you butter only one bite-sized piece at a time? One exception, if the bread or roll is hot you may butter all of it. Mmmm, yum.

SALAD Your salad presents practically no problems whatsoever because you can cut the lettuce with a knife. If you are left-handed, so much the better. In fact, it will be quite easy for you to eat it way over there on the left-hand side. For most of us the question, "Shall I or shall I not move it to the middle, or better yet to the right side?" Sorry. Oh, well, so I'll struggle with it and make it easier by keeping a small piece of bread in my left hand to use as a "pusher."

EUROPEAN AND AMERICAN CUSTOMS VARY SOMEWHAT In Sweden, one must keep both hands above the table all the while. Wonder why! In America, if the left hand is not being useful, it is placed in the lap. The Europeans eat their meat with the left hand, as you no doubt know. The fork is in the left hand and the knife in the right, a piece of meat is cut and popped directly into the mouth without changing the fork from its upside down position or anything. In America a complicated system is used of transferring the fork to the right hand, turning it prongs up and then eating (*of course the knife must be placed on the plate in the process*). It is not difficult to understand why connoisseurs prefer the Continental method.

TIME TO DANCE

The Man of the Moment asks you to dance, he comes around the table, pulls out your chair and off you go; but not before laying aside your napkin, bag, and gloves. Personally, I like the rule that says, "You never place a soiled napkin on the table until everyone at the table has finished eating and is ready to leave." If you like it too, you will place your napkin on your chair along with the other accoutrements.

REPAIRING YOUR LIPSTICK

Speaking of military gear, don't fight the Battle of the Bulge on social occasions; don't fight your Battle with Beauty at the dinner table either. You may just glance into a mirror at the table to see whether your lipstick is Niagraing down your chin, and you may gently replace what has come off. Major reinforcements are brought to the battle lines in the privacy of a powder room.

REMOVING AN UNMASTICABLE OBJECT

In spite of the well-laid plans of mice and men—and you, there may be the uncomfortable moment when you can't swallow what you have in your mouth. In this category would fall fish bones, gristle, olive pits, etcetera. This could happen to anyone, but it had to be you. As gracefully and inconspicuously as possible you remove the unmasticable object with your fingers and place it on the side of your plate.

WHAT TO PUT ON THE SIDE OF YOUR PLATE Also on the side of your plate are the sauces you dip things into rather than putting them on. Also is the salt for radishes and the butter, when there is no butter plate. Nothing is placed on the table cloth except the things you eat with or in. If you happen to spill something like a pea, this too is placed on the side of the plate.

VISUAL POISE FOR SOCIAL AFFAIRS

SPILLED FOOD If you happen to spill so that it becomes a tremendous mopping-up operation, you should send out an SOS and get help. Silverware that is dropped will happily be replaced as will food that is not what you ordered. As will food that is, by some saboteur, sabotaged. Pies with flies and waldorfs with worms will be taken back to the kitchen post haste in a restaurant. In the home of your favorite friend, it might be better for you to capitulate and let the fly have the pie. It's simply delicious, but with all the other wonderful dishes, you are just too full!

SERVING DESSERT

Did you notice that before being served dessert all the plates and silverware were removed? The only thing remaining of your place setting is your water glass. Here comes the dessert silverware—a fork and a spoon, sometimes just one or the other. After you have finished, the used piece is placed on the dessert plate just as the salad fork was placed on the salad plate, the soup spoon in the soup bowl (or on the coaster underneath if it was small), the butter knife on the butter plate, the coffee spoon in the saucer, the vegetable spoon in the vegetable dish.

Unused silverware remains as you found it. Dishes are not stacked. Finger bowls are utilized. Napkins are placed, crumpled, on the left side. It has been a delicious dinner, the company has been divine, the conversation has been bright and sparkling, the tab is paid, the waiter is tipped, your coat is on. You float toward the door that closes a chapter on "Dining With You is Delightful."

UNFORGIVABLE MANNERS

1. To show any signs of haste while eating.
2. To discuss morbid or unhappy topics.
3. To monopolize the conversation.
4. To not show up on time for a dinner engagement.
5. To not compliment your hostess on some phase of the dinner.
6. To not answer her written invitation with a note immediately.
7. To in any way attract attention to yourself with boisterous or uncouth behavior.

You will notice that the "unforgivables" have nothing to do with how you handle your silverware or whether you use your fingers to eat french fries. Knowing the techniques for the table will give you confidence and free your mind for the more important matter of winning friends and influencing people. Therefore, they are important but not something about which you need have a nervous breakdown. If you don't know what to do—ask.

UNIT THREE

WARDROBE PLANNING

Introduction

"If you have beauty he will admire you. If you are witty, clever or profound, he will respect you. But if you have charm he will adore you and lay at your feet the love that a man gives only to a charming woman."—Old Arabian Proverb.

Your personality is affected by the clothes that you wear. To realize this you have only to think of the time you were caught at your very worst—hair up in curlers, slip showing, dress torn. You probably apologized for your appearance only to find your self-consciousness growing with each word. Or how about the times you have gotten a run in your hose? Were you ever wholly unaware of it?

We feel our best when we look our best. To put it another way, a woman's self-confidence is in direct ratio to her physical appearance, her good grooming.

Although your clothes should never overshadow your personality, they should form an attractive frame for the picture that is you. If you are not yet convinced that clothes influence temperament and behavior, recall some plays that you have seen. A light musical comedy would be a complete failure without the gay, colorful costumes that add so much to its effect. On the other hand, a depressing drama dressed in somber hues has an atmosphere of gloom and apprehension even before the action has begun.

Yes, you must look the part, and inasmuch as you are the star in your own personal drama of life, you cannot afford to look any less than the leading lady. Some embarrassing clothing experiences in your life may have taught you the necessity of being well dressed on every occasion. This doesn't mean that you must spend more money than you can afford. Good taste is purchased with good sense rather than dollars. This lesson will be concerned with stretching your clothing budget so that you will always have "something" to wear.

CHAPTER 12

WARDROBE PLANNING

If you are one of those women who say, "I have absolutely nothing to wear," as you stand in front of a packed closet, there is something drastically wrong with your clothing habits. Let's begin at the beginning and stretch your clothing dollar, not by spending, but rather by salvaging for use anything that you might already have.

YOUR CLOTHING INVENTORY

The first step then is to make an inventory of the clothes you now own. For most of us there are two major divisions—summer clothes and winter clothes. Into the former will go your summer cottons, beach clothes, pastel shoes. Into the later category will go all the things you don't actually put away for the colder months.

Immediately you will be able to see the saving in buying for the fall, winter and spring seasons, clothes that will be suitable for all three. San Franciscans are noted for their beautiful, well-groomed appearance. This is partly due to their having twelve months in which to wear one wardrobe.

Because summer is only one-fourth as long as the other seasons, you should plan on a minimum wardrobe for this time of year. You will be able to save your money for the more social winter months if you can sew your own cottons. Summer cotton dresses don't usually require the fine tailoring technique of, say, a suit and this is a good time for you to put your creative talents into a constructive channel.

The inventory you are requested to make is for the purpose of ferreting out dresses, suits and coats that, with some clinical therapy, can be salvaged for a long life of usefulness. In a later lesson you will be shown how to accessorize and how to mix and match your clothes to get the ultimate value out of them. Presently, it is up to you to get all your clothes in shipshape condition.

If you come across dresses that make you feel inferior or apologetic, be critical of them. It might be best to discard them. Not, however, if this includes your entire wardrobe! Be patient, for in the next several weeks you will learn what colors, lines and styles are best for your figure. Then you will be able to go out and buy new clothes that will be a pleasure to you and to others.

WARDROBE PLANNING

YOUR CLOTHING UPKEEP

Right now, keep your clothes wearable. Mend and repair hems and seams as soon as you take a garment off. It's a mistake to put it in your closet thinking that you will get around to it later, only to discover that later is later than you think and you're out in the public with your hem down.

You can take a tip from retail stores where clothes are hung on display for your perusal and approval. They are hung on the correct type of hangers with enough distance between each garment for them to "air." All buttons are buttoned and the zippers are zipped. This is not just for appearance, but keeps the garment from sagging out of shape.

But enough of this chit chat. Go to your closet at the first opportunity and see if you are giving your clothes the attention and care they deserve.

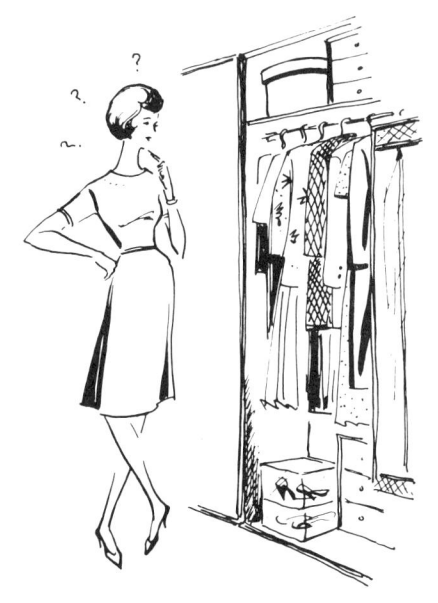

Lacking a jewelry box? Use the boxes your jewelry comes in. Simply take off the lids and place them in a neat arrangement in your drawer. There before your eyes is each necklace, bracelet or what-have-you. No hunting for jumbled jewelry.

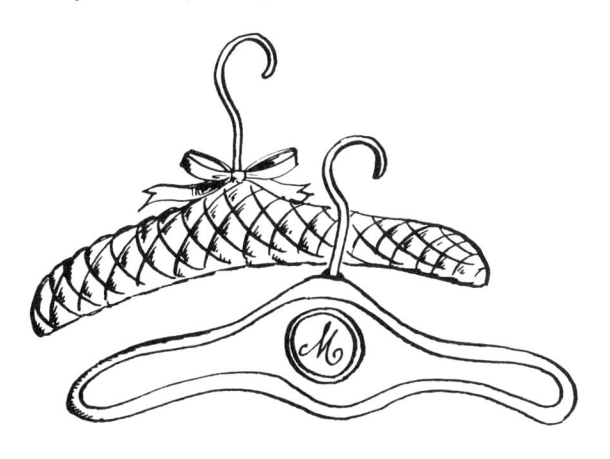

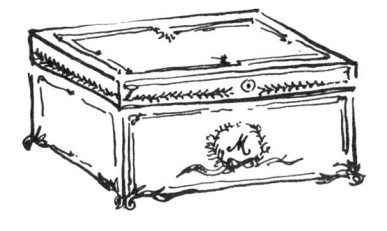

Jewelry Box

Padded Hangers

WARDROBE PLANNING

UPKEEP SUGGESTIONS

1. "Every Garment in Service" is a good slogan for one who wishes to make the most of a wardrobe. Make up that inventory and keep it on hand. New purchases may be added as made, and discarded garments crossed off.
2. "A Place For Everything and Everything in its Place" will minimize wear and tear on your clothes—and your nerves. Knitted garments should be folded in a drawer or box. Gloves should have their own special niche as should jewelry, hose, handkerchiefs, belts, undergarments and hats.
3. "Dust Destroys" as you will learn if you don't protect your out-of-season clothes in dust-proof bags. Fabrics deteriorate from dirt and perspiration; therefore, all clothes should be cleaned or washed before being stored.
4. "A Stitch in Time Saves Nine" is nowhere more true than in the literal sense. Repair your clothes as soon as the need for attention is noticed.
5. "All God's Chillin Got Shoes." The only question is, are they polished, are the heels kept straight, are they protected from rain and snow and dust?
6. "Cleanliness is next to Godliness" and you can keep rather close if you have three sets of lingerie, one to wear, one to wash, and one to spare.
7. It pays to "Be Prepared" for those unexpected emergencies. Be prepared too for the day-to-day care of clothes. Do you have at hand the following?

clothes brush	_____	mild soap	_____
spot remover	_____	water softener	_____
shoe polish	_____	mild bleach	_____
suede brush	_____	automatic iron	_____
sewing kit	_____	moth crystals	_____
pressing cloth	_____		

8. "Know-How" to care for the various fabrics in your wardrobe. Usually garments will come with a tag telling what the fabric is and how it should be cleaned or laundered. Read this carefully before throwing the instructions away.

Avoid the Extra Expense of:
   Dry cleaning fabrics when careful hand laundering would do just as well. Washing fabrics that *must* be dry cleaned.

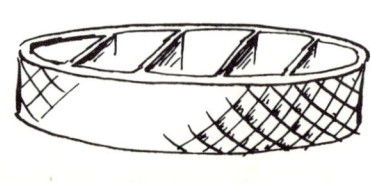

Belt Hoop

Handkerchief Box

Hosiery Box

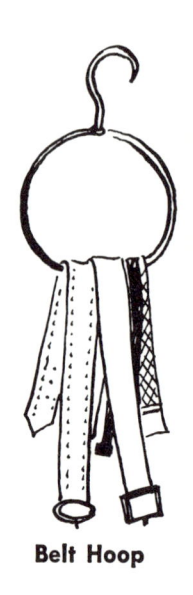

Skirt Hanger

WARDROBE PLANNING

HOW WELL DO YOU CARE FOR YOUR CLOTHES?

Giving your clothes the proper care contributes to longer wear and better grooming. You will find that the proper equipment makes caring for your clothing easier and more interesting. Do you have storage space well planned? Is your mending basket complete? Is your cleaning kit adequate? Do you have laundering and pressing conveniences?

CLOTHING CARE TEST

Check yourself on the care you give your clothes. If you score between 165 and 220, your clothes are a personality asset. If your score is between 110 and 165, you sometimes feel ill at ease in a group because of your clothing. Any score under 110—you should spend much more time on the care of your clothes!

Here we go then. Give yourself 5 points for yes or excellent, 3 points for often or good, 1 point for sometimes or fair, and 0 for no or poor.

Score Here

COATS, SUITS, AND DRESSES

1. Do you keep your skirts on hangers adapted only for that purpose? _____
2. Do you keep seldom-used clothes in dust-proof bags? _____
3. Do you send dark-colored garments to the cleaners as often as they should be sent . . . Frequently? _____
4. Do you have heavily padded hangers for coats and jackets? _____
5. Do you leave enough space between each garment in the closet so that they won't get crushed? _____
6. Do you close all zippers and buttons when you hang a garment? _____
7. Do you open all fastenings before putting a garment on? _____
8. Do you handle all your clothes carefully and hang them as soon as you take them off? _____
9. Are you careful so as not to ruin your clothes with perspiration stains? _____
10. Do you mend and repair your garments as soon as you notice they need it? _____
11. Do you remove spots and stains as soon as they appear? _____
12. Do you avoid using your better clothes for house work and lounging? _____
13. Do you properly "moth proof" your woolen garments at the end of the season? _____
14. Do you keep a clothes brush handy and use it? _____
15. Do you use a pressing cloth? _____
16. Do you rotate the wearing of your clothes so that each has a chance to "rest" between times? _____

Dust Proof Closet Bag

Skirt Hangers

HATS AND GLOVES

1. Do you keep your hats protected from dust between wearings?
2. Do you stuff the crowns with tissue to prevent their getting out of shape?
3. Do you size and press your veils when they become limp?
4. Do you brush your hats frequently?
5. Do you wash white gloves after each wearing?
6. Do you have a special place for your gloves so that they are put away flat and in shape?
7. Do you avoid wearing gloves that look shabby either because of too much wear or improper care?
8. Do you fold your gloves properly whenever you remove them?

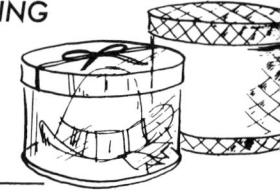

Hat Boxes

SHOES AND HOSE

1. Do you keep your heels even, not run-over?
2. Do you replace heel caps often enough to prevent ruining the heels of your shoes?
3. Do you keep your shoes brushed and polished?
4. Do you protect your shoes from dust when not in use?
5. Do you avoid getting your shoes wet?
6. Do you help them retain their shape by using shoe trees?
7. Do you use a shoe horn to avoid crushing the heel counter?
8. Do you wash your nylon hose after each wearing?
9. Do you roll your stocking to the foot when putting it on?
10. Do you wear gloves when handling your hose to prevent snagging your hose?
11. Do you rub your feet with cream to prevent roughness, and runs in hose?

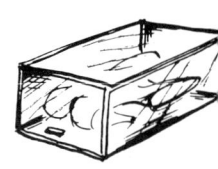

Shoe Boxes

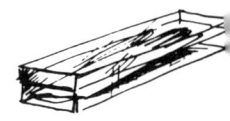

Glove Boxes

OTHER ITEMS

1. Do you empty your handbag once a week so as to brush and clean the lining?
2. Do you wash your girdle often enough to keep it fresh?
3. Do you have a special box for jewelry?
4. Do you give your jewelry an ammonia "beauty bath"?
5. Do you fold sweaters and put them in a drawer rather than hang them on hangers?
6. Do you follow the fabric care directions given with your clothing purchases?

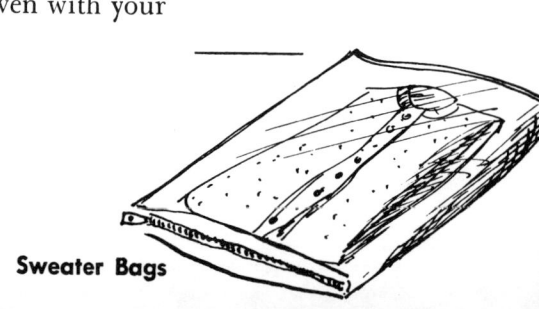

Sweater Bags

WARDROBE PLANNING

7. Do you allow your night clothes to air?
8. Do you keep flowers and scarves ready for immediate use?
9. Do you use the correct ironing temperature for your various fabrics?

TYPES OF FABRIC

You would be bewildered and panic stricken if you were to awaken one day to find yourself living before the discovery of synthetic or man-made fibers. You would look for your lovely rayon underthings and you would not find them. Your nylon hose would be gone too. What an adjustment you would have to make were you suddenly placed in the world of several centuries ago. You would not have safety pins, zippers, elastic, buttons or many of the items that add to your comfort today.

In order for you to plan your wardrobe, you need to become acquainted with the qualities of various fibers which are classified as either natural or synthetic.

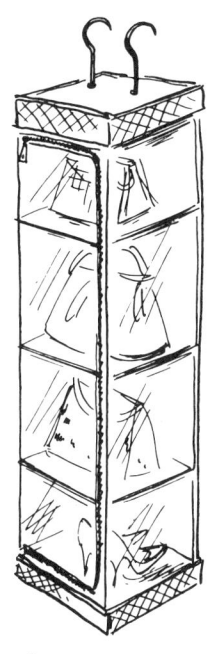

Accessory Closet

NATURAL

WOOL Warm, absorbent, elastic and long lasting especially when worsted. Other animal fibers include: Alpaca, Camel's hair, Mohair, Vicuna, Angora.

SILK Strong, lustrous, responds well to dyeing.

COTTON Dull, uninjured by heat, sunlight, and boiling.

LINEN Cool, uninjured by heat, sunlight, and boiling.

SYNTHETIC

RAYON Acetate rayon (e.g. Celanese); Cuprammonium rayon (e.g. Bemberg); Viscose rayon (e.g. Crown tested) weak, lustrous, easily dyed, affected by heat. Loses 30% of its strength when wet.

NYLON In hosiery the gauge and denier are designated. Denier: Size or number of filament or yarn. The higher the denier number, the heavier the yarn. Gauge: The number of stitches in a given unit of space. Usually the higher the gauge the lower the denier.

Other synthetics include: Lastex, Plextron, Visca, Vinylite, Vinyon, Fiberglass, Aralac.

AVOID INFERIOR FABRICS SUCH AS:

Dotted swiss that loses its dots because they are not woven or permanently printed.

Corduroy that becomes velveteen because the ribs were only pressed in.

Seersucker that washes to become gingham because the crinkle is only roller embossed.

Flannel that sheds due to excess flocking.

Colors that fade even in lukewarm water.

"Permanent" pleats that are not permanent.

CHAPTER 13

PLANNING PURCHASES

If, like most people, you have a limited amount to spend on clothes, then it is imperative that you make each purchase really count. You cannot afford to make mistakes. Your purchases must be well-planned and good values. Buy fashion-wise clothes, avoid fads that will be out of date in six months.

Don't be a "last minute" shopper who suddenly decides she must have a new dress for the party tonight. If you are planning ahead, you will be able to anticipate your needs and make purchases when it is most advantageous to you—end of season sales or when the new stock has just come in.

PLAN TO COMBINE YOUR ENSEMBLES

Two and three piece outfits are ideal for double-duty service since the parts can be combined with other pieces in your wardrobe to form new ensembles. This will be especially true if each new purchase is bought, not for itself, but for its adaptability to the rest of your collection. Make your large purchases first, like coat or dress, and build your small purchases around them. Select one basic color scheme per season around which to build your outfits—an excellent way to stretch the use of your accessories.

GETTING THE MOST FROM ONE HUNDRED DOLLARS

If you had just $100.00 for a new ensemble which would include the following items, how much of the money would you spend on each one?

	Fill in Price
Hats	_____
Bags	_____
Gloves	_____
Dress or Suit	_____
Shoes	_____
Jewelry, scarf, belt or other accessory	_____
Lipstick (color definitely an accessory)	_____

If you are a wise shopper you would spend not more than half on the dress or suit and the rest would do for the accessories. A dress or suit is only half bought until it becomes a complete ensemble.

THE ORDER OF PURCHASE

On the imaginary shopping tour for your new ensemble, which item did you buy first? The dress or suit, of course, and which purchase came next, and next? Cover the right side of the page as you fill in your answers.

1. Dress or suit	1. Dress or suit
2. _____	2. Shoes
3. _____	3. Bag
4. _____	4. Gloves
5. _____	5. Hat
6. _____	6. Other accessory
7. _____	7. Lipstick

IMAGINARY SHOPPING TOUR

Shopping can be fun when you know that your money will be well-spent with no regrets. It can be exciting too. Let's now imagine that we have decided to purchase a white cotton blouse with a Spanish flair. We have only $5.00 to spend and the blouse will have to be no more than this.

SELECTING A STORE

Our first decision should be to eliminate those stores not catering to our particular need—white cotton blouses for $5.00 or less. We select the store where we think we will find what we want right off the bat and walk in. Yes, they have white cotton blouses. For $5.00 or less? Yes, they think so. With a Spanish flair? Well, now it gets more difficult. Would you like to look at several? Yes, indeed. In size 34, please.

CONSIDERATIONS FOR MAKING AN INTELLIGENT PURCHASE

We have now decided on the size, color, fabric, price and style. But is this all we must consider in order to make an intelligent purchase? Let us see.

SIZE Don't let a sales person talk you into getting a garment that won't fit. Oh, yes, the store has an alteration department, but your purse has a bottom too. Unless you have a difficult figure, let them worry about fitting you.
A coat, dress or suit is almost impossible to alter through the shoulders. The shoulder seam should come out even with the outside of the shoulder bone, no matter what the clerk says.

PRICE You are on a budget and to step out-of-bounds now means skimping somewhere else. The clothes you give the hardest wear must be the most expensive. Other items that are principally ornamental needn't be the best. They must be the most for the least.
No sense in looking at $150.00 suits if your budget allows only half that amount. It will just make you unhappy. Anyway, original designs in America can be copied in a less expensive fabric, with a little less workmanship and for much less money than the original. This fact makes American women the best dressed in the world today.

FABRIC The upkeep of a garment can sometimes cost you more than your original investment. It is rather foolish to buy an inexpensive item that requires dry cleaning. Our white blouse is an example. Be sure to carefully read the fabric finishing and clothes-care labels.

WORKMANSHIP It may be that you can buy a real bargain and by going over the seams yourself have a dress that will last several seasons.
It is here that manufacturers of low-priced clothes save on their labor costs. You usually get what you pay for.

COLOR It is essential that each new purchase fits into the wardrobe you already have. To buy a navy blue dress when you have only black accessories can prove to be an expensive purchase indeed. It means buying accessories to match.
Small touches of bright color will give your ensemble a lively mood. These touches can be added with inexpensive scarfs, flowers and jewelry.

STYLE You know what lines you would like to have, and only you, not the clerk, know where you are going to wear it and with what. Don't accept substitutes.
It so happens that we need the white blouse to go with a Mexican skirt we bought in Mexico City. Surely the sales person does not know this unless we tell her and even then she may not be able to imagine it.

APPROPRIATENESS With your "Planned Purchase" Plan, you will select your clothes with their future life in mind. Your wardrobe will become a distinct social advantage when you choose clothes that fit the occasion.

To save money, if you are not a social butterfly, it might be wiser for you to rent a gown rather than buy one for those rare occasions that you need one.

MANUFACTURER AND DESIGNER Price may or may not be a criterion of quality. If a commodity is cheap, find out why it is so cheap, for it may not be a bargain. It might be a white elephant.

BUYING BY BRAND

Recently consumers have become interested in what is behind the labels on ready-to-wear garments. For years we women have relied upon "brands" to guide us in our food buying and, as a rule, we have found standard brands to be dependable. Now we can apply this same buying practice when shopping for our clothes. We can make a habit of asking for the brands and labels that have given quality and satisfaction.

Experts in the world of fashion are acquainted with most of the designers and their work. It is not necessary for you to have this extensive knowledge; however, it will be helpful for you to study fashion magazines so that you can recognize the designers of fashions that are your "type" and fit.

The ready-to-wear industry is highly competitive. Most houses specialize in one type of garment in order to manufacture dresses, coats, suits, or whatever for the lowest price possible.

MATCH COLORS

Another shopping commandment that will save time, effort and mistakes is to take the items to be matched with you. This is the reason for putting the hat fourth on the list. You will be able to select your hat for harmony of line, color and texture. It is advisable for you to see the hat from all angles as it looks on your head and then to view it in a full length mirror in relationship to the entire ensemble.

Colors can be very tricky, they look different in artificial light. Ask the clerk to let you take items out into the sunlight so that you can see whether or not they really match. Also, don't trust your memory when it comes to matching colors. If you have a color problem take a small piece of the fabric with you.

HOSIERY SHOPPING

Another item that must be considered is hosiery. You should select shades that flatter your legs and blend in with the ensemble. Hosiery styles and colors change from season to season. Try to keep up with the latest ideas on leg flattery. When making hosiery purchases buy at least three pairs at one time in the same shade and length. In this way you will have pairs long after the first stocking has developed a run.

PERSONALITY AND PURCHASES

Do you allow your personality to influence your purchases? No matter how well you may know what you want and the products that fill the bill, you will not be able to shop efficiently and effectively if you display the following shopper attitudes. If these descriptions mirror your personality, correct your consumer attitude so that you may be served more effectively.

BE HONEST IN YOUR APPRAISAL

The Timid Soul who stands on the edge of the crowd hoping to be waited on.

The Wise Guy who insists on letting the clerk know her place—she looks down her nose.

The Suspicious Shopper who must tear off the wrapper and examine the garment minutely no matter what the label said.

The Gullible Shopper who accepts anything, sight unseen.

The Individualist who refuses any help or suggestions from the clerk.

The Crack Shot who knows it all.

The Hesitant Shopper who takes half an hour to make up her mind.

The Conformist who buys just because everyone else is.

The Just-Looking Shopper who takes up a clerk's time with no intention of buying.

The Stubborn Shopper who refuses to buy a certain commodity because she doesn't like the clerk's attitude.

The Bargain Hunter who consistently searches for bargains regardless of need.

The Never-Satisfied Customer who asks for discounts and other special favors and who often returns the items she has purchased.

GOOD SHOPPING HABITS

Here are a few tips on shopping that will add to your shopping enjoyment. You will undoubtedly be able to add others that will guarantee satisfaction—or your money back.

1. Make out a shopping list. Keep a pad conveniently placed so that you can add items as you think of them. Organize your list according to stores and the departments in the store so that you will not have to retrace your steps.
2. Put your list in a convenient place in your handbag so that you will be able to refer to it without searching for it.
3. Shop at convenient hours. Avoid the noon and rush hours when city workers crowd the stores.

4. A clerk likes you to remember her name. Form the habit of shopping at certain places, the clerks will be more interested in you personally.
5. Shop for those brands which have given you satisfaction in the past.
6. Don't shop when you're tired. You may buy without good judgment just so you can go home.
7. State clearly and briefly to the clerk what you want. She is hired by the store to be of assistance to you, don't hamper her by confusing her with lengthy conversation.
8. Don't shop with a friend. This is no hard fast rule, but you will be able to shop more efficiently by yourself. Besides, clerks find a customer-with-a-friend the most difficult to serve.
9. Sales people will appreciate your patience. They have long trying hours.
10. Be pleasant and polite. The clerk's suggestions may be worth at least temporary consideration.
11. Know what you want and don't waste time looking at something you never intend to buy.
12. Ask no unreasonable favors unless you are prepared to pay for them.
13. Avoid arguments. Although "the customer is always right," you may not be.
14. Consider the rights of other customers. Women sometimes act at the bargain counter the way men do behind the wheel of a car. It will pay to give a few seconds to small courtesies.
15. Dress appropriately. A well-dressed person attracts the clerk's attention.

APPROPRIATE DRESS FOR SHOPPING

In small communities you may be forgiven for shopping in a pair of slacks; in downtown areas, never.

A woman is not dressed for the street until she is wearing a hat, suit or dress, gloves, hose and shoes, and is carrying a bag. It goes without saying that she wears cosmetics too as a part of her good grooming.

HOW TO FIND THE RIGHT FOUNDATION

An Undercover Story

It's true that the underclothes you wear are the foundation of your fashion. Therefore, it's important that you choose the ones that will do the most for your figure and your clothes.

A good brassiere will make for bosom beauty by lifting the breasts and supporting them. It will create an illusion of size for the too-small breast, give control to the large, so select brassieres that solve your particular bosom problem and that have the correct lines for the clothes to be worn over them.

A well-fitted girdle is a girl's best friend. It will flatten, firm, smooth out. The less control you need, the lighter in weight your girdle can be. But never fool yourself into thinking that you don't need to own any at all. If you do, you will miss the figure flattery that comes from controlling your silhouette with the proper undergarment.

TRY BEFORE YOU BUY, AND

1. *Be sure to wear dark underwear with dark dresses.* There's nothing worse than detecting very light underwear beneath dark clothes. Wear white under light.
2. Don't pin your underpinnings. Sew them. Hold your straps in place with strap catchers. Save your clothes and your silhouette.
3. Buy slips that fit. Wear them about one inch shorter than your skirts. Full petticoats for full skirts. Pencil slim with straight skirts. You might like to build-in a back panel of lining taffeta in your straight skirts, then you won't have to worry about an extra garment.
4. Own three sets; one to wear, one to wash, one to spare. You can't feel your best unless you are clean from the skin out.
5. Hand launder your precious underthings. They will last longer and retain their shape. Don't throw them into the washing machine.
6. Consider your figure first. Buy undergarments that really fit. Ask the corsetier to help you.
7. Non-stretch panels give firm control wherever you need it, on the tummy, derrierè, upper thighs.
8. Watch your posture. Good posture will do more to re-proportion your figure than the best undergarment.
9. Watch your weight. Losing excess is the best waist-cincher you can find.
10. Select the fabrics you like to feel next to your skin. It doesn't matter whether it's cotton or dacron, nylon or lastex. Take your choice.

BUYING BRAS

A brassiere should support the breasts from underneath, not with tight shoulder straps. It should be purchased in a cup size that is adequate. If you have a bosom that is not large enough to give balance to your figure, don't hesitate to cheat. Wear falsies. Make sure your bra doesn't cut under your arms or over the top of your breasts. Give yourself breathing room too. This means that it is wiser to buy a bra that has stretch panels than one that doesn't. As you probably know, A B C indicates cup size running from small to large. But do you know that 34, 36, etc. indicates the inches around your diaphragm, but not really any more than a 34 blouse means you have a 34 inch bustline? Don't insist that you wear a 32 when a 34 might fit better.

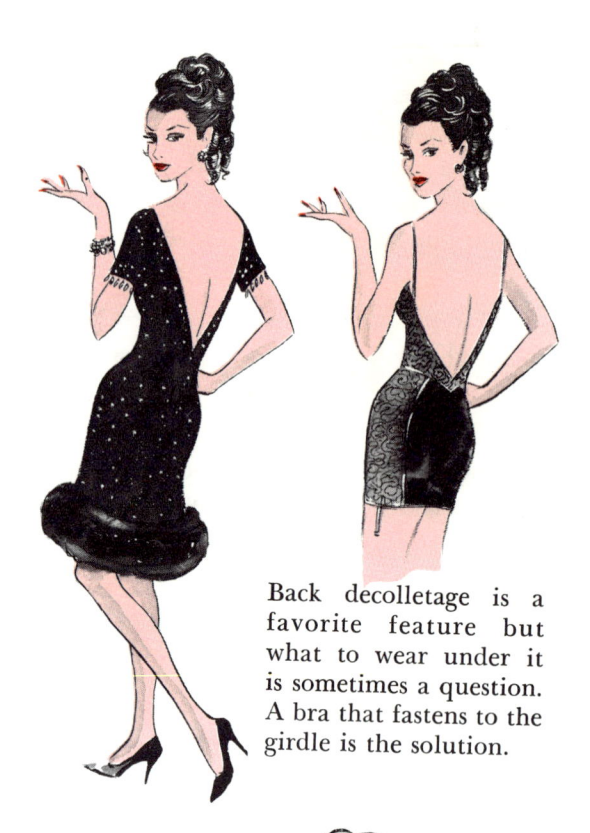

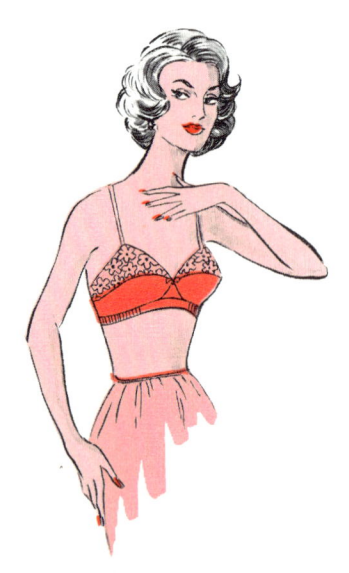

Back decolletage is a favorite feature but what to wear under it is sometimes a question. A bra that fastens to the girdle is the solution.

A heavier bosom requires not only a larger bra but more support both under the bra and under the arms. Buy a fairly wide body band, it will be more comfortable.

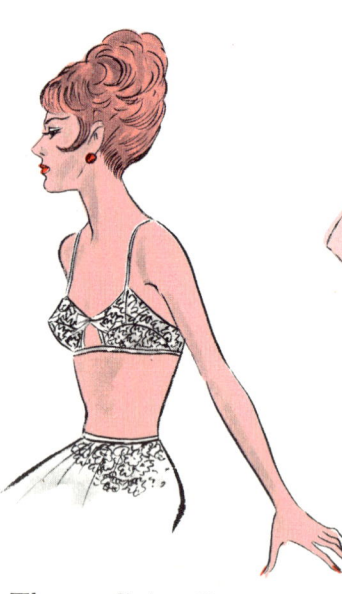

The small bustline requires a minimum amount of support and control.

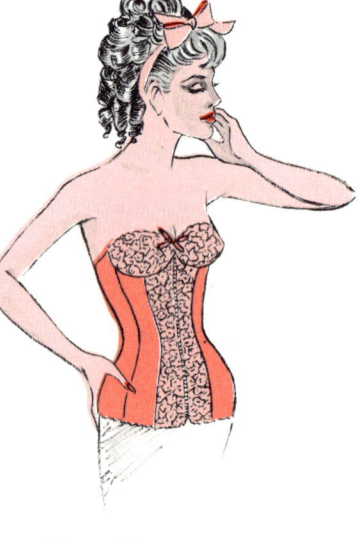

A long-line bra is a must for those pretty party dresses that have fitted bodices.

PLANNING PURCHASES

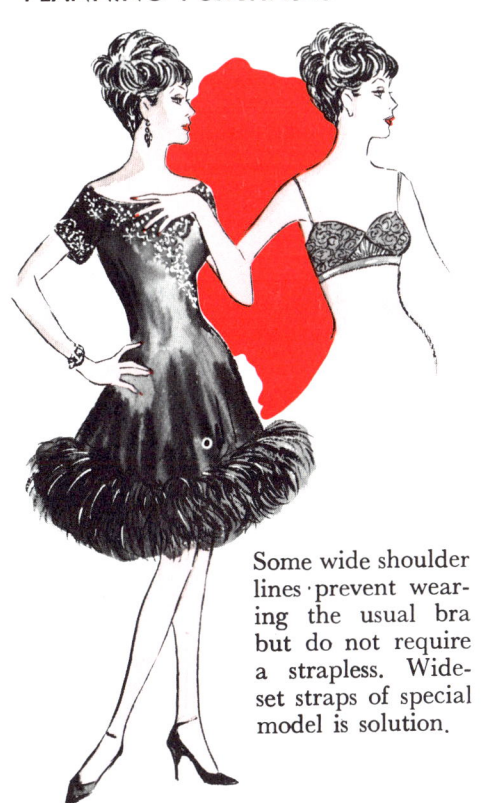

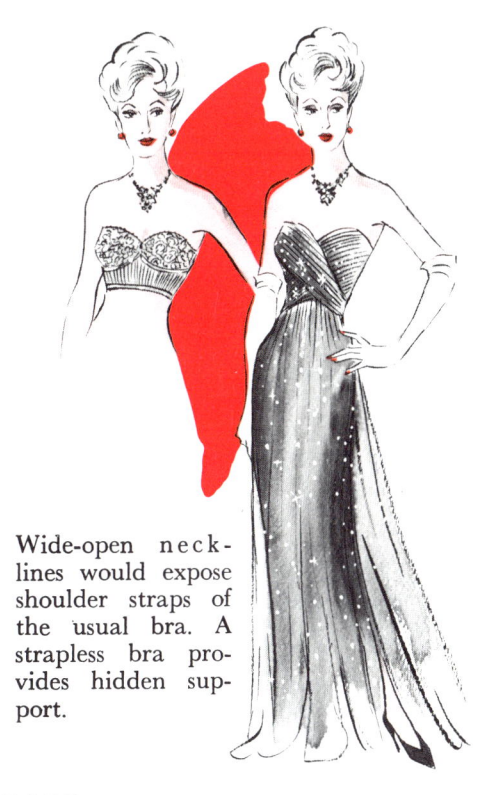

Some wide shoulder lines prevent wearing the usual bra but do not require a strapless. Wide-set straps of special model is solution.

Wide-open necklines would expose shoulder straps of the usual bra. A strapless bra provides hidden support.

BUYING GIRDLES

When you're beginning to think about new girdles, take a good long look at yourself in a full length mirror. And not through rose colored glasses. Admit the bumps that are there. Just as you would consider your face shape when you select a hair style, so you must be honest with yourself about the foundations you will need for the basis of your fashions.

The girl who thinks she can cut corners when it comes to the right foundation couldn't be further from the truth.

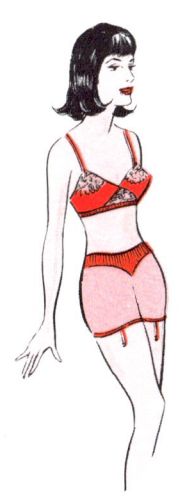

The young, slim figure can best use this type girdle. It gives freedom of action, at the same time, a flat, smooth silhouette.

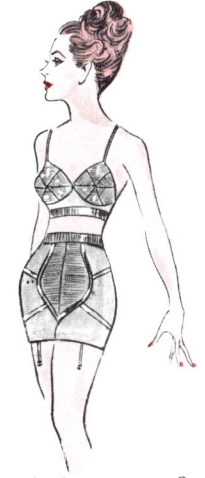

The in-between figure needs a high riding girdle to smooth out waistline bulges.

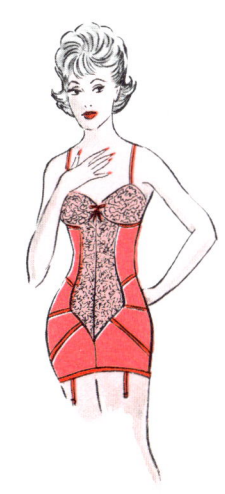

Girls of any age who have a real figure problem need this "all-in-one" for full figure control.

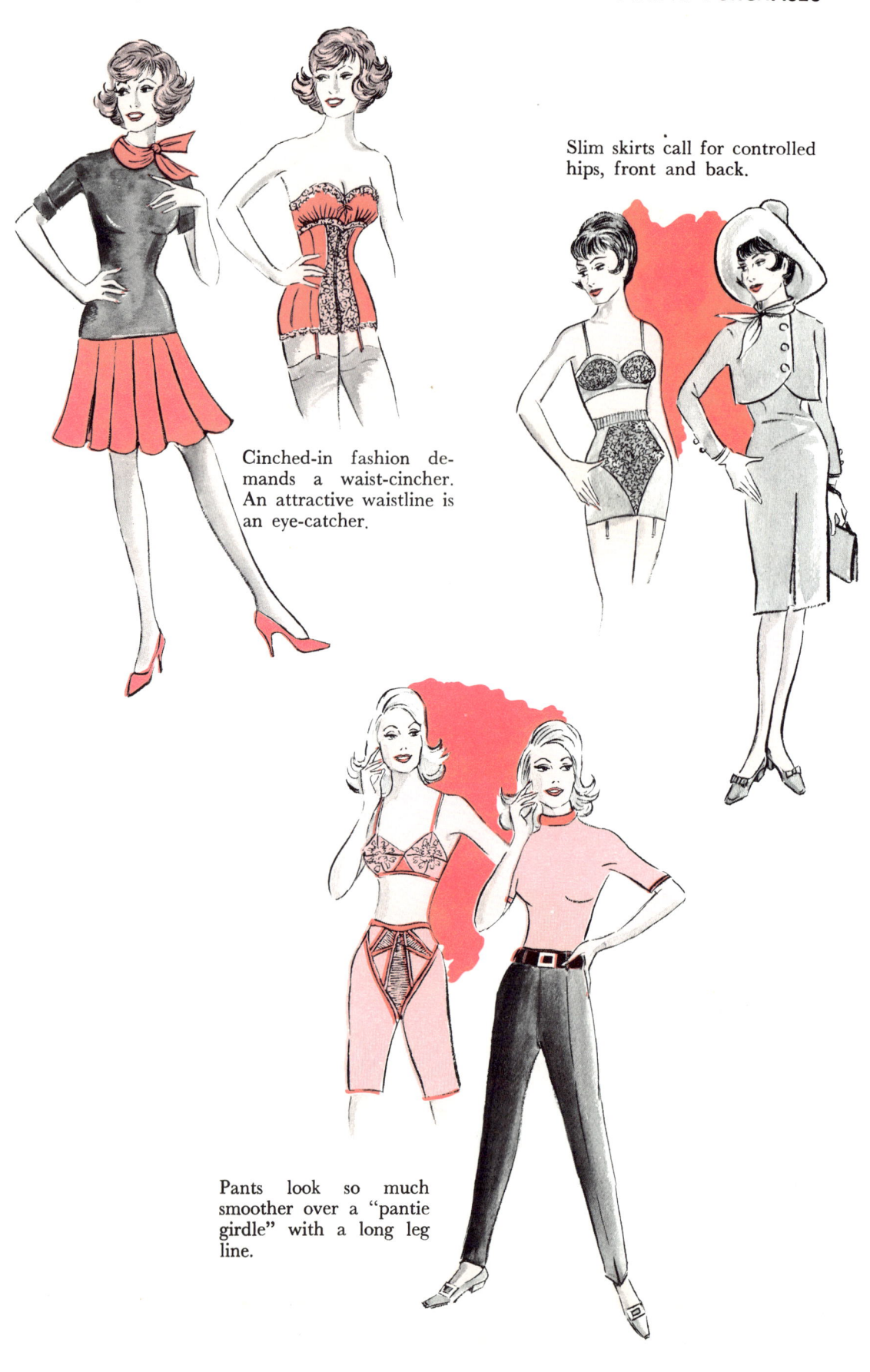

Cinched-in fashion demands a waist-cincher. An attractive waistline is an eye-catcher.

Slim skirts call for controlled hips, front and back.

Pants look so much smoother over a "pantie girdle" with a long leg line.

CHAPTER 14

THE BASIC WARDROBE

Introduction

A *basic* wardrobe should be the outcome of careful wardrobe planning. If it is really true that women in America can have original designer's styles for one-tenth the original price, why don't more look like a million dollars? Because the average woman doesn't plan ahead for clothing purchases, she buys on the spur of the moment. Her colors, fabrics and accessories aren't as well coordinated as they might be. Her wardrobe is not carefully selected for her kind of life so that it is appropriate for every social and business engagement. In other words, she has clothes, but not a basic wardrobe.

WHAT IS A BASIC WARDROBE?

A basic wardrobe is a coordinated series of clothes designed to go around the seasons, twelve months a year, and around the clock, twenty-four hours a day.

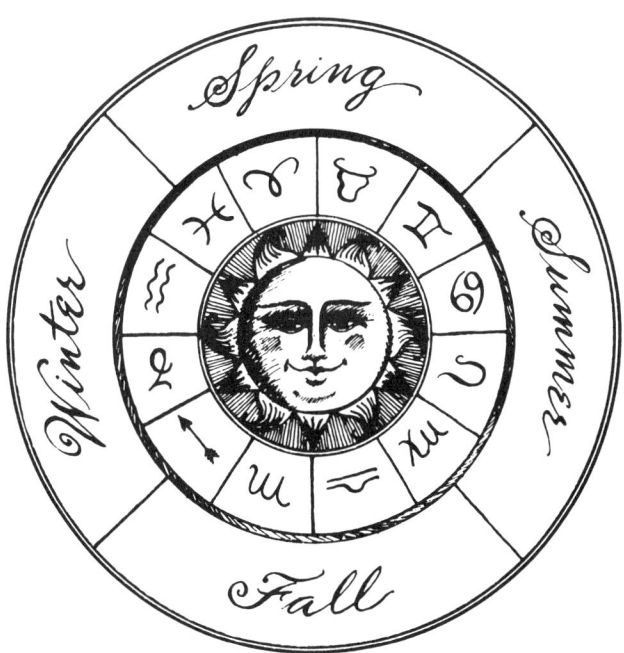

A carefully executed basic wardrobe plan will provide any woman, no matter what her mode of life, with a minimum number of coordinated clothes to wear for any social or business occasion.

BASIC CLOTHES ARE APPROPRIATE

Learning about the basic wardrobe plan will make it possible for you to always have something to wear that will be appropriate and in good taste whether you are going out for a job interview or out for cocktails and dinner at eight.

BASIC CLOTHES ARE PLANNED FOR

A basic wardrobe is like an heirloom chain that is carefully preserved and in which any missing or broken link is promptly replaced. These replacements must be planned for so that those items that require more money can be of the best fabric, style and workmanship. It would be folly to skimp on a basic coat or suit that will last, if wisely selected, for five to ten years. Even with the roughest wear they should last three years and should be budgeted into the wardrobe no more often than this.

It may be necessary to vary the fabrics somewhat to fit the climate in which they are worn, but the principal theme will remain the same. A truly basic wardrobe consists of fashion, not fad. It consists of clothes that have been collected over the years, of clothes that are in style even though they may not be the most stylish.

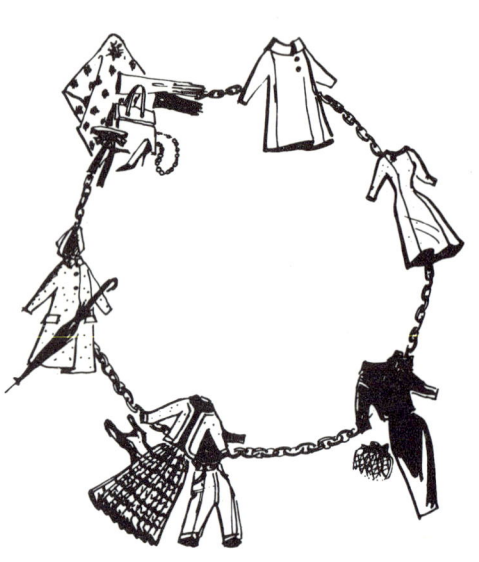

BASIC CLOTHES ARE FASHION-WISE

Fashion-wise clothes do not tell the world what season they appeared on the clothing horizon. In fact, they are so understated that it would be difficult, if not impossible, to date them with a tag of vintage 1960 or whatever.

Fads, on the other hand, are attention-getters and should be purchased only after all basic clothes have been accounted for. The sac dress of 1958 is a good example of the rapid birth and demise of a fad.

Yes, fads are eye-catchers and, as such, are to be avoided unless you have an abundance of ready cash. Beware of finding yourself without the basic wardrobe requirements and then rushing out to buy something for a special occasion. Under the excitement and heat of the race against time you are bound to be caught in the trap of a fad. It will prove to be a money waster.

BASIC CLOTHES ARE SERVICEABLE

Print dresses, red shoes, spring-a-lator mules are just a few of the bad buys. Even knit dresses and sweaters can prove to be money down the drain because once a knit, always a knit. Can they really fill more than one obligation in a busy schedule?

THE BASIC WARDROBE

If you buy items just because you are drawn to them like a moth to a flame and not because they will be serviceable, you will not be able to afford to look as well as you might. For instance, a sweater would probably cost you in the vicinity of ten dollars and, for the sake of a hypothesis, let's say you will wear it thirty times before it goes into the rag bag. At this rate, it cost you thirty cents (.30) every time you put it on.

Compare this bargain with some of the clothes that are hanging in your closet. You will be shocked to discover that your seldom-if-ever-worn clothes are lazy and not worth their keep. It's the basic items that are the work horses of your wardrobe and make it possible for you to have something to wear each and every day.

It is obvious that your affection should go to the "work horses." And there's a moral to this story. Put the major portion of your clothing dollars on those clothes that are worn most often. Find original and ingenious ways to get by for special occasions that would otherwise deplete your clothing budget.

Good taste has never been purchased with money, but good fabrics and good workmanship have. If you are going to look well in your clothes, how much better for you to spend every cent you can afford on the items where quality counts. Buy the best you can afford when you shop for a basic coat, a suit, a basic dress and the accessories you will wear with them. It will pay off in more pleasure and longer wear.

PURCHASES FOR THE BASIC WARDROBE

As stated before, a basic wardrobe consists of a minimum number of coordinated clothes to fit every business and social occasion. When planning your purchases, three specifics must be kept in mind. These are:

1. **COLOR** The basic colors are black, dark brown and navy blue. Sometimes beige, gray or tan serve as alternates.

2. **FABRIC** Must be wearable throughout the year. Silk, light-weight wool, synthetic copies of these.

3. **STYLE** Must be fashion-wise and not extreme.

Each item for the basic wardrobe is listed and will be considered separately taking into consideration the three specifics. Keep in mind that fabrics might need to be adjusted because of climate.

A BASIC COAT

Color: A basic coat must be either one of the three basic colors; black, dark brown or navy blue, or it may be a neutral that will blend with every color in the wardrobe.

Fabric: The fabric should be of a fine quality and should not be a novelty weave or texture. The fabric could be cashmere, worsted wool, baby llama or velveteen.

Style: The style should be unadorned, with slit pockets, no attached belt, preferably no buttons. If there are buttons these must be covered with the fabric of the coat. The collar should be softly rolled. The sleeves may be convertible, no cuffs. There must be no saddle stitching or contrasting trim. The coat must be full length and one inch longer than any of the skirts over which it will be worn.

A Basic Coat

A BASIC DAYTIME DRESS

Color: This dress must be one of the three basic colors: black, dark brown or navy blue. If, however, the wearer looks bad in all of these, she may select a neutral. It is to be understood, of course, that if she goes into a neutral, each item must match each other item. This is true of the basic colors too so that if you want a black coat, your dress must also be black.

Fabric: This may be a fine worsted wool, wool jersey, wool crepe or a dull silk.

Style: It is essentially a covered-up style with a simple neckline that will take to scarves, jewelry or collars. It must have sleeves, preferably elbow or three-quarter length. Any belt must be self-covered including the buckle, so must any buttons be self-covered. There will be, of course, no braid or trim attached. The skirt should be of a cut most suitable to the wearer but not extremely full.

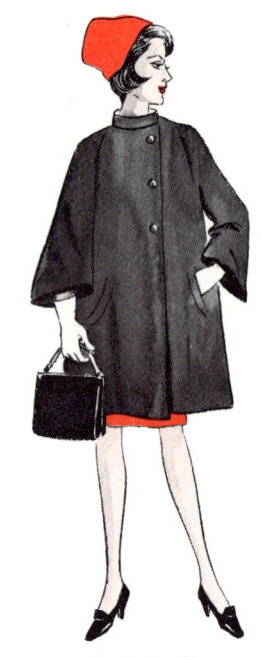

A Basic Dress

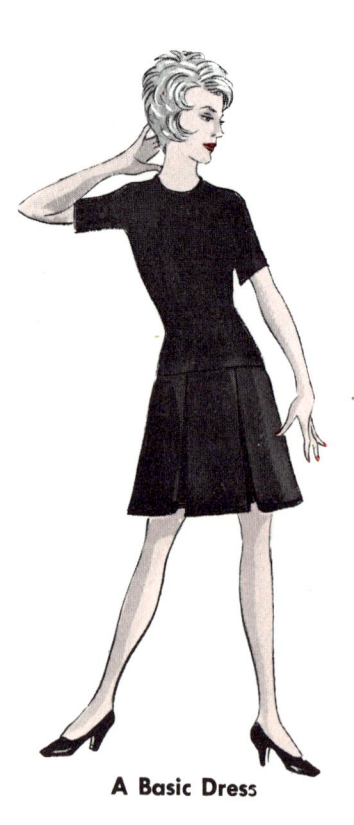

THE BASIC WARDROBE

A BASIC AFTER FIVE DRESS OR SUIT-DRESS

Color: It is not absolutely necessary that this dress be a basic color. However, it must blend in with the basic color selected. If it is not a basic color, it is suggested that it be a muted color tone and not bright enough to attract attention so that people recognize it.

Fabric: Should be really rich and lovely. It might be a brocade or peau de soie or silk shantung or faille or velvet.

Style: This should be essentially bare with a cover-up jacket. The dress may be short sleeved or sleeveless unless the arms are a problem. The neckline should be cut lower than the daytime dress.

There should be no contrasting buttons—they must be self-covered as must the belt, if there is one. The jacket must also have self-covered buttons and should be softly styled. The collarline of the jacket should be soft so as to allow necklaces, flowers or pins.

A Basic After Five Suit Dress

A BASIC SPORTSWEAR COSTUME

Color: This need not be in a basic color but must go with the basic color selected. It may be in two pieces that mix or match.

Fabric: A knit fabric is good for this, or a tweed skirt in combination with a sweater.

Style: Essentially tailored. A simple sportswear dress might be a better selection for some figure problems than a two-piece sweater and skirt outfit. It would be wiser for the overweight girl to have a costume all one color rather than breaking her figure in two with a skirt one color and a top another.

Basic Sportswear

A BASIC RAINWEAR COSTUME

Color: Bright for gloomy days but coordinated with the basic color.

Fabric: No see-through plastics. Otherwise any rainproof material. "Drax" is a finish that may be put on a fabric by a dry cleaner to make it waterproof. This works on almost any fabric.

Style: Jaunty. There must be a raincoat, a rain hood or hat to protect the hair, an umbrella and a pair of boots or galoshes. Again, no see-through plastic.

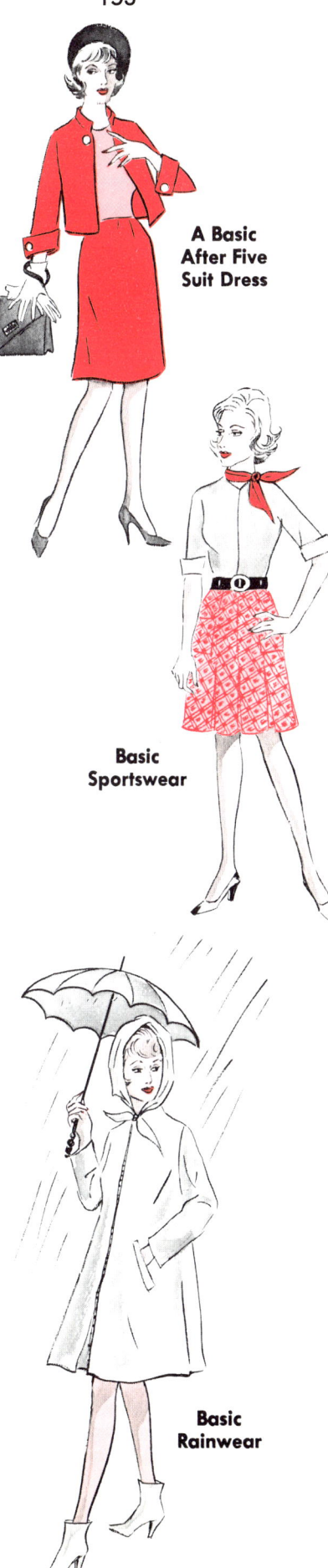

Basic Rainwear

THE BASIC WARDROBE

BASIC ACCESSORIES

A scarf has been called the missing link in a woman's wardrobe. There should be at least one in the basic wardrobe of every woman. This may be used under her coat in the neckline or it may be tied over her hair or used anywhere on her basic dress to add flair.

It should be 36" square in a solid bright color that blends with hair, skin and basic clothes. It should be silk and hand rolled.

This scarf might be black or one of the other basic colors for a very young girl, but it will probably be more flattering in a color that contrasts excitingly with the basic wardrobe color. It might be white.

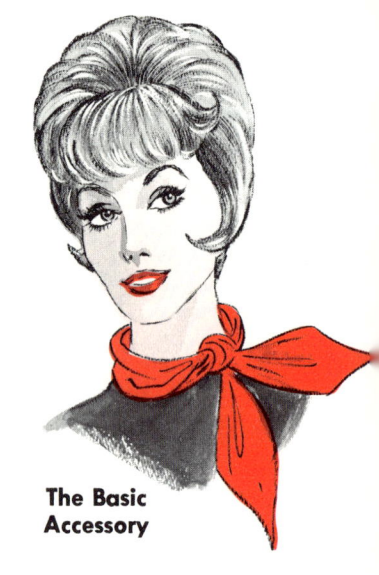

The Basic Accessory

DRESS-UP, DRESS-DOWN ACCESSORIES

Basic accessories must be divided into two categories: those that are appropriate in the daytime with either basic or sport clothes, and those that are appropriate for after-five wear or for special occasions in the daytime. These two categories are "dress-down" for daytime and street wear; and "dress-up" for evening or special daytime occasion wear.

SHOES

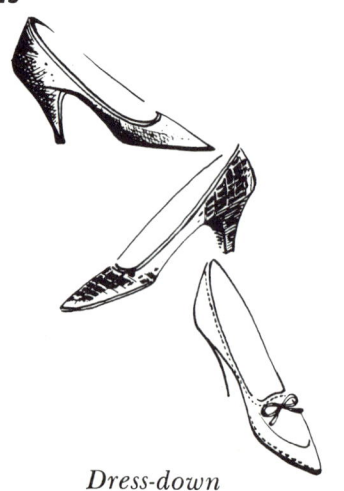

Dress-down

A pump in leather with closed heel and toe is always appropriate.
The leathers that are dress-down include:

calf	lizard
kid	reptile
pig skin	
alligator	

Fabrics would include:
some tapestry fabrics
burlap

Dress-up

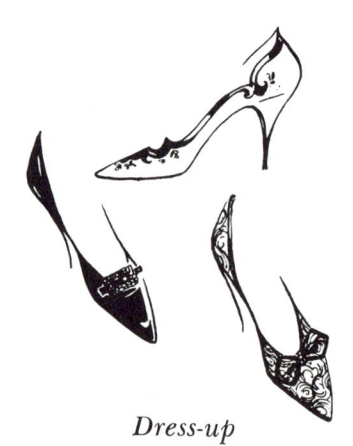

A pump in a dress heel height is always appropriate. Beware of open shoes unless you have beautiful feet and are prepared to buy special hosiery for a "bare foot" look.
A dress-up leather is suede.
Most fabrics are dress-up:

peau de soie	
velvet	shantung
faille	satin

THE BASIC WARDROBE

BAGS

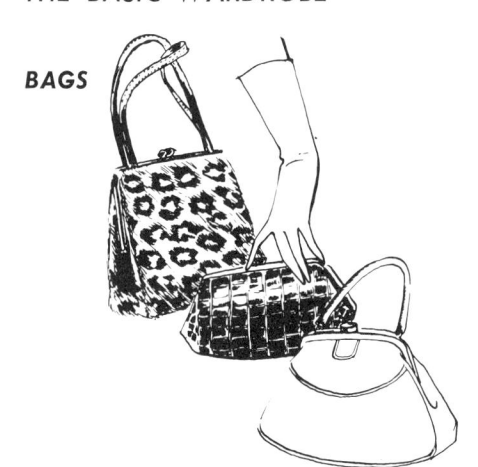

Dress-down

The same as for shoes. However, although the bag and the shoes may match, it is not absolutely necessary that they do so. For instance, a pair of alligator shoes might be worn with a calf bag.

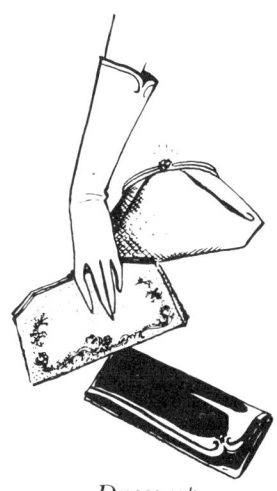

Dress-up

The same as for shoes. However, it is not necessary for the bag and the shoes to be in the same fabric. Other bags for after-five wear would be those made of the following:
- mother of pearl
- sequins
- pearl beads
- metallic leathers or fabrics

GLOVES

The perfect basic glove is the eight button length kid-skin glove with inside stitching. This may be worn either in the daytime or in the evening. It is complementary to almost every type of garment except the most casual.

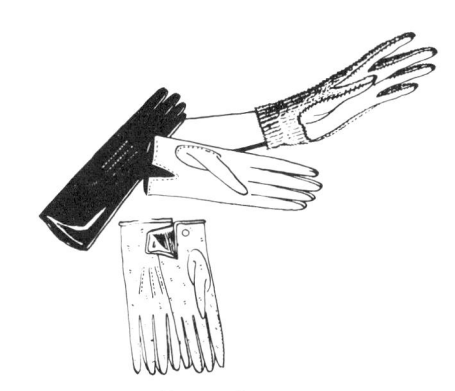

Dress-down

Casual knit gloves with outside stitching. Combinations of fabric and leather such as driving gloves. Beware of gloves that come with fancy stitching in bright colors. They are not basic and have no place in a basic wardrobe.

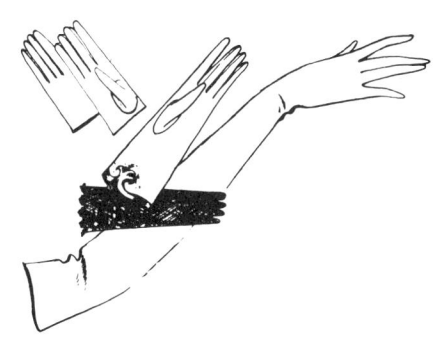

Dress-up

All dress-up gloves have inside stitching. For formal wear they may be either mitt (to the wrist) length or they may be formal (above the elbow) length.

Basic dress-up gloves would **not** have beading or sequins. The most decoration they would have would be small pearl buttons at the wrist.

JEWELRY

The perfect basic jewelry is pearl. It is appropriate with a sweater or with a formal gown. It is always in good taste.

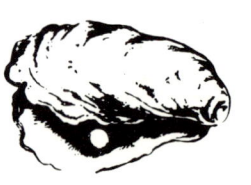

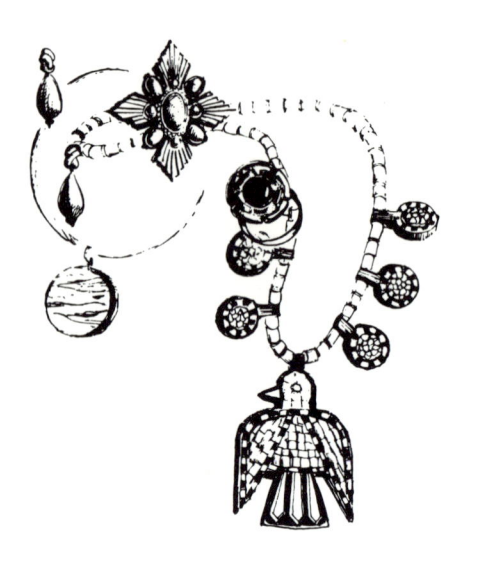

Dress-down

In the dress-down category should be included all jewelry that seems right with sports clothes. This would include:
- semi-precious stones
- gold
- silver
- copper
- Indian jewelry
- turquoise
- wood

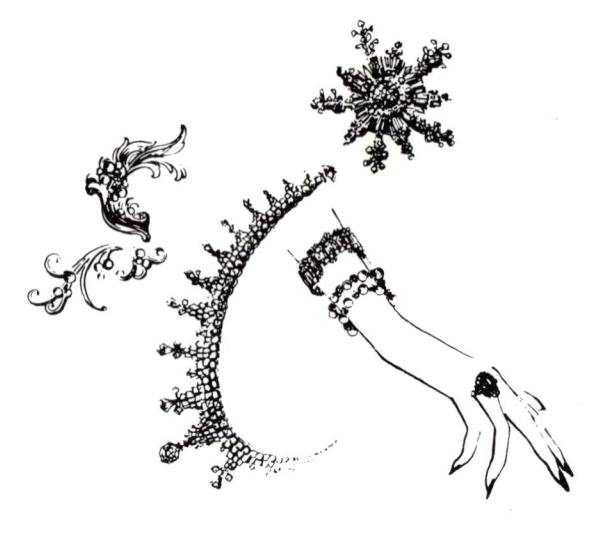

Dress-up

In the dress-up category should go all jewelry that seems precious; such as:
- rhinestones
- crystal
- aurora borealis
- ruby, sapphire, diamond
- emerald
- cut glass that looks like precious gems

THE BASIC WARDROBE

HATS

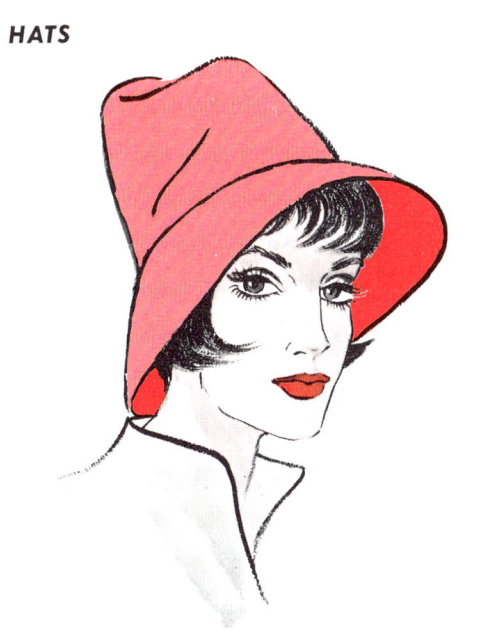

Dress-down

Keep in mind that a hat is appropriate for any daytime occasion and that a woman does not attain a "finished" look until she is wearing a hat.

Basic fabrics include:
  Felt
  Velour
  Velvet
  Feathers

Leather is essentially dress-down to be worn with tailored clothes.

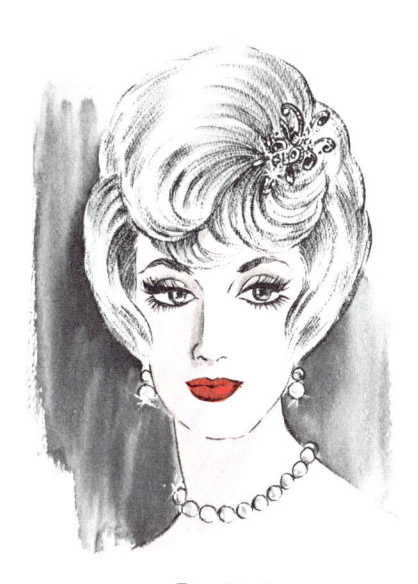

Dress-up

For a stunning appearance after five, a woman should have something in or on her hair. This does not have to be a hat. It may be one of the following:
  Fake or real flowers
  A veil
  A velvet ribbon
  A jewel

Of course this must be chosen to go with the costume with which it is worn but it need not be expensive.

SEASONAL ITEMS

You may be wondering how it is possible to wear some of the basic wardrobe items in the middle of the summer when the weather is so hot it would seem foolish to put on a velvet hat, for instance. The answer to this dilemma is to have a few strictly summer clothes. Just keep in mind that the less money you spend on these, the more you will have to spend on the other three seasons of the year.

Following is a list of seasonal items. Read them through. It may be that the ideas given do not apply in your area but, the advice is offered with a broad intent to make you appropriately dressed almost anywhere in the world.

FABRICS FOR SUMMERTIME ONLY

Linen and *cotton* are considered summertime fabrics. They might be designed to be worn for either daytime or evening in bright, festive, vacation colors. They will look dress-down with basic dress-down or summer dress-down accessories. They will look dress-up with fabric accessories dyed to match. Exception: Some cottons are dyed dark to be worn during the early fall season. Others are so colorful that they may be used to advantage around the Christmas Holiday season to add a gay note.

SUMMERTIME ACCESSORIES

Dress-down

Into this category will fall patent leather shoes and all other patent leather accessories. These are to be worn any time between Easter and Labor Day. This is one leather that cannot be mixed with any other. If one accessory is patent leather all other leather accessories should be patent.

Patent leather is dress-down and because it is shiny, it is to be worn with dull cottons. Straw hats and other straw accessories are to be worn only during the summer months. They are for daytime wear.

Dress-up

In some vacation resort areas it is proper to go without hosiery—a suntan taking their place. Bare foot sandals in metallic leathers are used for evening wear.

Shell or seed jewelry is used for both daytime and evening in colors to match or contrast.

A beautiful chiffon scarf may be all the wrap necessary to cover bare shoulders.

This is the time for bright colors, light-weight flowing fabrics—and romance.

Chiffon hats that are light as a breeze are more dress-up. However, they may be worn in the daytime as well as in the evening for party time occasions.

FABRICS FOR WINTERTIME ONLY

Some fabrics are so *heavy* that they would be worn only during the coldest months. Such a fabric is wool felt. Again, unless you have an unlimited clothing budget, it is wiser to collect clothes that can be worn throughout the various seasons.

Exception: A fine fur stole may be worn all year round. Never in man's history has fashion been sacrificed for comfort. If you want to wear a lovely fur even though the weather is too warm, go ahead.

WINTERTIME ACCESSORIES

Dress-down
Woolly-knit headgear
Woolly mittens
Woolly scarves

Dress-up
Usually those accessories that are dress-up may be worn all year round.

INGENIOUS WAYS TO GET BY

If you are going to get the most out of the following chapters on Wardrobe Planning, you must begin to think of yourself as a rather clever innovator. It has been said that necessity is the mother of invention, and if you are on a limited clothing budget, goodness knows, you have plenty of necessity.

Here are a few suggestions that are real "penny pinchers," but don't look that way.

CHANGES FOR A BASIC DRESS

Fake *fur* belt

Fake *fur* weskit (wear only one at a time)

Fake *fur* collar and cuffs

Net over-skirt. May be in same color as dress. It takes only 1½ yards gathered at the waist, sewn to a piece of velvet ribbon and cut the same length as the dress. Sew irridescent sequins or pearls to the skirt and you have a really "lush" look.

Flowered polished cotton apron worn in the back or on the side.

A scarf tied around the neck with a matching flower to hold it.

A velvet belt with a velvet handbag and suede shoes.

An inexpensive, oblong silk scarf tied ascot fashion with dime store pearls used to trim the edges.

A velveteen or slipper satin stole. 36" material may be sewed double instead of lining.

A cardigan sweater trimmed with grogram ribbon the color of the dress and worn in place of a jacket. The tape is sewed around the collar and down the front.

These are just a few ways to wear a basic dress. Let your imagination run riot as you invent ways to wear flowers, scarves, jewelry, jackets and overskirts.

MORE INGENIOUS INVENTIONS

EVENING BAG So you can't afford an evening bag. Get a dime store cosmetic bag and cover it with sequins or that broken strand of pearls or inexpensive scatter pins. Or, buy a quarter yard of satin in a tone to go with your dress, buy a zipper and some buckram and make your evening bag.

A PARTY DRESS FOR CHRISTMAS What are you going to wear to the Christmas party? How about a basic black dress with perky red and green bows tied all over the skirt? If you already have the dress, the investment will be about thirty cents and a little time. Or, take a print summer cotton and doll it up with colored sequins to match the flowers. These can be sewed as outlines on the flowers in no time.

FOR SPORTS Going boating, bowling, sport car riding or just for a walk through the park? Buy several pieces of striped fabric and make your own colorful headbands to hold your hair in place.

FOR EVENING WEAR A drapery fabric skirt in combination with a velveteen scoop-necked blouse makes a wonderful "evening" combination.

Drapery balls of fringe make an interesting addition to any scooped neckline.

FABRIC COMBINATIONS

Some of our most famous designers have come into the limelight by their unusual use of fabric combinations. Denims now have diamonds. Sweaters now have beads. Let your wildest idea have a try. All of them won't be good, but some of them might set a new trend. Whatever the results, your fashion will be more fun when you add some touch that is uniquely your own.

USING THE QUICK-CHANGE Sometimes changing the buttons will do the trick, or cutting off buttons that are superfluous. Removing an inexpensive piece of costume jewelry and replacing it with something of your own may take a dress right out of the bargain class.

A hat can be made to complement more ensembles if the trim is easily changed.

A limp hat veil can be made like new again by pressing it lightly with a hot iron between two pieces of wax paper.

An inexpensive basic hat can be made to look like much more money by trimming it with a lovely artificial flower or a fine feather or a beautiful chiffon scarf.

BEAUTY BY ACCENT

You have undoubtedly heard that Parisian women are famous for their beauty. What is this beauty? It is beauty achieved by "accent." They study their best features and accent them with carefully selected "pieces" of fashion. You can do the same.

For beautiful hands, a ring.

For creamy skin, a strand of creamy pearls.

For bright eyes, earrings in a matching color.

For slender legs, a pleated skirt.

For a tiny waistline, a contrasting cummerbund.

For a beautiful back, low decolletage.

Don't read another line until you have started a list of things you can do to be better dressed on less money. Individualized beauty accent is your goal.

CHAPTER 15

LINES FOR FIGURE FLATTERY

Introduction

The most fundamental factor in correct dress, is line. When lines get together, they cause optical illusions and it will be the purpose of this lesson to instruct you in the ways and means of using lines to create an illusion of symmetry. Applied to your clothing, this means the lines forming the silhouette must be nicely proportioned and that any other lines, a pocket or yoke, must not detract from it.

From time to time, the ideas surrounding the perfect feminine figure change so that today's ideal is tomorrow's ugly duckling. On the whole this is good, for it satisfies our natural desire for variety. It fires our imagination and gives us the chance to turn over a new leaf. But whatever the ideal of the day, it behooves us to adapt the current lines of fashion to our silhouette so that they compliment our figure type.

Not so long ago, shoulders began to melt away. Concurrently Dior attempted to melt the bustline away, unsuccessfully, we are happy to report. Skirts have ascended and descended, and time after time, our concept of the figure beautiful does a right about face. This is fine, but some of us must stick to certain line combinations no matter what fashion dictates. Not that you can't have your fashion and your figure too. You can when you capitalize upon "line" and use it as a tool in your own behalf—to emphasize your good features and minimize your poor ones.

OPTICAL ILLUSIONS IN DRESS

Optical illusions happen when the lines of your clothes mingle with those of your figure. It is reassuring to know that certain lines can be depended upon to perform specific functions. Vertical lines give the appearance of height or length; horizontal lines add width and make you look shorter. Used in any one part, they add bulk. Curved lines add roundness or fullness. Repeat a line and you multiply its prominence.

ILLUSIONS CAUSED BY LINES

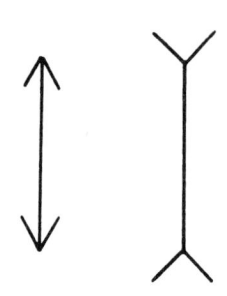

The right line looks longer than the left, in truth, they are the same length without the prongs.

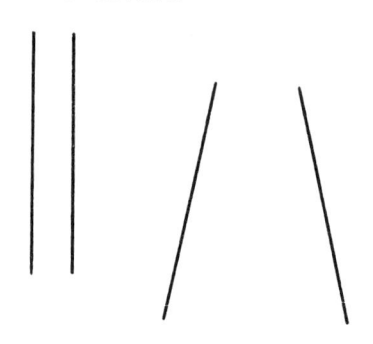

Parallel lines appear to be longer than two lines of the same length that angle toward one another.

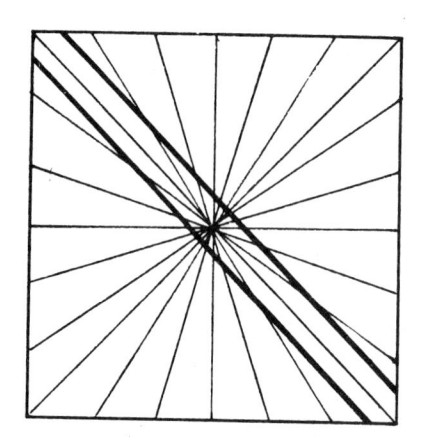

The two darker lines are straight.

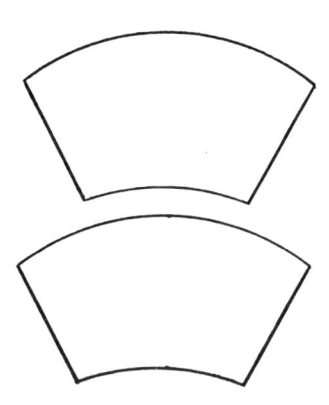

Both are the same size, although the lower one looks largest.

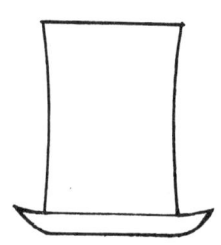

The top hat seems to be much taller than its brim is wide, but this is not so, its height is the same as the width of the brim.

LINES FOR FIGURE FLATTERY

SELECT FLATTERING SILHOUETTE LINES

Learning what lines will do is like learning the A B C's of dress. It is the beginning of learning to create a lovely background for yourself with the clothes you wear.

If you are overweight or have a figure imperfection, don't wait until you've remedied the defect; start wearing becoming clothes and improve your figure now, the line way.

Select the most flattering silhouettes for your figure from the eight basic silhouette lines.

EIGHT BASIC SILHOUETTE LINES

1. Plain Silhouette — Accents outline

2. Vertical Line — Adds height

3. Horizontal Line — Adds width

4. Diagonal Line — Adds interest

5. Asymmetrical Line — Disguises figure faults

6. Multi-stripe — Adds height and width; therefore, bulk to the figure.

7. Princess Line

It does a number of things.
1. It nips in the waistline.
2. It expands the hip and bustline.
3. It adds height.

For the young under-developed, teenage figure.

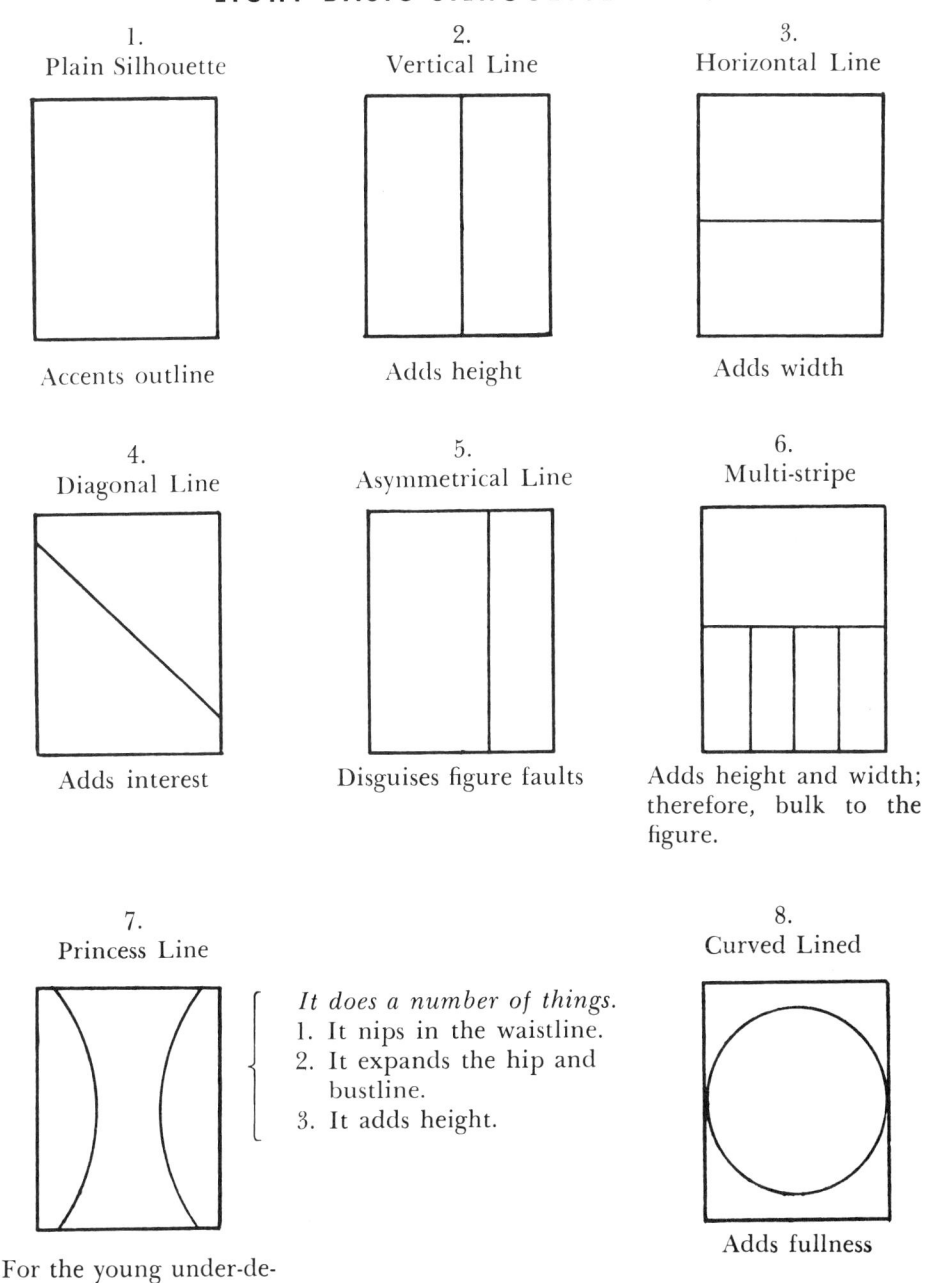

8. Curved Lined — Adds fullness

LINES FOR FIGURE FLATTERY

WHAT'S YOUR LINE?

The following is a list of do's and don'ts for the four major figure variations. They infer that you may be above average in height or shorter than average, or too thin or too stout; hence can benefit by some clothing camouflage.

TALL

WEAR *Horizontal lines*—wide belts, yolk lines, circular trimming, peplums.

Hip length or three-quarter jackets.

Contrasting colors.

Large accessories—heavy jewelry and large handbags.

Soft, rounded shoulders.

Dolman sleeves of three-quarter length.

Heavy, bulky fabrics; large prints.

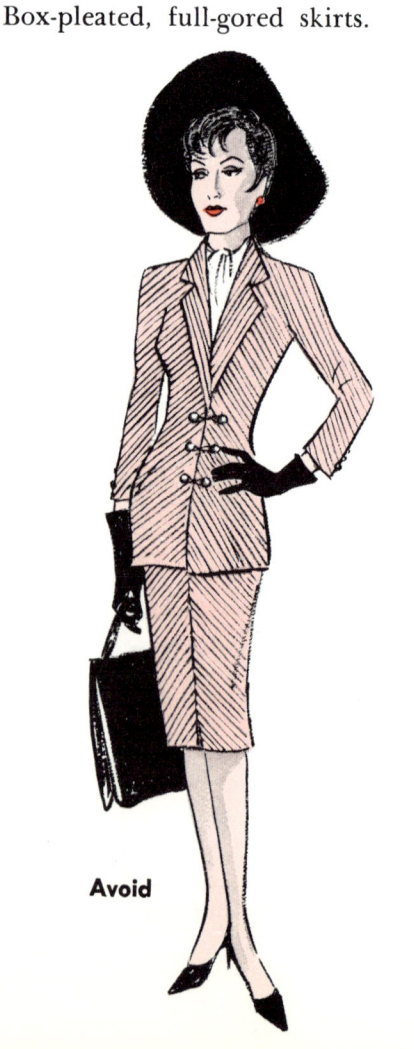

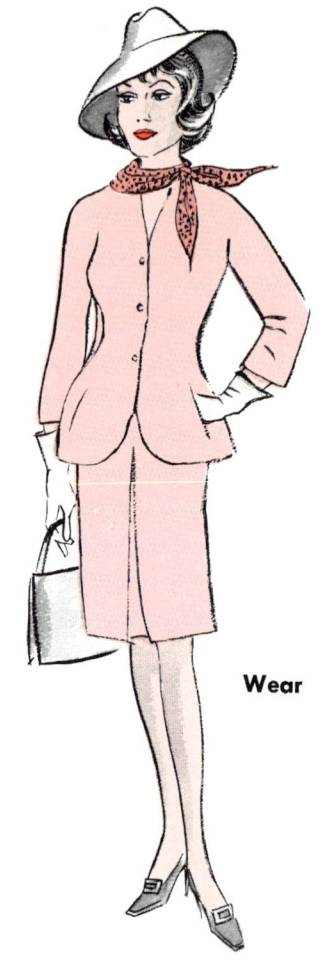

Box-pleated, full-gored skirts.

Wear

AVOID *Pencil lines,* narrow belts vertically placed tucks or buttons.

Medium-length jackets.

Angular trimming, continuous pleats.

High, pointed crowns on hats.

Small jewelry and accessories.

Exaggerated shoulders.

Tightly fitted full-length sleeves.

Flimsy fabrics, such as organdy small patterns.

Tight, tubular skirts.

Avoid

LINES FOR FIGURE FLATTERY

SHORT

WEAR *Vertical lines*—princess style or with trimming from neck to hem.

Bolero jackets, short jackets.

Easy fitted sleeves, full-length or short.

Delicate trimming.

Small accessories—small brimmed hats, small pocketbooks, lightweight costume jewelry.

Soft, lightweight fabrics. Small collars.

Self-belts or no belt.

Medium-full skirts.

Slightly longer hemline.

Simplicity in detail.

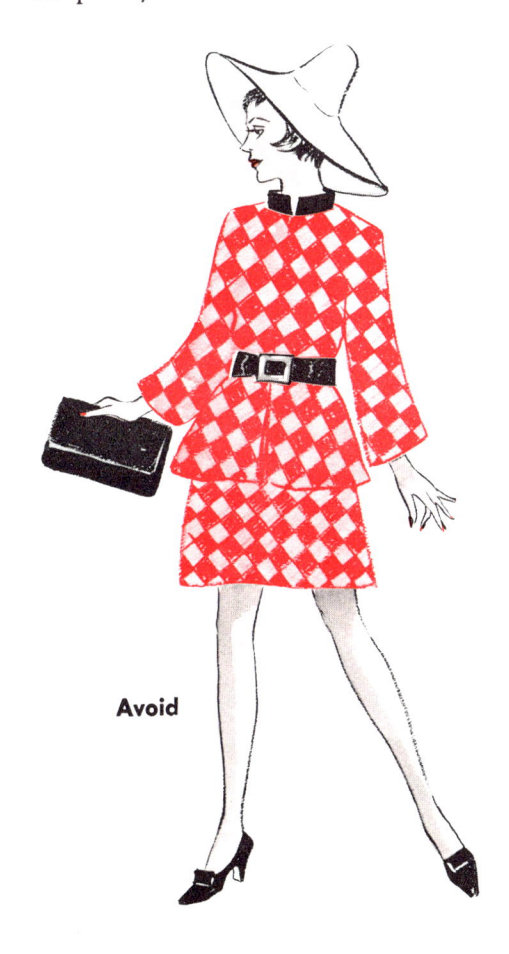

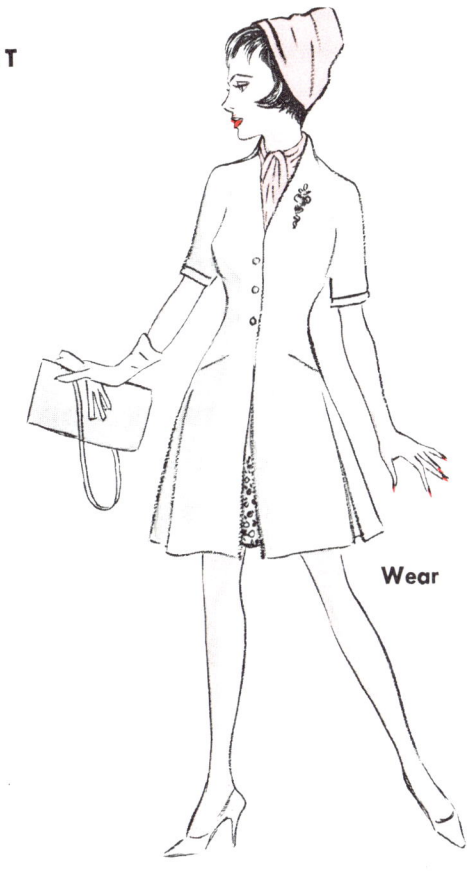

AVOID *Horizontal lines.* All exaggerated lines.

Overlong jackets.

Sleeves chopped at the elbow.

Massive trimming such as large belt buckles.

Large muffs, picture hats, bulky furs.

Large plaids and prints.

Bulky fabrics.

Wide cuffs.

Wide or contrasting belts.

Box pleats.

Conspicuous hems—contrasting borders and embroidery.

Lines that break the figure into definite parts.

LINES FOR FIGURE FLATTERY

STOUT

WEAR *Vertical lines*—center panel and buttons down the front.

Simple dresses with half-belts.

Dull finished, straight hanging fabrics of medium weight.

Diagonal trimming, such as pockets.

Medium-gored skirts with center stitching or pleat.

Set-in sleeves.

V necklines and pointed collars.

Jackets not longer than two inches below the hipbone.

Narrow, self-belts.

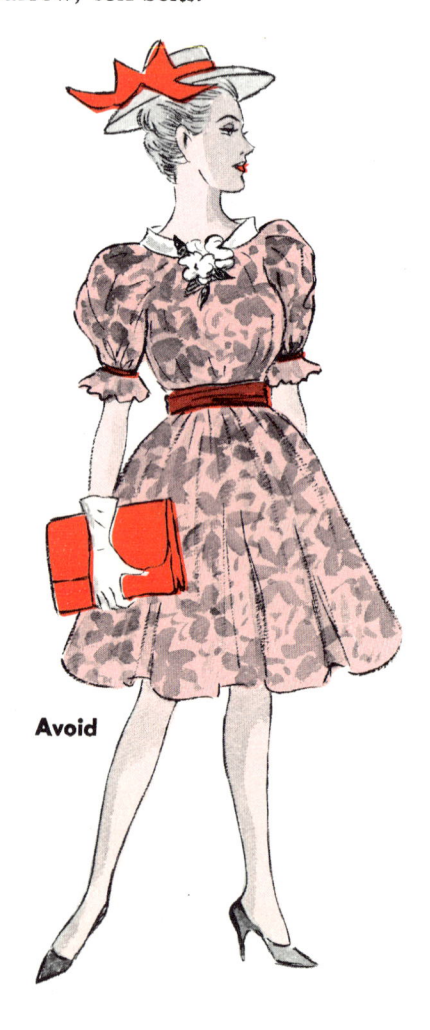

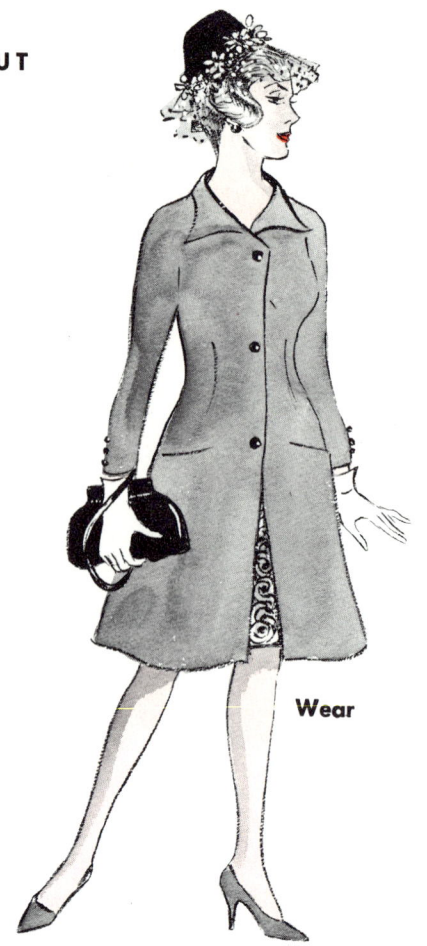

AVOID *Horizontal lines,* round necks and collars.

Two-piece dresses.

Clinging fabrics or heavy fabrics.

Round trimming or curved lines.

Skirts with all-around pleats, wide gores or peplums.

Puff sleeves, droopy sleeves, tightly-fitted sleeves. All round necklines.

Very long or short jackets.

Set-in belts, wide or contrasting belts.

LINES FOR FIGURE FLATTERY

THIN

WEAR *Horizontal and curved lines.* Modified vertical lines.

Two-piece dresses, suits with peplums.

Bright but subtle colors.

Full-bodies, crisp fabrics.

Large pockets, modified according to height.

Full skirts, yoked or circular.

Size of accessories should be in relation to height: Short and thin—small accessories; tall and thin—large ones.

Cummerbunds of contrasting color.

Soft, rounded shoulders with puffed sleeves or kimono.

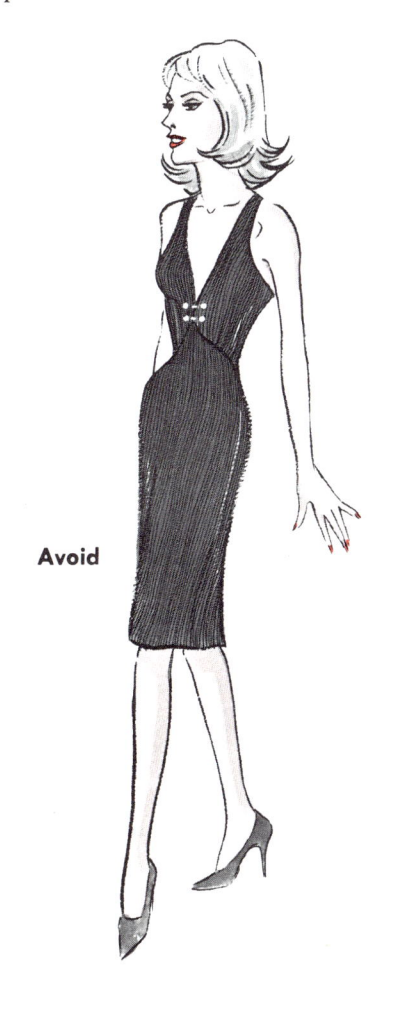

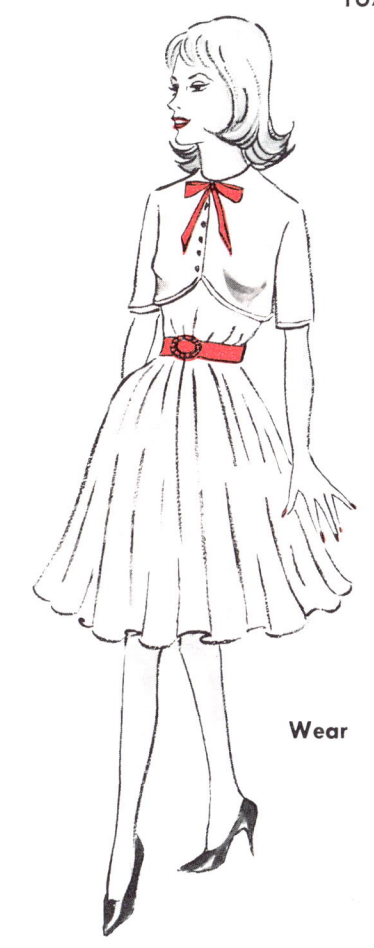

Wear

Avoid

AVOID *Vertical lines.* Exaggerated lines.

Deep V necklines.

Tight-fitting clothes.

Low-keyed colors.

Clinging fabrics. Flimsy fabrics.

Tight, tubular skirts.

Pencil-slim skirts.

Those accessories not in proportion to your height.

No belt unless you are very short.

Exaggerated shoulders.

Tight-fitting sleeves.

HOW DOES YOUR FIGURE LOOK?

The full length mirror once again becomes your best ally. Disrobe and stand at least ten feet away and really look at your figure. Forget about measurements and judge it according to the way it looks. With the help of a hand mirror, examine your figure from the back and sides as well as the front. If you wear a corset or girdle, wear it for studying your proportions; it will affect the lines of your figure to some extent.

Nature, in her enthusiasm for variety, has given women an endless combination of shoulders and waists and hips. But as different as they are, figures can be classified when considered from the standpoint of comparative proportions.

SHOULDERS

All shoulders are either medium, wide or narrow in comparison with the hips that go with them. Waistlines, too, will appear to be medium, wide or narrow in comparison to shoulders and hips.

HIPS

Hips have to be medium, wide or narrow compared to the shoulders. In addition to this, for the purpose of deciding how your figure looks, your waistline will be placed medium, high or low in comparison with the rest of the body. Your legs too will appear to be medium, short or long.

WAISTLINE

A waistline that would seem tiny, to believe the tape measure, can look wide in comparison to the rest of the body, while a waist that measures a generous number of inches can look narrow if one's hips and shoulders are definitely wider. Hips can look wide if they are combined with narrow shoulders.

THE BASIC FIGURE

The basic figure then, we will say, has medium proportions.

1. *The shoulders* are neither too wide nor too narrow when compared with the *hips*.

2. *The waist* is neither too high nor too low, nor unusually wide, compared with the rest of the figure.

3. *The legs* are neither decidedly short nor long.

4. *The basic figure* is slender or medium of weight and medium in height.

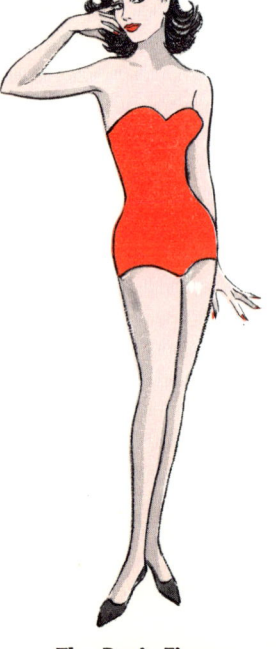

The Basic Figure

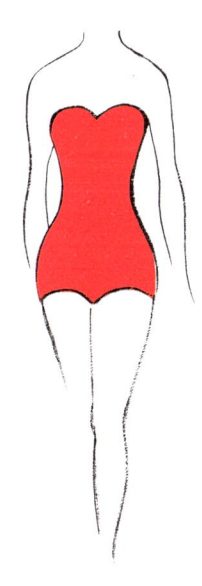

LINES FOR FIGURE FLATTERY

THE THREE HIPLINES

ROUND HIPS The medium proportions of this type gives a verdict of "not guilty," it sets you free to wear a larger variety of clothes than any other figure type. While your hips are not wide compared with the rest of your figure, neither are they narrow. Lines that accent the width of your hips combined with lines that make your shoulders look narrower make your hips too prominent. Lines that widen the hips should be balanced by those that widen the shoulder.

Round or Medium

SQUARE HIPS This type of hipline looks better in pegged skirts than either of the other types. If there is fullness in the skirt it is better to have the flare come below the upper hip (no gathers at the waistline). Crisp shoulder lines are best combined with sleeves that are loose enough at the underarms to allow the silhouette to widen out gradually from waist to shoulders. Waist-slimming lines are generally flattering to your figure and you can wear wide belts successfully if you are slender and if your waist is not too high. Waist-slimming lines, beltless effects and long torso lines are excellent.

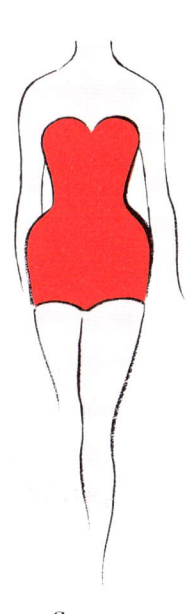

Square

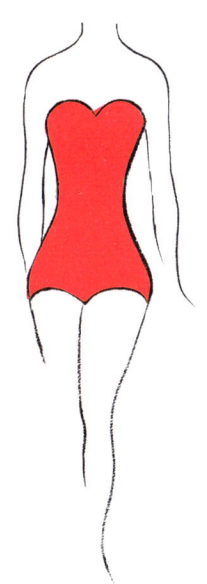

TRIANGULAR HIPS Flared skirts that widen gradually from waist to the hemline are far more graceful on a triangular hipline figure than any other kind. Avoid accenting your lower hipline with jackets, short coats or horizontal detailing. Your figure will look best in suit coats and jackets that come just below or just above the waistline. Clothes with lines that accent the width of the shoulders are flattering to triangular hips because they balance low hip width. If your hipline is unusually long, as is often the case, wear raised waistlines or lowered waistlines, wide belts, horizontal lines across the upper hip. Fullness above or below your waist, if you are slender, is flattering.

Triangular

On with the Beauty Brigade!

CHART YOUR FIGURE FOIBLES

Using the basic figure as your yardstick, chart your proportions as you stand in front of the mirror. You will want to put in whether your neck is long or short, slender or wide because, combined with the shape of your face, it will determine the necklines you should wear for the greatest flattery.

There are other figure foibles to consider, such as bustline, abdomen, back, arms and the slope of your shoulders. These individual features sometimes distort the beauty of an otherwise attractive figure.

CHECK ONE:

Shape of face	Round	___	Square	___	Long	___	Oval ___ Other___
Width of neck	Medium	___	Wide	___	Narrow	___	
Length of neck	Medium	___	Long	___	Short	___	
Slope of shoulder	Medium	___	Square	___	Very sloping	___	
Width of shoulder	Medium	___	Wide	___	Narrow	___	
Bustline	Medium	___	Large	___	Low	___	Flat ___
Length of arms	Medium	___	Long	___	Short	___	
Width of arms	Medium	___	Heavy	___	Thin	___	
Width of waist	Medium	___	Wide	___	Narrow	___	
Length of waist	Medium	___	High	___	Low	___	
Width of hips	Medium	___	Wide	___	Narrow	___	
Shape of hips	Round	___	Square	___	Triangular	___	(See Three Hiplines)
Abdomen	Flat	___	Round	___	Protruding	___	
Back	Flat	___	Curved	___			
Length of legs	Medium	___	Long	___	Short	___	
Height	Medium	___	Tall	___	Short	___	
Frame	Medium	___	Slender	___	Heavy	___	
Weight	Normal	___	Light	___	Heavy	___	

FLATTER YOUR FIGURE

You will want to accent the good features of your figure and camouflage those you wish to remain unseen. No matter what your figure foibles, there is no cause for despair. Once more fashion and fabric hie to the rescue. By wearing the lines recommended for each problem, there is no doubt you will derive greater satisfaction from your clothes and the way you look in them.

THE EFFECTS OF COLOR AND PATTERN

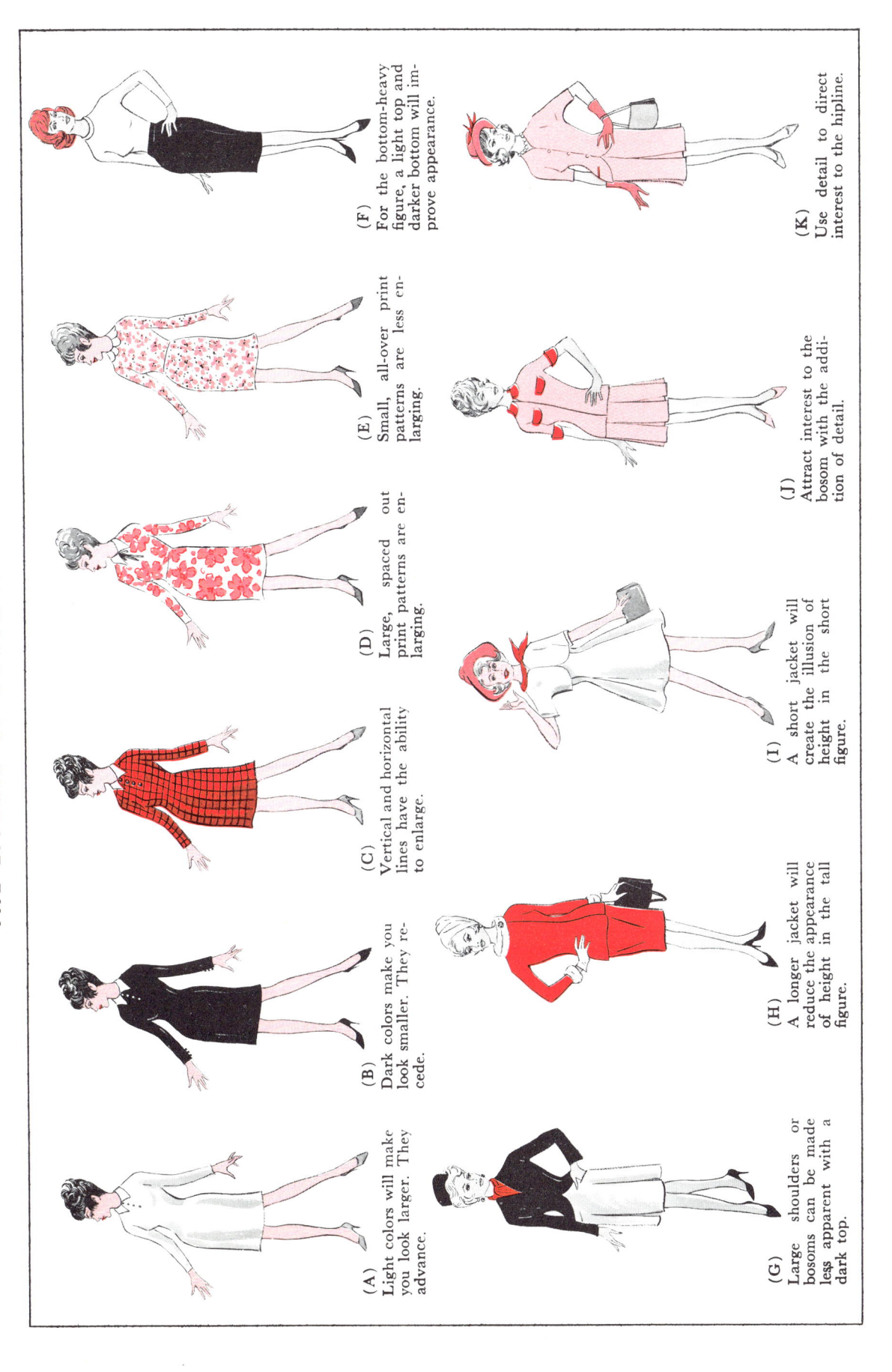

LINES FOR FIGURE FLATTERY

(A) Light colors will make you look larger. They advance.

(B) Dark colors make you look smaller. They recede.

(C) Vertical and horizontal lines have the ability to enlarge.

(D) Large, spaced out print patterns are enlarging.

(E) Small, all-over print patterns are less enlarging.

(F) For the bottom-heavy figure, a light top and darker bottom will improve appearance.

(G) Large shoulders or bosoms can be made less apparent with a dark top.

(H) A longer jacket will reduce the appearance of height in the tall figure.

(I) A short jacket will create the illusion of height in the short figure.

(J) Attract interest to the bosom with the addition of detail.

(K) Use detail to direct interest to the hipline.

STYLE SELECTOR FOR FIGURE TYPES

IF YOU HAVE	WEAR	AVOID
A round face	V necklines	Turtle necks
A square face	Round or V necklines	Square
A long face	Turtle necks, chokers, ascot ties, scarves	V neckline
Oval face	Anything, you have no neckline problem	
A narrow neck	Ascot ties, scarves, chokers, turtle necklines, stand-up collars that are high, frou-frou ruffs, softly draped necklines	Thin, clinging fabrics Skimpy bodices Bony exposure
A broad neck	Man-tailored V necklines, bateau collars, wide square necklines, rounding neckline with no collar	Turtle necklines Ruffles Dainty fabrics Chokers
A long neck	Square necklines, hats and hair fairly low in back. Ascot ties, scarves, high stand-up collars	Long dangling necklace, V-shaped necklines, Low necklines without a horizontal line around the neck (choker, scarf)
A short neck	Low V neckline, roll-back collars, picture necklines. High necklines that are dropped a little in center front. Hair off neck, short. Brimless hats	Bulky jewelry, chokers, wide shouldered clothes and built-up shoulder lines. High round necklines. Hair that comes to the shoulders. Turned down brims on hats
Square shoulder	Dolman sleeves, cap sleeves, sleeves that fit loosely at the armhole, saddle shoulders	Shoulder pads Halter necklines Large collars Set-in sleeves
Very sloping shoulders	Wide V necklines Square necklines Small shoulder pads	Strapless gowns, spaghetti string shoulder straps Sleeveless dresses
Wide shoulders	Usually no problem	

LINES FOR FIGURE FLATTERY

IF YOU HAVE	WEAR	AVOID
Narrow shoulders	Wide lapels, stiff shoulder lines, leg-of-mutton sleeves, yokes across chest, built-up shoulder lines	Small collars, droopy shoulders, tightly-fitted sleeves, vertical lines
A large bosom	Fullness across the bustline is best, wide armholes and sleeves, loosely-fitted bodices, long swagger coats	Fussy details, bows, pockets, tight sleeves, tight armholes, fitted coats
A flat bust	Padded bras, ample fullness above and below, amusing bodices, details—pockets, ruffles, lace	Tight bodice, heavy accessories, bodices without detail
A low bust	Wear good uplift, brassieres correctly fitted	
Long arms	Full, loose fitting bracelet-length sleeves, large cuffs, gauntlet gloves, sleeves that end just below the elbow	Long, tight sleeves, sleeveless clothes, extremely short or full-length sleeve
Short arms	Full-length sleeves, loosely fitted	Color accents, such as contrasting cuffs
Plump arms	Slack-fitting sleeves, clothes with full armholes, full-length sleeves, sleeves that end just above the elbow	Short puffs, skin-tight sleeves, soft shoulder lines
Thin arms	Draped, full sleeves, long balloon sleeves, puffs, raglan sleeves	Sleeveless dresses Tight sleeves Sheer fabrics
A wide waist	Partial belts, lines that direct the eye downward and inward below the shoulder, fullness above the waistline, narrow self belts, princess lines that break the figure into 3 parts	Contrasting colors at waistline, wide belts, narrow skirts, especially bias
A narrow waist	This seldom poses a problem	

IF YOU HAVE	WEAR	AVOID
A high waist	Vertical lines, unbroken by yokes, beltless clothes, dropped waistlines, lines that break the middle hip area	Yokes, unless high on the shoulder, raised waistlines, contrasting belts
A low waist	Raised waistlines, bolero jackets, horizontal lines above the waistline, wide belts if you are slender, three-quarter length sleeves, contrasting collars	Lowered waistline, long suit coats, vertical torso lines, large oversized pockets on skirts, sleeves with contrasting cuffs at wrist, detailing on bodice that ends below waist
Wide hips	Accented shoulders, bloused effects above the waist, gathers at waistline, diagonal pockets, contrasting colors above the waistline, peplums and tunics that come below the widest part	Lines that narrow the shoulders, tightly-fitted skirts, horizontal pockets, horizontal lines across hips, change of color at hipline.
Narrow hips	This is a problem?	
A rumble seat	A little fullness below waist at center back, garments loosely fitted at the small of the back, full skirts, shirtmaker lines, over-blouses	Tight skirts, tight belts, too short bolero jackets, plaid skirts, cut-away jackets
The diaphragm problem	A little extra width in skirt below the waist, partly belted effects, closely fitted gathers over diaphragm, draped effects over diaphragm	Bunchy bows at waistline, thick gathers either above or below waistline, tight belts
An abdomen problem	Skirts with front fullness just below the waist, gathers to either side of center, suit jackets that end below widest part, partial belts	Form-fitting garments, bias skirts, too plain front, short jackets, built-in belts

LINES FOR FIGURE FLATTERY

IF YOU HAVE	WEAR	AVOID
Long legs	Tiered skirts, slightly shorter hemline, conspicuous hems, tunic jackets	Vertical lines, long hemline, color sameness, short jackets
Short legs	Vertical lines, Princess styles, slightly longer hemline	Horizontal details below hips, short hemline, hemline borders
Fat legs	Seam hosiery, neutral-dark colors, slightly flaired skirts	Seamless hosiery, pencil-slim skirts, too short skirts
Thin legs	Seamless hosiery, skirts that are narrow to medium in width, light-colored hose	Dark seamed hose, extremely full skirts, dark-colored hosiery

CHAPTER 16

THE PSYCHOLOGY OF COLOR AND COLOR MAGIC

Introduction

Consciously or unconsciously you are aware of color. It is so closely keyed to your daily living that you often refer to your moods in color terms. You are so angry you "see red" when things irritate you, you "feel blue" when you are lonely, you turn "green with envy" when the neighbors drive by in their Cadillac; your outlook is "black" because trouble is brewing, you feel "in the pink" today, the sun is shining.

Have you ever stopped to consider how much your moods are in tune with the weather and the changing seasons? In the spring when nature bursts forth in riotous color your interests are accelerated and you, as well as the budding trees, are given a new lease on life. As summer approaches there is an atmosphere of peace and joy, warmth and plenty, it is difficult to work or concentrate and summertime becomes "siesta" time. Autumn is heralded by such vivid colors that, if the season were longer, we would tire of them. It is as though Nature wishes to remind us that though winter is coming, lovely spring is not far behind. Winter too holds her own unique color palette with which to clothe the landscape and enchant the soul.

It is difficult to name a color that you do not associate with something else, hence we have colors named for metals such as copper, silver, gold, and aluminum; for precious stones such as amber, ruby, emerald, pearl and sapphire; for fruits and vegetables such as maize, lime, lemon, plum, orange, apricot, wheat, avocado, cherry, and eggplant; for flowers such as orchid, rose, violet, and larkspur; for other various things we find in our surroundings such as sky blue, coral pink, charcoal gray, winter white, oyster white, robin's egg blue, forest green, mustard yellow, and moss green.

SIGNIFICANCE OF COLOR

All of these expressions have arisen from significant experiences that have been associated with color. You will be able to gear your colors to you and to the occasion like a master craftsman when you are guided by the traditional associations that every color has.

1. **RED** the color of blood and fire is exciting to the mind and the appetite. It has meant gaiety, vigor, bravery, sensationalism and danger.

2. **YELLOW** signifies gaiety and is associated with sunlight—the source of wisdom. This color is more often associated with mental activity than with cowardice.

3. **GREEN** is the color of growing things and signifies the peace of all outdoors. It is a youthful color representing life, hope and faith.

4. **BLUE** the color of the sky, is a conservative color and stands for love, honor, dignity, fidelity and truth.

5. **ORANGE** is the color of plenty and is associated with abundance (maybe that's why we should wear it so sparingly).

6. **PURPLE** is the regal color, note "Royal" purple, and stands for wisdom and silence.

7. **WHITE** is the symbol of virtue. It is no accident that the bride traditionally wears white to her wedding. The white dove is the dove of peace and the white flag indicates humility.

8. **BLACK** indicates sophistication and mystery. It is the color of the night—aloof, wise and silent.

9. **GRAY** the somber color, is indicative of old age, decay, retirement and indifference.

10. **BROWN** the color of earth, is a conservative color that symbolizes autumn and atonement.

Color is the dimension that will work miracles. It can paint radiance on your face and enliven or subdue your temperament and tempo. It is the flowering of your personality in fabric. If you have not dabbled with a paintbox since you were in grade school, a refresher course in color harmonies will be helpful, for a sure eye is invaluable when combining colors in an ensemble and coordinating them in a wardrobe.

THE PSYCHOLOGY OF COLOR AND COLOR MAGIC

THE COLOR WHEEL

We must be aware of the twelve bright colors of the color wheel, but they must not blind us to the endless variations of color tones and their use, along with white and black, in our wardrobe.

There is nothing supernatural about the way color works its magic, for you can apply rules in color as you can in mathematics. There is a reason for every trick that color plays, its powers can be captured, harnessed, and employed to produce a gleam of admiration in the eyes of your personal audience.

THE COLOR WHEEL

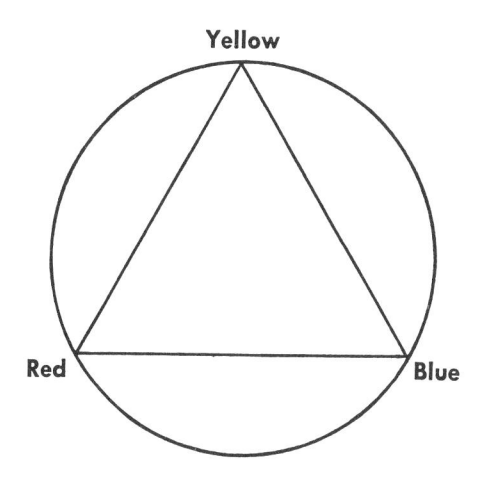

PRIMARY COLORS

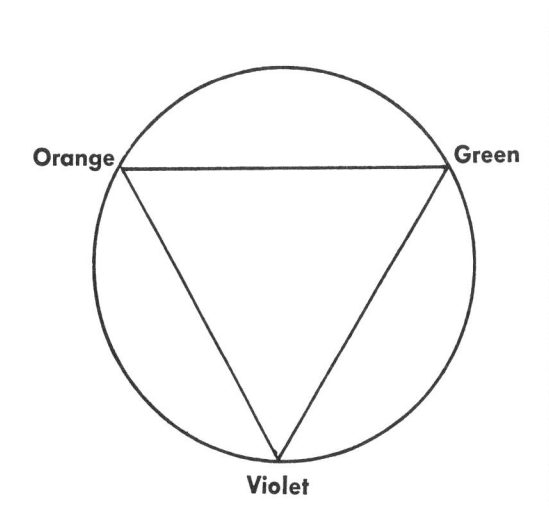

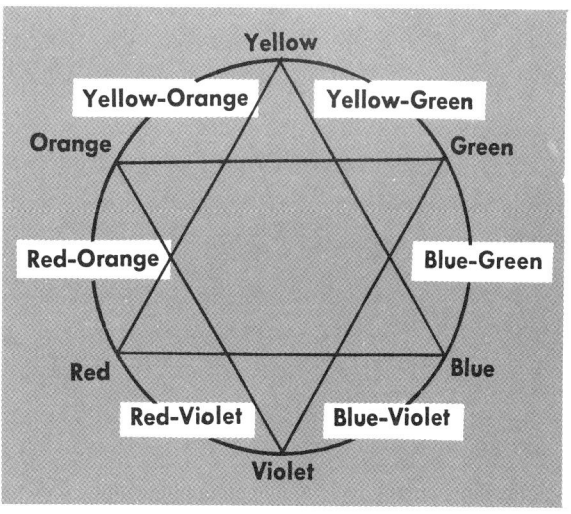

SECONDARY COLORS

TERTIARY COLORS

COLOR HARMONIES

RELATED COLOR HARMONIES are those produced from colors that lie near to each other on the color wheel. You will present a lovely picture if you combine only those shades that bear the same undertones such as yellow-green and yellow-coral. This is *analogous color harmony,* a combination of neighboring colors with one color in common.

Another handsome costume can be created of various shades in the same color. Light, medium and dark blue illustrate this type of color harmony. It is *monochromatic color harmony* . . . "mono" meaning one and "chroma" meaning color.

CONTRASTING COLOR HARMONIES are produced by combining colors that are far apart on the color wheel. You will have the most success with these when you obtain the maximum contrast in the intensity of the colors used. For example, a dress of bright yellow adorned with a cluster of violets might have a harsh effect. However, if the yellow were dulled, to say, a yellow beige, the effect would be quite pleasing.

NEUTRALS are colors of very low or grayed intensity. These are colors that receive a shot in the arm when combined with bright, intense colors. A harmony of this kind is an "accented" neutral and the Law of Areas suggests that you wear the dullest colors in the largest areas, the medium colors in the medium areas and the intense or bright colors in the smallest areas.

This rule will solve your figure problems inasmuch as you will be able to wear any color that is flattering to your skin and hair simply by toning it down, and not have to worry about what it is doing to your hips. A dark and dull color decreases size, makes one appear smaller. On the other hand, bright, light colors increase size and reveal contours. Both of these facts can be applied when and where needed—to your advantage.

You are probably beginning to wonder how you are going to work this magic with color that we promised you so that you compliment your personality, figure, eyes, hair and skin simultaneously. Don't give up the ship, we have set sail for "Beauty Yours for Sure," let's not stop until we get there.

It may clarify matters considerably if we take up each one of these factors separately.

COLOR AND PERSONALITY

You have already learned that colors have clearly defined significances, that these associations can be used to dramatize the mood of any event. Your sensitivity to the atmosphere you create with colors can make a highly effective Lorelei of you, your appearance and personality.

Psychologists say that your color like and dislikes reveal a great deal about your personality. The dominant person likes to wear bright intense shades with definite color contrasts. She is the gregarious, impulsive, stimulating person who is often sought to lead others. Those who prefer pastels, tints, and soft colors are retiring by nature, letting the world go by. They are the soothing type who is demure and just plain sweet. Which type are you?

Do you think your color preferences in any way overshadow your personality? You cannot afford to divorce your appearance from your personality, both will suffer. If you decide that you are not willing to give up a pet color, no matter how unflattering, you can satisfy your color hunger by using it in small touches in jewelry, buttons, gloves, handkerchiefs, flowers.

By the way, your wardrobe will be more versatile when its colors are occasion-keyed.

FIGURE YOUR COLORS

It is quite easy to remember that light and bright colors are advancing and make one appear large, and that dark and dull colors are receding and make one appear smaller.

If your figure requires subdued, slenderizing colors and you need a vivid touch for your face, wear a dark dress and have the bright color close to your face in a small area. The addition of a scarf, flower, collar or costume jewelry will turn the tide—and the eye.

Whenever there is a face and figure color conflict, you should not forsake one in favor of the other. Not for all the rice in China! Flatter your figure with the face-flattering shades in lower intensities.

COLORS FOR YOUR EYES

Hazel eyes are Chameleons that reflect any color you might wear, but other eyes are emphasized when you wear a color that matches them or is slightly darker. Brown eyes are emphasized by brown, blue eyes by blue. When wearing contrasting colors, be careful they do not rob your iris of its color.

All this brings us to color "thieves" and how they rob one another. Let's investigate some of the things that colors do to one another, so that we will be prepared to use this pilfering for our own advantage.

The tricks of color are the result of various effects that colors have on one another; and inasmuch as your skin and hair have color, they are not exempt from these pranks.

THE FOUR RULES OF COLOR MAGIC

Get on your thinking cap, your magic carpet too, if you have one, and we'll be off to the Land of No—it isn't what you think it is. Take red, for instance, if it's placed next to orange, it will seem to be redder. Just as your face gets redder when you try to figure out why. But then we aren't interested in whys, we're just interested in wherefores. Therefore,

1. **STRAIGHT COLORS** Any straight color (red, yellow, blue) will drain self-color from another that consists of itself and something else.

    Red drains red from orange making it appear more yellow. Blue drains blue from green making it appear more yellow. Yellow drains yellow from yellow-green making it appear more green.

This rule is important inasmuch as your skin has a mixture of red, yellow, and brown pigment. You can get rid of the yellow "jaundiced" look by wearing colors that "pull" out the yellow such as green, orange-red and turquoise. All these colors have a touch of yellow as the "stealing" agent.

Do you get it? Then we can go on.

2. **REFLECTING COLORS** Some colors will reflect back more color than they take away.

    Ruddy complexions are made redder by bright red clothes.

    Blue eyes are enhanced by blue.

    Bright yellow makes an ochre-toned skin more yellow.

You have only to think of the times as a child that you held a buttercup under your chin to see whether or not you liked butter. You did if your chin went yellow, which it invariably did. This was reflected color.

Whether it's good or bad to accentuate the yellow or red pigment in your skin depends upon its own color balance and this balance in relationship to the color of your hair.

3. **INTENSITY OF COLORS** Colors intensify their compliments.

    Red—green
    Red violet—yellow green
    Red orange—blue green
    Orange—blue
    Yellow orange—blue violet
    Yellow—violet

If you refer to the "Color Wheel" you will be reminded that the complementary colors are those across from each other. This rule means that violet will emphasize, unflatteringly, the yellow-toned skin. It also explains why blue is almost universally popular, it emphasizes light flesh tones. And how it flatters blonds! Have you ever noticed that red heads love to wear green?

THE PSYCHOLOGY OF COLOR AND COLOR MAGIC

4. COLOR TONES When a light tone is placed next to a medium tone, it makes the light tone seem lighter. Ash blond hair will turn "dish water" next to a beige, but will turn golden next to cinnamon.

The same medium tone will seem lighter when placed next to a dark tone.

Red hair is enhanced by rust.

If you place a medium tone next to a dark and a light tone, it will draw toward the one it is most like. Light-toned skin will seem lighter when seen with dark clothes and brown hair.

When colors start stealing the lime-light from each other, the medium color (man in the middle) always loses. He gives up the fight and simply sides with the color most like himself. In the example above, the skin would steal the show and the hair would play second fiddle to the dark-toned clothes.

Never, Never, Rule: allow the brilliance of your clothes to out-shine the intensity of your hair if you are blond, medium blond or titian.

SKIN COLORS CLASSIFIED

We are now ready to classify your skin so that you can get busy on applying the four rules. We mentioned that your skin had three pigments, red, yellow, and brown; these are found in various amounts in different skins so that some appear to be:

White—very little pigment
Cream—with an equal combination of red and yellow
Pink—with an overbalance of red pigment
Yellow—with an overbalance of yellow pigment
Tan—with an overbalance of brown
Olive—a cool type skin
Brown, Copper & Ebony—an abundance of pigmentation

SKIN COLORS AND THEIR COMPLIMENTS

TRANSLUCENT SKIN A light-toned skin that seems to have a translucent quality may be so lacking in pigment that the owner has a sickly appearance. This can be remedied by the application of color-heightening make-up and clothing shades that add color to the complexion. These would include all the deep reds and red-red violets, red-oranges that are deep or bright, dark greens, dark and bright blue-violets and blues, and white which intensifies the skin. Blue grays are lovely in medium tones.

CREAM COLORED SKIN The possessor of cream colored skin is particularly lucky in that she has a wide variety of colors to choose from, especially colors that won't dull her hair—bright yellow and yellow beige are culprits.

A PINK COMPLEXION Is usually associated with titian hair, to offset the "blushing" of this type, grayed-down fashions are suggested. These would include the palest tints of yellow, pink and apricot; moss, olive and avocado greens; charcoal and banker's gray; oyster and chalk white; a whole gamut of blues, powder, paste, french, and midnight. This type looks lovely in ebony black too. So you can see, even the woman with the most difficult color problem of all, titian with florid skin, does not have to confine herself to an uninteresting monotony of color sameness.

A TAN COMPLEXION Is inclined to look "muddy" when it is worn with dull, uninteresting colors. It needs the enlivening effects of bright, intense colors. It is flattered by the yellows, orange-reds, true reds. It is complemented by the greens and blue-greens so long as they are not too dark or too grayed-down.

AN OLIVE COMPLEXION Has very little intensity of its own and is inclined to look sallow if it is worn with tones that are too bright in contrast to it. It blends with beige and medium brown tones as long as they are not too close to it in value. Because it is a "cool" complexion it is flattered by the cool greens and blues, such as; avocado green, olive, moss, and gray-greens; blue-grays, teal, the blue-green blues. Usually dark brown and black should be avoided unless they are worn with color accents.

BROWN, COPPER AND EBONY Complexions are flattered by bright colors that have the same underlying tones. They are complemented by colors that are as intense as themselves. The extremes of black and white are not as good as the dark grays on the one hand and the eggshell white on the other.

TO ENHANCE ANY SKIN The colors worn must be lighter or darker than it, in value. This is true of every skin no matter what its balance. Those of you with a yellow cast will find that your skin is most flattered by colors that contain the same underlying tone. Hence include in your wardrobe: grays, or natural colors, eggshell white, yellow beiges, lime and turquoise, mahogany and british tan.

WHEN YOUR HAIR HAS TURNED TO SILVER

You can still be lovely to look at if you wear the colors that complement your hair and skin. Naturally you will not be able to wear some of the colors that you wore when you were sweet sixteen, but then sweet sixteen cannot wear the lovely, dignified colors that are now for you. These include almost everything except yellow, brown and beige. No need to content yourself with navy blue and black when all of these are flattering: *In the reds,* mauve, raspberry, burgundy, coral, shocking pink; *in the blues,* teal, slate, ultramarine, mulberry, midnight, aquamarine and orchid; *in the grays,* bankers, steel, smoke and battleship. You will be wonderfully pleased if you choose shades that are darker than your skin and hair.

COLORS IN COSMETICS

You have examined your skin and found it not to your liking, or perhaps you have decided that your flattering color range would be widened if the tone of your skin were changed slightly. Well, this miracle too is within your reach through the judicious use of color in cosmetics. In order for powder, foundation, rouge and lipstick to seem a natural part of you, each must contain a trace of the same underlying tone as that in your skin.

COLORS IN ACCESSORIES

Now we have come to the point where we must consider the importance of correctly chosen accessories. Your becomingly styled costume can be ruined by bag, hat, shoes, gloves or jewelry that is wrong for you, the time of day, or the "feel" of the clothes being worn.

It is with imaginatively selected accessories that you can express your own personality with distinction. Therefore, it is wise for you to not only choose the correct accessories but to choose those that give your ensemble a flair and an air. For example, a navy suit would be correctly accessorized with navy purse, bag and gloves, but it would be discriminatingly accessorized with navy bag and shoes, wheat colored gloves, yellow earrings and a slightly lighter blue hat.

There are rules for assembling accessories and although current fashion may come up with ideas that contradict the rules, they are safe to follow when in doubt.

ACCESSORY COLOR RULES

1. When wearing bright colored accessories with the basic colors (black, brown, navy) do not wear more than two that match.
2. These two should be neither too far apart nor too close together.

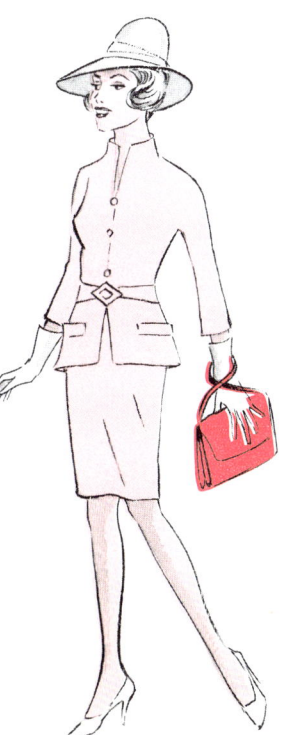

Correct	Incorrect
bag—shoes	shoes—hat
shoes—belt	shoes—jewelry
belt—hat	belt—bag
hat—gloves	hat—earrings
gloves—earrings	gloves—bag
earrings—bracelet	

By this rule, it would be incorrect to use more than two bright colored accessories with a dark suit or dress and these two should be placed so as to give accent without confusion.

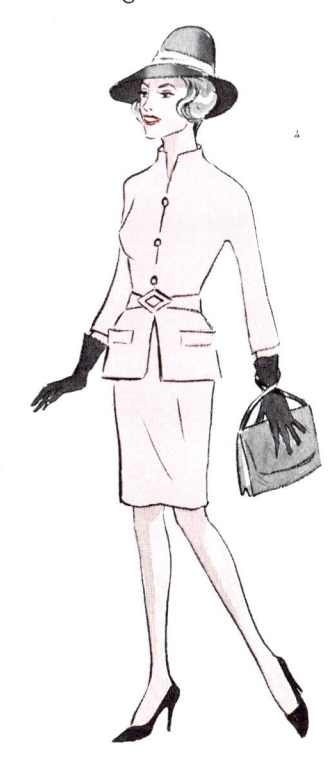

3. *It is advisable not to use more than three different colors in accessories and these must all have some relationship to the basic costume and to each other.* For simplicity we will divide color into three categories.
   1. *Basic colors* include black, brown, navy blue and sometimes wine and dark green.
   2. *Neutral colors* include white, beige, gray and tan.
   3. *Bright colors* include all others.

With a basic suit we could use the following:

Basic suit	Hat	Bag	Gloves	Shoes	Flower
Navy blue	White	Navy	Navy	Navy	Red

This example combines white (a neutral) in one accessory; navy blue (a basic) in three accessories; and red (a bright color) in one accessory.

4. We must never combine two basics in the same ensemble except Dame Fashion decrees that brown–black are ultra chic.
5. If your costume is in a dark color and your hat is the bright accent, dark shoes and bag are indicated.
6. Pastel and white shoes may be worn with white or pastel dresses. However, these shoes are for resort or home wear and are not fashion-wise for street wear in the city.
7. Hosiery that is sheer will reduce the size of the leg. It is always safe to wear stockings in a color that blends with the costume.
8. It is desirable but not absolutely necessary to have the texture of the bag and shoes match. A leather bag should be worn with leather shoes. Suede shoes, however, may be worn with a fabric bag such as broadcloth.

TO SUMMARIZE ON COLOR SELECTION

1. Do the colors you have in mind for future purchases fit into your present wardrobe?
2. Are you thinking in terms of flattering your face and figure?
3. Will these colors be fashion-wise in twelve months?
4. Are these colors occasion-keyed to fit into your way of life?
5. Will these colors dramatize your personality and enhance it?

CHAPTER 17

ACCESSORIES

Introduction

A woman is never completely dressed for the street until she is wearing her hat and gloves; these in addition, of course, to her dress, shoes, hose and bag. On some occasions you may wish to wear gloves without wearing a hat. This would be entirely proper to informal summer gatherings or in suburban areas where hats are an exception and not a rule.

HATS

If you would add fillip to your wardrobe and a look and then a second look, here are some suggestions.

CHAPEAUS THAT ATTRACT BEAUS

1. Repeating similar shapes in your accessories complements the dress and makes for harmony, i.e., a straight-lined tailored dress should be worn with a hat that has "sharp" rather than round or droopy lines.
2. Your hat should tend to ovalize your face; therefore, never repeat in the lines of the hat those that you do not wish to emphasize in your face.
3. Every hat must be proportioned to fit your head, your height and your figure.
4. Stand up in front of a full-length mirror and examine the effect of the hat from the front, sides and back before making your final decision.
5. Your hat must be suitable in color, line and texture to the type of dress it accessorizes.

HAT SHAPES

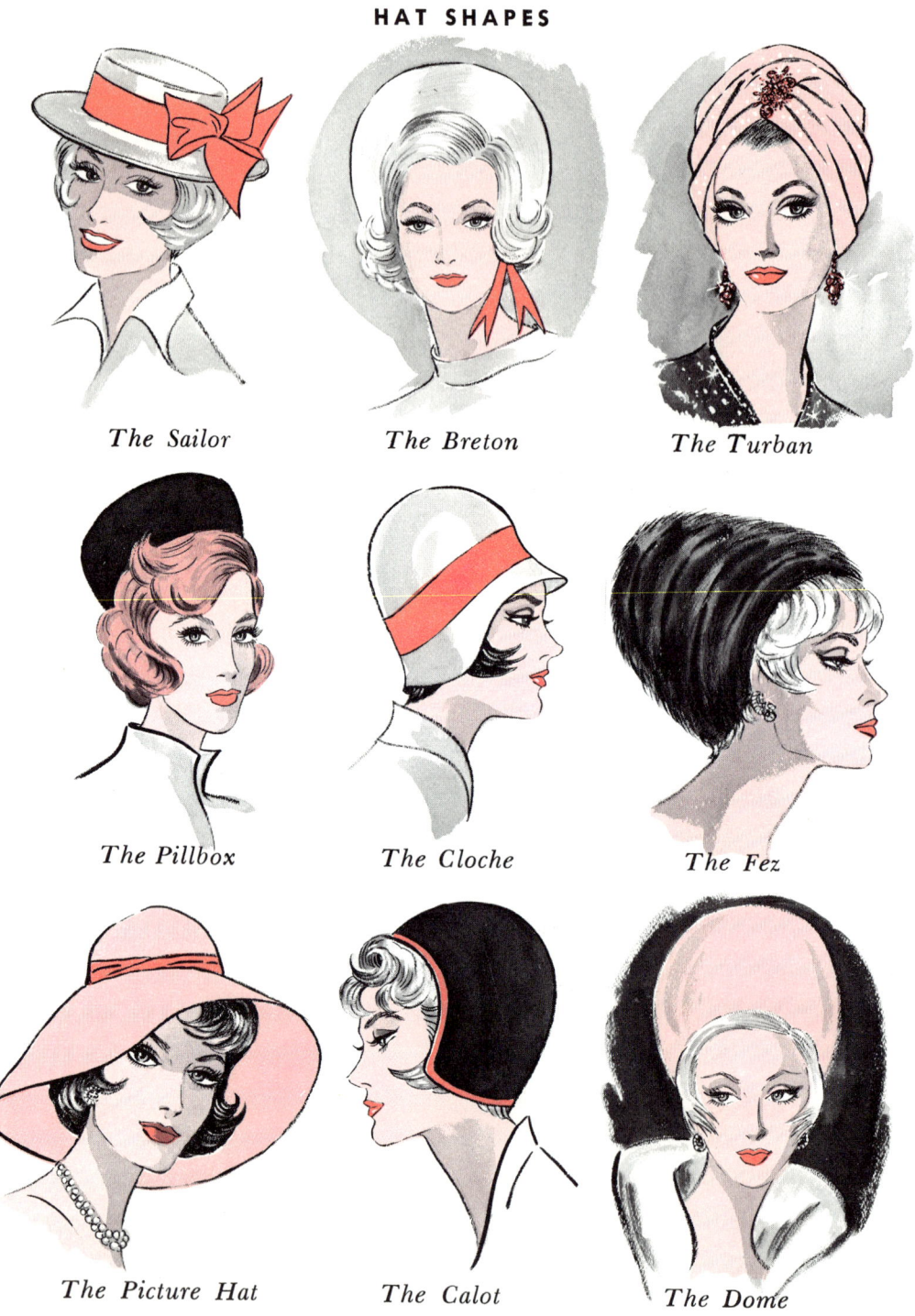

The Sailor   *The Breton*   *The Turban*

The Pillbox   *The Cloche*   *The Fez*

The Picture Hat   *The Calot*   *The Dome*

Remember these points: vertical lines *slenderize and lengthen*. horizontal lines *add width;* curving lines *round the face and figure;* diagonal lines and asymmetrical balance *diminish those aspects of appearance that you wish out of existence*. A large picture hat is fine for the young, romantic type but its sorcery ends where maturity and lined skin begins. Veils? They veil a thousand faults when properly chosen. You can prove to be a veiled-threat to Dan Cupid when you are stunningly attired.

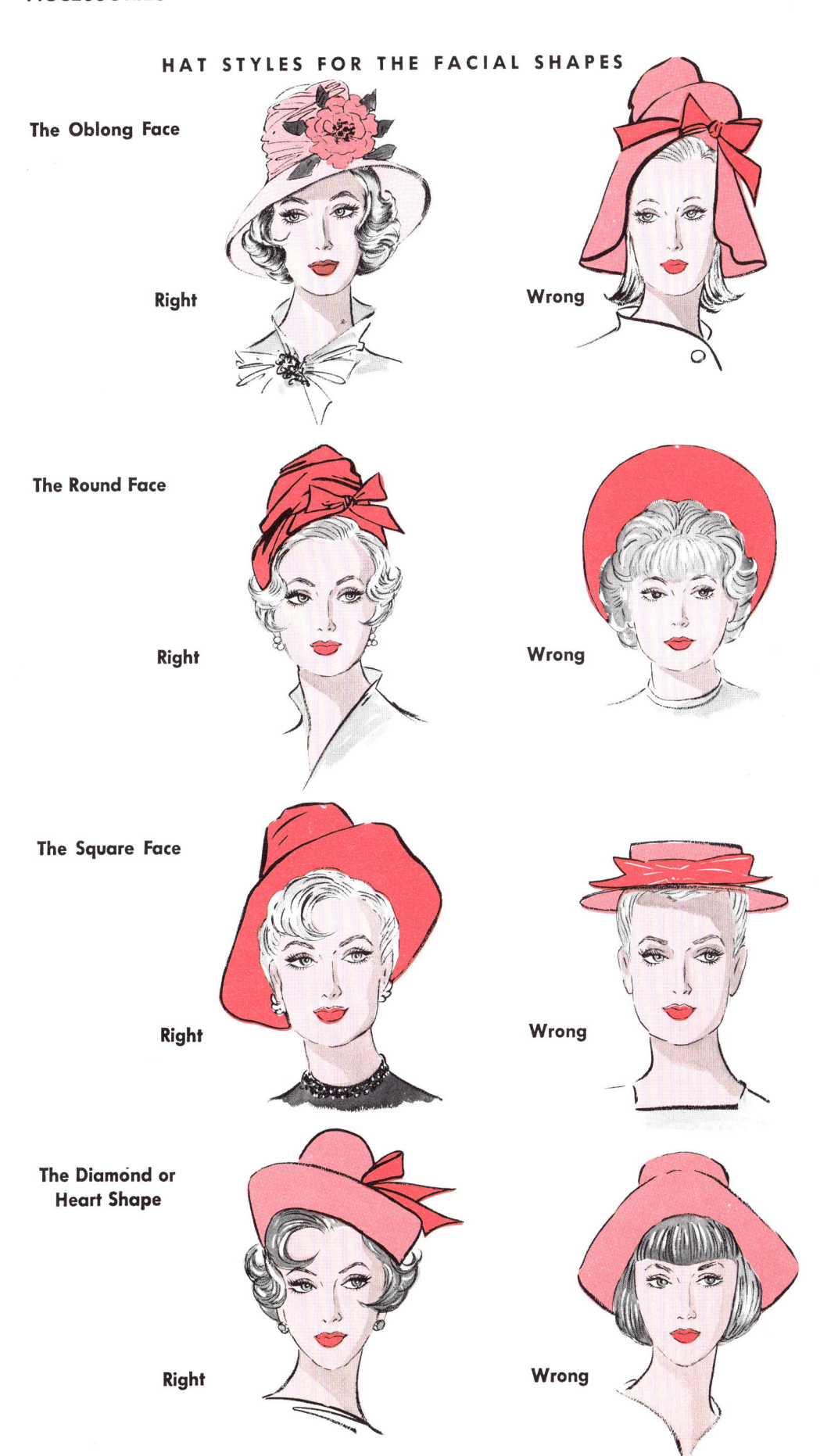

ACCESSORIES

HAT STYLES FOR THE FACIAL SHAPES

The Oblong Face

Right — Wrong

The Round Face

Right — Wrong

The Square Face

Right — Wrong

The Diamond or Heart Shape

Right — Wrong

JEWELRY IS SO PERSONAL

Too often jewelry is selected for its sake alone without thought to the woman who will wear it. Even though you possess a vault of precious gems, you will not add glamour to your jewels or to yourself if you do not wear them with discretion. Each piece must be appropriate to the costume and to the time of day. It must be in a size that is becoming to the proportions of the figure, the face and the hands.

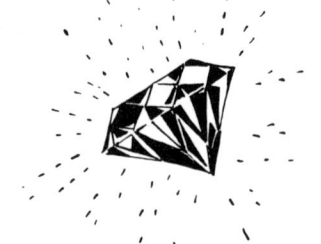

JEWELRY FOR DAYTIME WEAR:

Pearls

> Earrings with hats are inconspicuous and achieve a quiet, restrained air for the street, office or shopping.
>
> Necklaces should be selected in a length flattering to you.
>
> Bracelets that don't jangle are understated jewelry and proper.

Silver and Gold

> Earrings with a corresponding necklace speaks of good taste.
>
> Necklaces must match the earrings so that silver is worn with silver and gold with gold. This applies to other metals as well. Copper and aluminum bespeak the tailored look.
>
> Bracelets can be used in abundance if they fit you and the costume.

Rhinestones

> May be worn after twelve o'clock noon providing they give brilliance to an already dressed-up outfit. This would imply hat, hose, heels, etc.

A *watch* is appropriate at any time of day as are *brooches* and *simple clips*. Costume jewelry is worth its weight in gold for the lift it will give your costume.

JEWELRY FOR AFTER FIVE:

Pearls

> Their lustre can continue to contribute to your loveliness all through the night.

Fake Stones

> Wonderful for all jewelry.

Real Jewels

> Adorn yourself so that the jewels in no way compete with each other or your beauty. Don't sacrifice quality to quantity.

Rhinestones

> Do not buy matching sets of earrings, necklace and bracelet. Let your individuality and good taste be sparked in the selection of these sparkling baubles.

ACCESSORIES

NEVER, NEVER RULES:
1. Never combine one metal with another unless the mixture is within the jewelry itself.
2. Never combine pearls and rhinestones unless the mixture is carried out so that the jewelry looks as though it belongs together.
3. Never wear colored "fake" gems that sparkle in the daytime.
4. Never wear an ankle bracelet after eighteen.
5. Never wear jewelry that does not complement the color and the type of the costume.
6. Never wear rhinestones with essentially tailored clothes.
7. Never wear too much jewelry—it's worse than none.
8. Never wear jangly bracelets to the office.
9. Never wear jewelry that is not in proportion to your own size.

JEWELRY TO FIT

Too often jewelry is selected for its own sake alone with little thought as to its suitability for the woman who is to wear it. A woman with extremely long, slender fingers, for example, should wear a ring with the stones set with greatest width across the fingers. This minimizes the extreme length of the hand. *Rings* with stones set lengthwise down the finger help to make short fingers look more tapered.

TIPS FOR PRETTIER HANDS

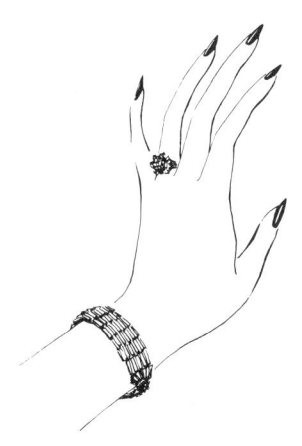

IF YOUR HANDS ARE LONG AND SLIM, a flexible mesh bracelet or several slender circlets are becoming. Rings should have large settings, round or horizontal, as wide as the finger. Dark polish is lovely on these hands.

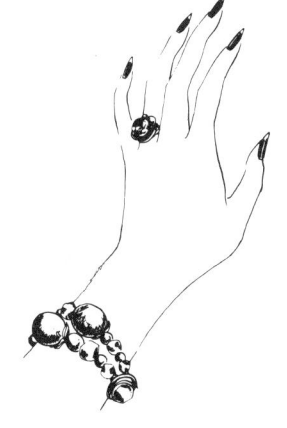

ON LARGE HANDS, wide rings or those with high, dome-shaped ornament are good. Wear a massive bracelet with high ornament, pushed up on arm. Lacquer nails with dark or medium polish; show clear moons and tips.

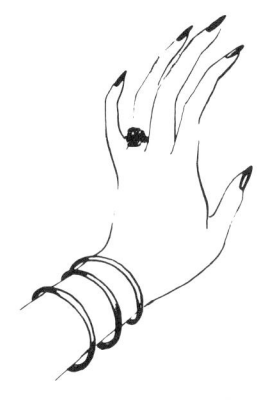

FOR THE SLIM LITTLE HAND, choose narrow bracelets and rings with rosettes of gems.
FOR THE BROADER HAND, pick more solid bracelets, pushed up on arm; rings with elongated settings. Wear light polish.

EARRINGS

As for earrings, the woman with a large, round face should wear massive, bulky ear clips for better proportion. Little ones will look lost. There are lightweight metals, such as paladium, that make large-sized earrings comfortable to wear. Ear clips triangular in shape—with the base at the lowest part of the lobe and the point at the top give a more becoming oval look to the long, thin face.

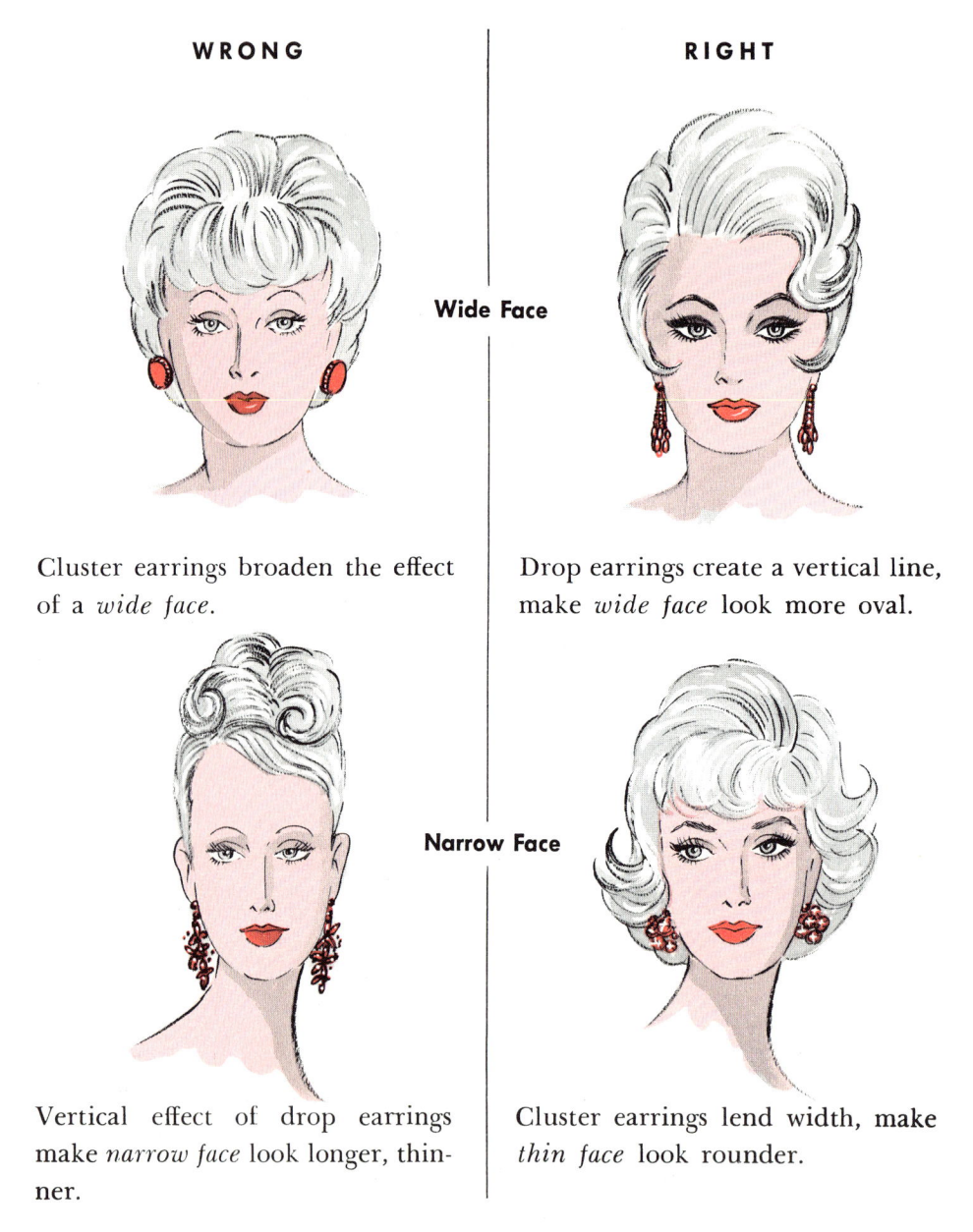

WRONG		RIGHT
	Wide Face	
Cluster earrings broaden the effect of a *wide face*.		Drop earrings create a vertical line, make *wide face* look more oval.
	Narrow Face	
Vertical effect of drop earrings make *narrow face* look longer, thinner.		Cluster earrings lend width, make *thin face* look rounder.

Colored stones in earrings are devastating if chosen to go with a girl's coloring. If, for example, the object of a man's affections is a girl with fair hair and blue eyes, a gift of earrings set with sapphires or aquamarines would show that he's really thought about his love. It's thoughtful, too, to match earrings to jewelry a girl already owns.

ACCESSORIES 193

NECKLACES AND CHOKERS

Necklaces and chokers—Always classic in pearls, real diamond jewelry, in metal and stone costume jewelry, too. But extra care must be used in selecting these. A high choker, for example, is not for the woman with a short neck, for it tends to make the neck appear even shorter. A brooch or clips are more flattering ornaments in this case. But, if a necklace is really wanted, it should be long enough to fall well below the base of the throat.

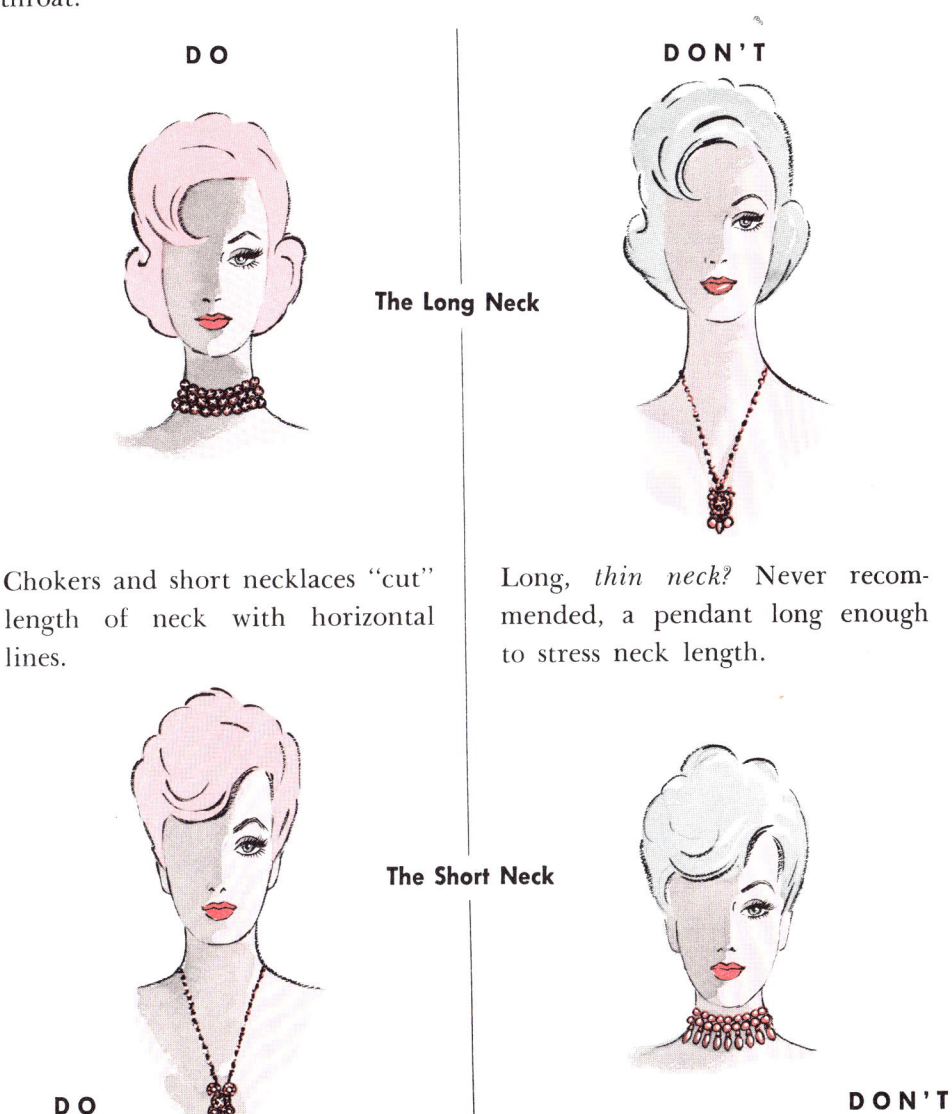

DO — *The Long Neck* — **DON'T**

Chokers and short necklaces "cut" length of neck with horizontal lines.

Long, *thin neck?* Never recommended, a pendant long enough to stress neck length.

DO — *The Short Neck* — **DON'T**

"Add" length to a *short neck* with long necklace that draws eye downward.

A choker really seems to choke a *short neck*. It almost makes it look like no neck at all.

THE GALLANT GAUNTLET

Your gloves are not only a protection for your hands, but also an opportunity for you to add dash, chic and flair to your costume. The type of glove you select will be determined by the size and shape of your hand as well as its appropriateness for the costume. Outside stitching is associated with the dress-down look so that gloves of this type are most appropriate with tailored clothes. Inside stitching is for the dress-up look and small mitts of this variety are perfect for short-sleeved cocktail dresses.

SELECTING YOUR GLOVES

There is another interesting rule that you might use for experimentation. It is this: the shorter the sleeve the shorter the glove, the longer the sleeve, the longer the glove. For three-quarter length sleeves the perfect glove is eight-button length.

FOR LARGE, SLENDER HANDS: Their size will be minimized by dark colors, their length by outside stitching on the fingers and horizontal stitching on the back of the hand.

FOR LARGE, BROAD HANDS: Their size will be minimized by darker colors, inside stitching, vertical stitching on the back of the hand.

FOR SMALL, BROAD HANDS: Lighter colors, perfect fit, light-weight fabrics.

FOR SMALL, SLENDER HANDS: Lighter colors, perfect fit, light-weight fabrics. The addition of jewelry on the outside of the glove will add bulk and the illusion of opulence.

FOR AVERAGE HANDS: The hands will look larger in light shades, especially if the gloves have outside stitching.

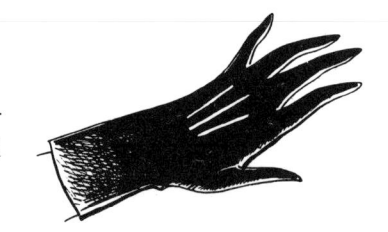

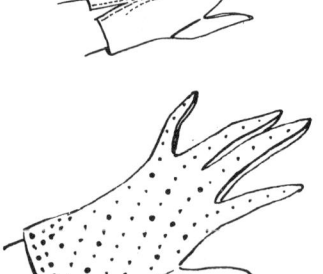

ACCESSORIES 195

BEAUTIFUL BAGS

No other accessory in your wardrobe stands out for the inspection of others as does your handbag. May it pass the rigid test. In order to do so it must be fastidiously kept both inside and out.

For daytime wear a bag tailored in shape of long-wearing leather or fabric is appropriate. Generously sized, it will allow you to keep all of the items you need in neat order.

For evening wear a bag of luxury fabric delicately fashioned will give an inexpressible air of femininity. The clutch type is convenient because it is small and easy to carry—even on the dance floor. Your bag for formal wear need not be expensive, only expensive looking. Its contents too should reflect credit on you. A jewelled compact, lipstick and comb are a delight to own and to behold.

Let your size govern the capacity of your bag.

FOR THE TALL-THIN AND TALL-HEAVY:
A suitcase type will not seem oversized.

FOR THE MEDIUM FIGURE:
Anything goes that is in keeping with the costume.

FOR THE SHORT-THIN:
Petite bags of an unbulky design.

FOR THE SHORT-HEAVY:
Medium sized bags of flat fabrics.

For the Tall-Thin and Tall-Heavy Figure

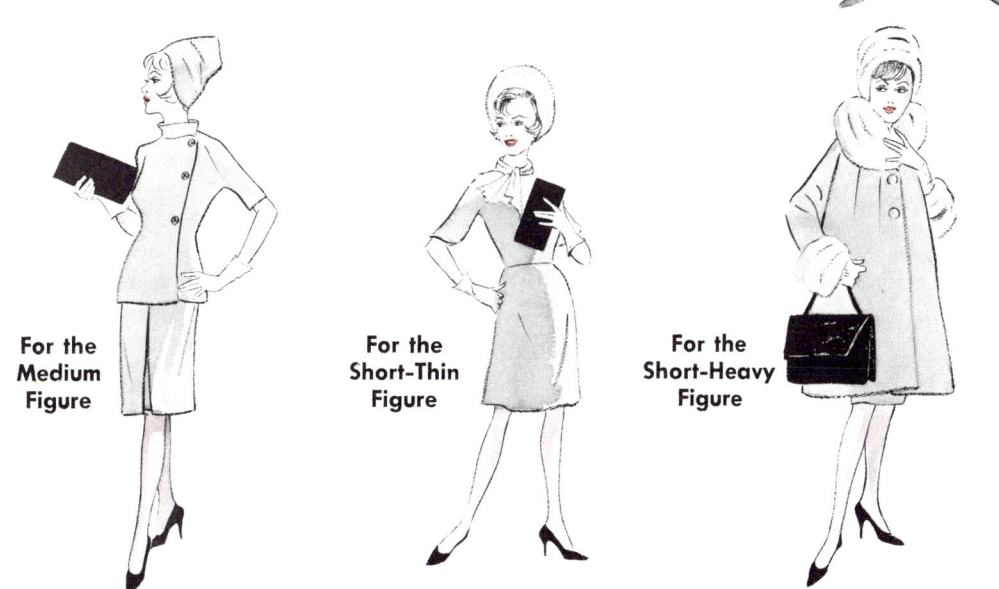

For the Medium Figure

For the Short-Thin Figure

For the Short-Heavy Figure

Unless you can afford a wide variety of bags, you will be wise to select those that are basic in fabric and style.

SHOES FOR SURE

The most versatile of styles for woman's ever-widening circle of activities is the classic opera pump with a closed toe and heel. The height of the heel will depend upon the use to which the shoe will be put and the preference of the individual. However, the pump is considered proper with almost all clothes for both daytime and evening wear. It has a dress-down look when in kid or calf and a dress-up look when in suede or brocade. A fabric shoe is the perfect accessory for a pastel gown when dyed in the same color.

Patent leather is considered to be a spring and summer leather although once again Dame Fashion may decree a change. If you enjoy novel and different accessories, keep in mind that ankle straps, loud colors and unique fabrics are not recommended for daytime, urban wear.

Most shoes for sports and for hard wear will have a tendency to make your feet look enormous. For this reason select a style that has slenderizing details.

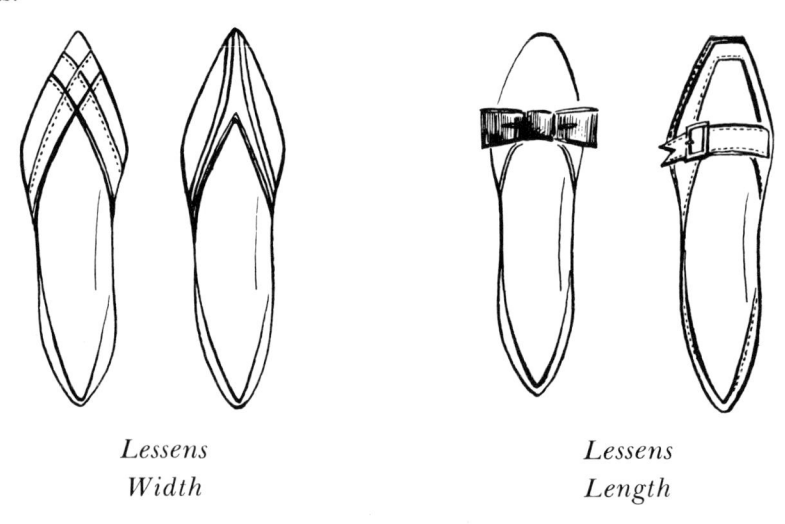

Lessens Width

Lessens Length

To lessen width: Vertical and diagonal stitching, low-cut at the instep, a moderately rounded toe.

To lessen length: A bow or narrow strap across instep, a rounded vamp, a rounded toe.

If you wish to hide your feet, avoid loud colors, fancy, flimsy footwear, platform soles and ankle straps.

Your feet will be more comfortable if you insist upon shoes that have correct fit, designed for your type of feet, a firm shank, soft uppers, kid lining that "breathes," a firmly fitted heel, and an inner lining that acts as a shock-absorbing cushion.

ACCESSORIES 197

SCARVES THAT SCORE

A couple of arrangements that really don't score are the peasant headgear type and the bulky bandage type. Other than these, a scarf can complement a costume with a stroke of dash.

There are many other uses for a scarf than the ascot and the bow. You will add a "theater" air to your costumes if you will learn to tie and arrange your scarves with a deft hand.

SCARF ARRANGEMENTS:

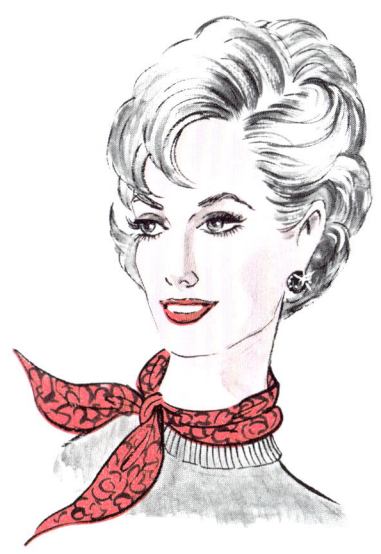

36" scarf rolled or folded in half. Ends brought through loop. (Cowboy style)

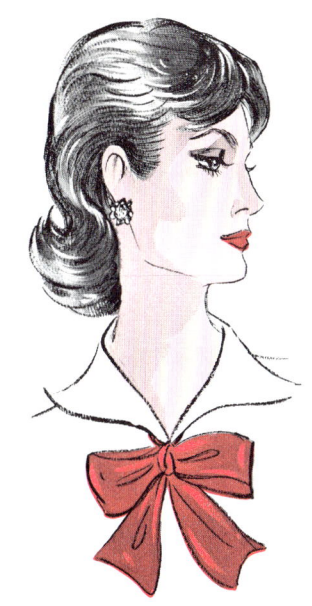

Long scarf about 6" wide tied into bow and pinned at neck of suit, dress, blouse.

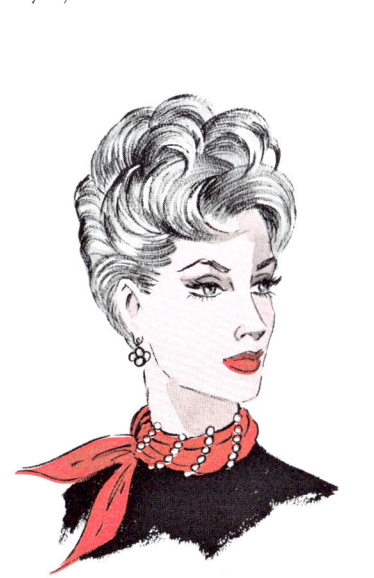

Tie scarf around neck of sweater or blouse, then wind pearls around scarf.

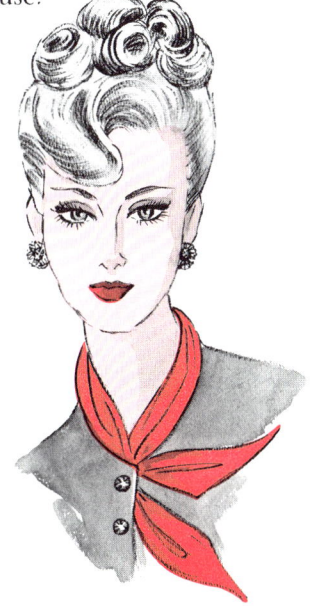

Scarf around neck of suit or dress and used to cover buttons.

A narrow or a 36″ square tied in a half bow and loop.

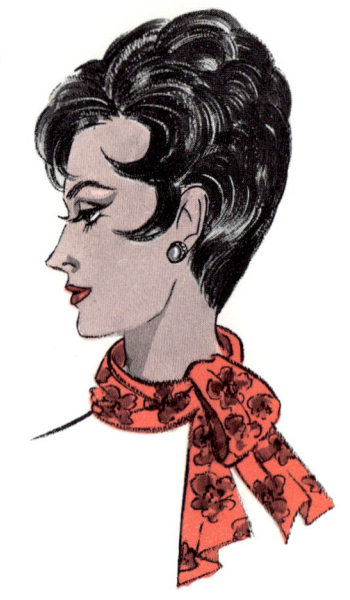

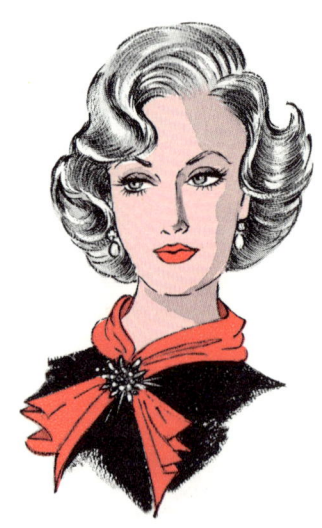

Scarf criss-crossed, (not tied) and secured with pin or flower.

ADDITIONAL SCARF ARRANGEMENTS

Envelope fold 36″ square under collar with a half-knot in front.

Scarf looped over belt.

Wide, long scarf used for cummerbund.

Three scarves braided. Wonderful as a belt with "skinny" pants

Always cover curlers. An Aunt Jemina tie will do nicely.

Acceptable version of the "babushka." The ends are crossed under the chin and tied in back.

For the beach, a colorful addition.

Under suits, a 36″ square folded in triangle with ends tied at back of neck. Other two ends tied around waist.

Scarf cascades casually from pocket. Any size may be used. Shake out folds by holding center of scarf.

6″ wide scarf cut on diagonal used in place of belt. Should be approximately 54″ long.

"Gypsy" tie. 36″ square folded in triangle and tied on one side.

Strip of cotton fabric 36″ long and 4″ wide when sewed, to be worn over the hair.

For "special" occasions, a lovely lace handkerchief.

For sunback dresses, a bolero of 36″ scarf tied over shoulders. Use "square" corners.

BOUTONNIERES

A woman who wears imaginative flowers is a feast for the eyes. Don't be afraid of the original. If you are given a corsage that won't harmonize with your dress you can pin it on your bag or gloves or coat. You might also wear it in your hair, or you can attach it to a ribbon and wear it like

ACCESSORIES

a bracelet. But whether you wear flowers fresh from the florist or artificial posies, they must lend a striking note of color and give a lift to a costume. You must choose them carefully so that they accentuate the positive.

Usually a flower is worn in the direction that it grows. Also, it will have added meaning if it is worn at the proper time of year. A boutonnier of fall leaves has a great deal of meaning around Thanksgiving time just as a daffodil plucked from the garden will give "oomph" in April.

If you look like one of the following types then the flower indicated is appropriate.

Exotic	—orchid
Athletic	—carnation or chrysanthemum
Ingenue	—sweet pea, lily-of-the-valley, field flowers
Romantic	—pink camellia
Voluptuous	—red rose
Matronly	—violet
Young Matron	—talisman rose

HANDKERCHIEFS

A wisp of snowy lace can symbolize your femininity on formal occasions. A gay dash of color can accompany your mood and mode in the daytime. You can either let your hankerchief make a public showing or a private one in the confines of your handbag. Whatever or wherever, its impeccable cleanliness and freshness will heighten your attractiveness. This will be especially true if it wafts your favorite fragrance.

EYEGLASSES

Better vision, increased good looks, *eyeglasses* can deliver both. The wearer should ask herself some quite relevant clothes questions before she makes her choice. Does she want to wear glasses that are decorated to the point of being a piece of costume jewelry in and of themselves? Does she wear a hat often? If she does, obviously a simple style will be best. And what about glass frames that are color coordinated with her wardrobe? Won't a neutral color that can be worn with everything be her best buy?

Of course if a gal can afford more than one pair her problem is cut in half. She can buy a basic pair to wear in the daytime and a more ornate pair for evening. If she has that much money to spend, she might seriously consider contact lenses. They will eliminate the need to shop for complimentary frames entirely.

Exception: For sunning, do wear dark glasses.

FRAMED FOR BEAUTY

Refer to the Face Shapes and select for your face the most flattering frame possible.

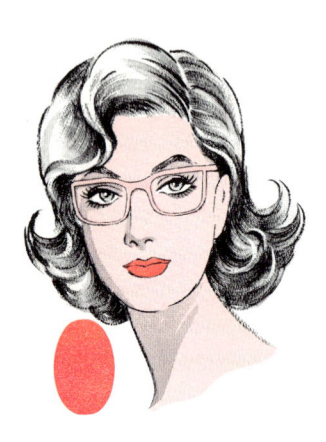

OVAL FACE — Frames that preserve the perfect balance of the face are indicated. These should follow the curve of the brow allowing some of it to show above the frames.

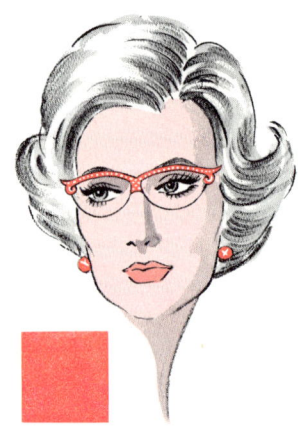

SQUARE FACE — The eyeglass lenses should be medium to large in size, not petite. The frames should have curved lines, not square.

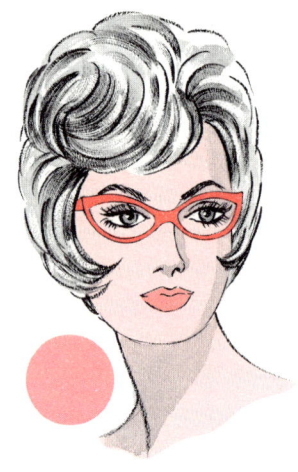

ROUND FACE — A frame with a low nose bar will allow the glass frame to sweep upward. Keep the lenses rather narrow, not round.

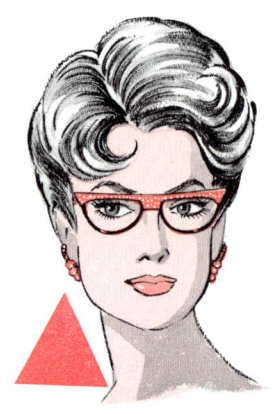

TRIANGULAR FACE — Frames that are medium to wide in a dark color will give needed weight to the upper part of the face. The shape should be wide enough to create an illusion of width across the temple.

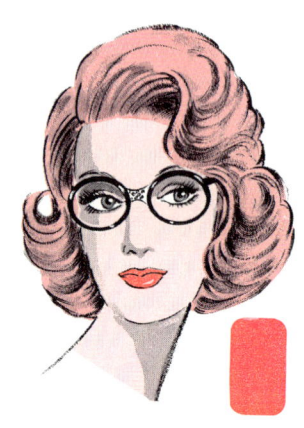

OBLONG FACE — A wide frame that has no up-curve will give an illusion of width to this narrow face. The lenses should be deep enough to minimize the length of the face.

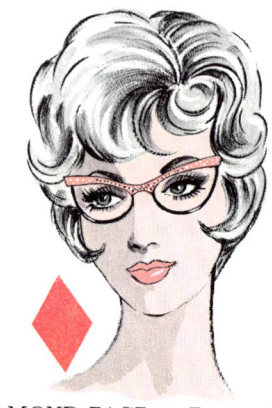

DIAMOND FACE — Frames that are widely flanged on top and narrowed at bottom will give width at the brow, but will detract from wide cheekbones.

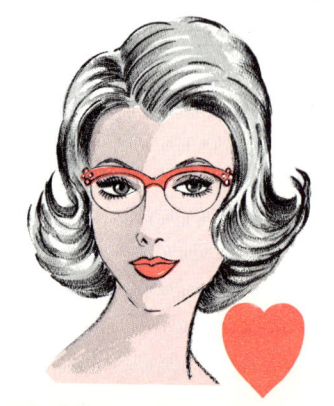

HEART-SHAPED FACE — Frames that have no sharp angles will detract from a pointed chin, as will frames that follow the line of the eyebrows.

Additional hints for eyeglass shoppers:

Wear sufficient eye make-up, enough to make up for the eyeglasses. Select a "basic" pair if you can afford only one. Be sure it is color-keyed to your wardrobe. Let an expert assist you in your selection. Try before you buy. Experiment with a number of pairs before making up your mind.

CHAPTER 18

THE TWELVE PERSONALITY TYPES IN DRESS

Introduction

Personality—that which constitutes distinction of person—what are its qualities, what is its price?

There are no two persons exactly alike. Perhaps that is why the world is an interesting place to live! If we all wanted to be (and could be) young, slim and blondly alluring, how tiresome life would be! Thank goodness we have variety—variety produced by the different natures of women and by the varying moods of each woman.

Some women show a distinct personality and she who is definitely one type is easy to analyze and to dress. Usually, she knows just how she wants to appear, selects the right type of costume, and commands admiration by the subtlety of her dress. Occasionally the definite type person does *not* know how to select suitable clothes. Then she appears absurd and seems incongruous in her garments because she completely ignores her personality; or, by overdoing the dressing of her type, she appears more like a caricature than a masterpiece.

Some women have more complex natures than others. In such persons the combination of personality qualities can be charming because of their variety. In fact, in most cases a personality is a combination of qualities, and the clothes worn should show this.

Some girls look terrific in tweed and others look terrible. Aside from build, the way a person acts and moves has a great deal to do with the type of clothes that are in "character" for her.

By reading through the Twelve Personality Types, you will be able to identify yourself with one or more of them. You will discover that each type has its own particular fabric, color, flower and perfume. If you are young, still in your teens, don't be too concerned if you don't seem to fit anywhere. It may be that you have not had time to develop your own clearcut set of personality traits. Perhaps you are still groping to learn just what kind of a person you are. Let your instructor and the other members of your class help you decide.

DRESSING TO TYPE

Whether you know it or not, your clothes always express your personality. But do they express the personality you WANT them to show?

A woman's charm is often concealed by the wrong type of clothing, whereas her personality can be brought out and enhanced when she is correctly dressed.

The object of this lesson is to teach *you* how to let the world know the best that is in you. How to bring out your best personality by your clothes.

It is never necessary to be a slave of fashion! Make it your slave instead. Use it as a medium of expression for your personality, charm and beauty by dressing to type.

ANALYSIS OF THE PERSONALITY TYPES

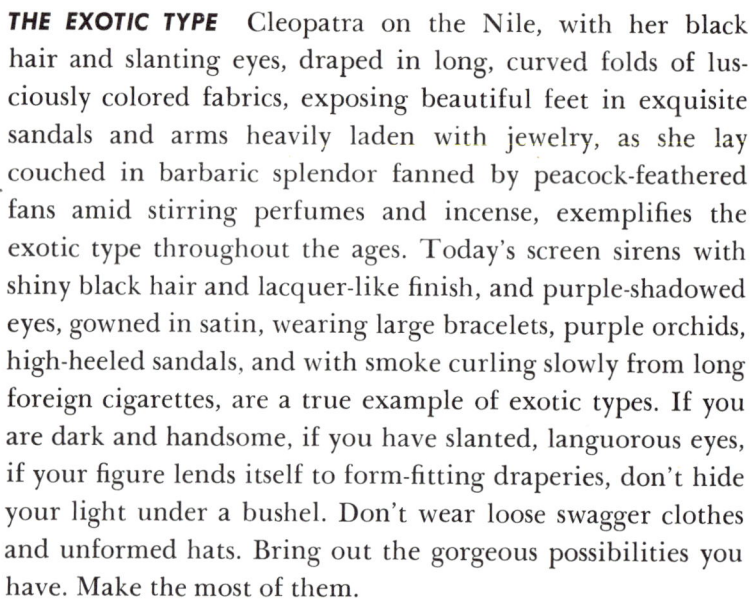

THE EXOTIC TYPE Cleopatra on the Nile, with her black hair and slanting eyes, draped in long, curved folds of lusciously colored fabrics, exposing beautiful feet in exquisite sandals and arms heavily laden with jewelry, as she lay couched in barbaric splendor fanned by peacock-feathered fans amid stirring perfumes and incense, exemplifies the exotic type throughout the ages. Today's screen sirens with shiny black hair and lacquer-like finish, and purple-shadowed eyes, gowned in satin, wearing large bracelets, purple orchids, high-heeled sandals, and with smoke curling slowly from long foreign cigarettes, are a true example of exotic types. If you are dark and handsome, if you have slanted, languorous eyes, if your figure lends itself to form-fitting draperies, don't hide your light under a bushel. Don't wear loose swagger clothes and unformed hats. Bring out the gorgeous possibilities you have. Make the most of them.

Don't wear bright red satin to the office or around the house. But have your tailored clothes so simple and so sleek in the daytime, your neck scarfs so white, and your one bracelet so barbaric, that your face and personality will show over the clothes. In the evening, don't throw your exoticism into everybody's face, but have your evening dress so well fitted, and your jewelry so gorgeous that your costume will make you look like the subtle, mysterious person you are. (Beware of seeming the "vamp on the leopard skin.")

Small turban-like hats are good for you if you are of this type. They show the size of your eyes. Heavy satins that hang and drape in voluptuous curves are excellent for your long, exotic gowns. Black chiffon underwear and very sheer dark hose, high-heeled sandals when appropriate, will add to

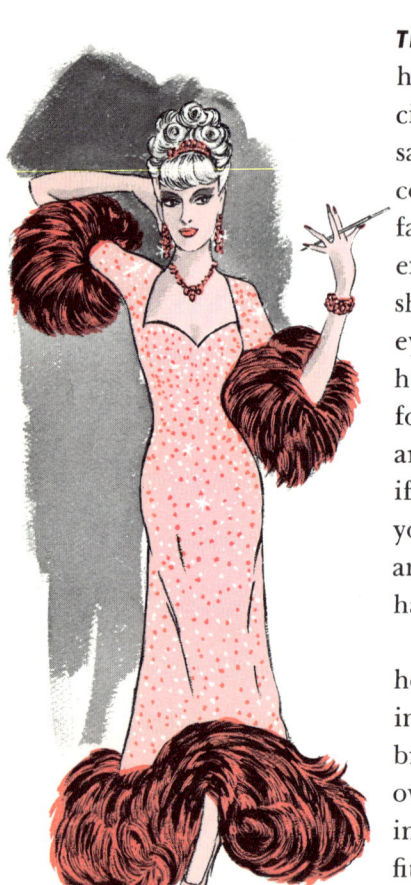

THE TWELVE PERSONALITY TYPES IN DRESS

your type of charm. Musky amber perfumes, deep purple orchids—you can wear all of these without having them overwhelm you as they might some other types. Your best colors, when you are not in black, are deep reds, burgundies, strong and turbulent shades, oriental and slightly mysterious tones. During the day, be very, very subtle. Never wear more than one exotic accessory. *Your time is night.*

THE INGENUE Marie Antoinette of Versailles, playing at milking, pampered and petted, young and playful, wearing panniers and puffs in pinks and blues, dainty, feminine, and oh, so young, given to flowery phrases and flowery perfumes— is a historic example of the ingenue type. Today, young women with curly brown or golden hair and big blue eyes, dressed in fragile fabrics, dainty slippers and hats, typify the ingenue.

If you are petite and youthful, if you are light and sweet, stay that way. You, of all people, can indulge in ruffles and dainty materials. You can tie little ribbons around your head and look trustingly at the world. Don't try to be exotic or sophisticated. Don't wear black or wine reds. Beware of jewelry for if it is at all heavy or ornate it will weigh you down. Make the most of the young years, be gay and personify the spirit of youth to all. Wear small, brimmed hats. Your ruffly dresses should be of dainty, light materials in pinks, blues, or pastel shades. Your underthings should match. Your hose should imitate the color of your skin, your small slippers the color of your costume. Dainty seed pearls or inconspicuous jewelry, lilac perfume and sweet pea are for you. You can grow up to be the young matron later. If you work you can be almost the American girl type in the office, but more dainty. You can be romantic in the moonlight. But always be the sweet young person that you are.

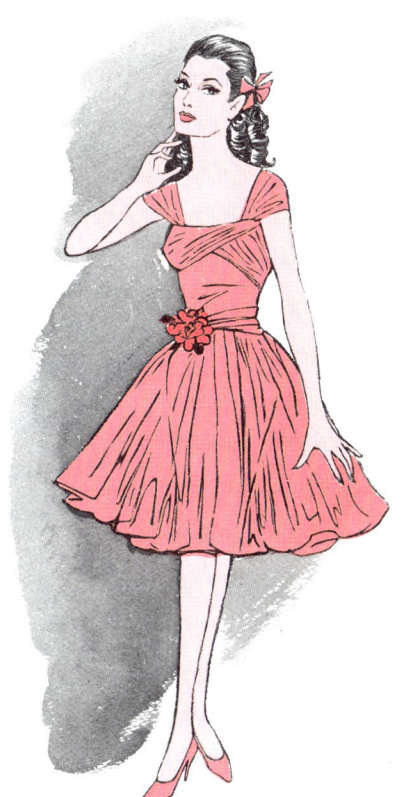

THE TWELVE PERSONALITY TYPES IN DRESS

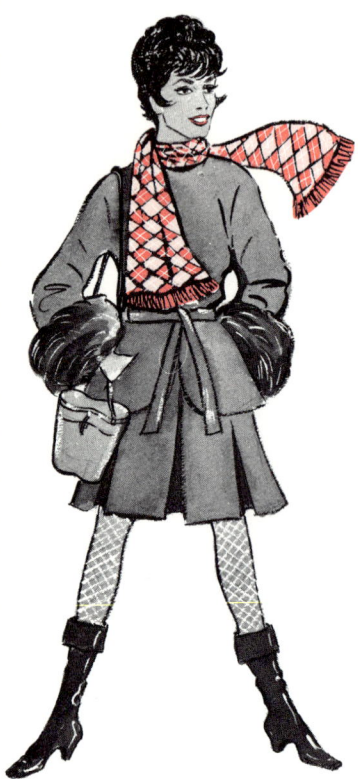

THE ATHLETIC TYPE Spartan women, living a rigorous and hardy life, with their trained muscles, perfect carriage, healthy natural color and sparkling eyes; are the best examples of this type. They were large or small, but never fat. And they always wore severely-styled garments. If you are athletic "looking," if your golf swing is a pride and joy, your swimming form a miracle, remember that there is nothing more incongruous than a tanned muscular arm emerging from a lot of fluffy ruffles.

Wear tailored lines even in the evening when you have to doff your sports clothes. The long, simple lines will show the fluid movement of a trained body. Yards of ruching around your feet will look worried and harassed by your firm stride. Don't try to be petite; don't let anyone talk you into trying to imitate romanticism. Be yourself! Wear strong, straight-forward clothes that will move with grace as you walk with forceful stride across the floor.

Whenever you can't wear sports clothes see to it that your wardrobe is carefully styled. Movements that otherwise would be graceful, may seem awkward in the wrong type of clothes. Don't let yourself appear too masculine, but don't ever wear "frou-frous" or slinky clothes. You, athletic woman, from your swagger hat to your sports shoes, should be trim and smart. Your linen dresses and chic sweaters and scarfs, your sporty-looking clothes designed in short straight lines, unadorned lingerie that fits for freedom of movement, jewelry that looks as sporty as yourself, all spell love of muscular activity and the evasion of the sometimes overdone subtleties of indoor life. Evening clothes should allow the body freedom and should not demand any extra care. Your perfume is heathery, or perhaps faintly reminiscent of pines and great open spaces. Your flower is the carnation. Your colors those of Mother Nature in both its summer dress and that of fall—greens and yellows and browns—for you are part of Mother Earth and *very wholesome.*

THE TWELVE PERSONALITY TYPES IN DRESS

THE ROMANTIC TYPE Helen of Troy, "divinely tall, divinely fair," beloved of many men, buffeted about by the winds of fate but always beautiful and charming to the end. From her classically curled hair to her sandled feet, Helen expressed the "essentially feminine." Her beautiful throat rose from the soft folds of her chiton.

> "O'er her fair face a snowy veil she threw
> And softly sighing from the loom withdrew."
>
> *Illiad, iii.*

A beautiful description of Helen, the epitome of romance.

If you are slender and large-eyed, if the waltz is your favorite dance, if you are gentle and sweet and very charming, you should show this delightful femininity in every way. Your picture hats, whenever it is possible for you to wear them, cast a becoming, shadowy glow on your lovely features. When you are at home your chiffon hostess gowns in pastel shades shimmer in the lamplight. Your lacy lingerie is a particular joy to you. Your sheer hose and your high-heeled slippers are dainty and fit your arching foot to perfection. Your jewelry is significant, each piece surrounded with memories of love and romance. Pale pink camellias at the breast of your gowns are your special flowers. And an aura of sweetness, jasmine or rose is always about you.

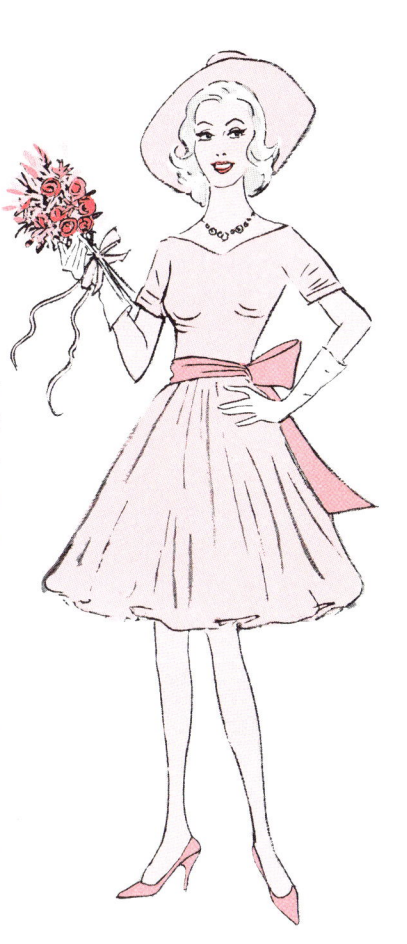

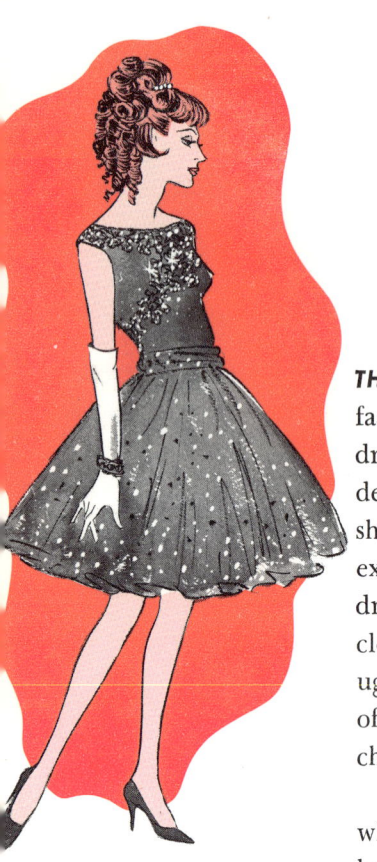

THE WOMAN OF FASHION Empress Eugenie, the most fashionable woman of her day, was the sponsor of the modern dress designers and French dress houses. Wearing clothes designed for her by Worth, or originating her own fashions, she was always in the lead. No wonder we select her as the example of this type! Today, those highly publicized well-dressed women, wearing the latest lines and ornaments, clothes that are sometimes becoming and sometimes almost ugly in their extraordinary lines and handling, are examples of this type. These women set the style and then hurriedly change before the style has a chance to become common.

For them everything must be "the latest," no matter what rules of becoming clothing fall by the wayside. Their hats are the most extreme and the very newest. Their gowns use lines, textiles and colors of the latest mode, no matter how unbecoming they may be. If you are wealthy enough to pay for the constant change in costume, if you like extreme things and can wear them with dash, you can be "a woman of fashion" type. Your posture must be perfect, and you must have complete assurance and self-confidence. You must be alert and enjoy novel things.

All that you wear, hat, gown, wrap, shoes, lingerie, hose and perfume, must be of a style a little ahead of that worn by anyone else or you will miss your mark. The very latest wrinkle, the newest bow, the most daring hat, you must keep your eyes open to have these before they are copied everywhere. You must be ready to don the shortest skirts or the longest trains or the broadest shoulders. You must keep ahead of the crowd or you will be swamped. You will have no claim to distinction if you are at all late in your choice. Your clothes need not suit you very well. Their only claim is their newness. If *fashion* is what you want, if that is the type which appeals to you, you must hurry, hurry, hurry to sense new styles.

THE TWELVE PERSONALITY TYPES IN DRESS

THE VOLUPTUOUS TYPE Lilith, the seductive, a woman men dream of, an angel to some and a demon to others, symbolizes the temptress. She went her own way, dressed ever to show her womanly charms that she might ensnare the thoughts and dreams of men. She was mysterious, elusive and consciously female, and her appeal was to the physical nature.

The voluptuous type wears clothes merely to give her body all its value. Satin, sequins and highlights emphasize every curve. This type of woman must be perfectly groomed at all times. She must constantly beware of "letting go," of getting too plump, too languorous in movements, or a little vulgar.

If you have exuberant curves, come-hither eyes and luscious lips you can dress to this type, but you must be very careful not to appear vulgar or common. There must *always* be simplicity of line in your costumes. The body and face must speak for themselves. Don't gild the lily. If you have the figure to show, and you wish to show it, do so in the privacy of your home where you can wear all the alluring and seductive garments you desire. When you are out during the day, try to be sophisticated in your clothes. Fussy or swagger things are never for your type. Your clothes should always be close-fitting but *never* obviously voluptuous.

Don't over-dress or you will lose all the charm that comes from the mystery, one of the most important attributes of your type. Men enjoy voluptuousness, but not when it lacks dignity and discrimination. In the evening you can wear low-cut, form-fitting gowns. Keep the lines simple. Make the garments you wear gorgeous only in the luscious materials you employ in making them. Rubies and diamonds, luxuriant as your type, are the stones for you. Satin shoes to match your gowns, with high heels to make your legs long and slender, are especially designed to fill your needs. Hose that are so much the color of your skin that they merely give the leg a sheen of silk and are not obviously stockings, add to your attractiveness. Vivid colors go with your vivid personality. You probably love bright hues and, in most cases, your type can carry them. Luxurious flower odors, lotus, heavy sweet peas, perhaps a little musky odor as well, are the perfumes for your type. Dark red, velvety-looking roses bloom for you alone.

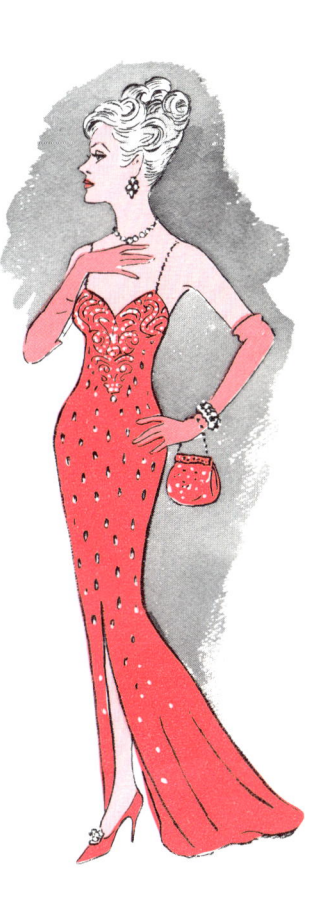

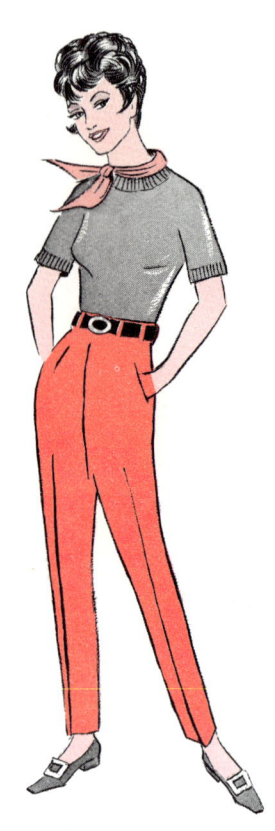

THE BOYISH TYPE Joan of Arc, in worn boy's clothes, her short hair free, a sword by her side, riding a horse, leading her troops to victory, young, alone but with her mind and soul leading her to the stars, was essentially the boyish type. Jo, in "Little Women," miserable in ruffles and hoops, her white gloves showing the masculine size of her hands, impatient of fashion, desiring freedom and comfort in clothes, conscious of her angles and her elbows, hating feminine styles, was truly boyish.

If you have a nice cheerful grin instead of a sweet smile, if you don't care about being feminine and delicate, if you feel dithery and all arms and feet in dainty fluttery dresses, *be yourself. Be comfortable.* Wear the clothes you wish. By being honest, straight-forward and happy in your clothes, your poise and your wit will attract people to you. Don't force yourself to wear clothes just because they are in style. Make *your* style the aim of your dressing. Be individual. If you have an unpretentious taste in clothes, your mind and wit must show constantly that clothes are merely a neutral background for your busy mentality, otherwise you may seem dowdy and uncouth. If you are not well groomed, your clothes will be merely the confession of an erratic and haphazard mind. But if your casual looking clothes carry the mark of *good breeding and taste,* they will complement your busy mind and unfeminine body. If you wish, you may go hatless wherever possible. You may wear loose, straight swagger-type clothes, but they must be well cut, fitted, and of good materials. Low-heeled shoes and stockings that go with your clothes must be selected. You can wear colors that are neutral or mixtures, but blues and browns are symbolic of your type. In lingerie that is primarily for comfort, and with only the perfume of a well-soaped skin, you can move with all the vigor and speed you wish.

Don't slouch! Bad posture so often accompanies loose, comfortable, casual looking clothes. Your leadership must show in the way you stand or your entire appearance will be slouchy instead of carefree.

THE TWELVE PERSONALITY TYPES IN DRESS

THE SOPHISTICATED TYPE Ninon de L'Enclos, social leader of Paris and friend of the greatest wits and poets of France in the 17th century, whose distinguishing characteristic was neither beauty nor wit but perfect evenness of temperament, is the most vivid example of this type. The hair arrangement named after her attests to the charm and simplicity she desired. The sophisticate is the woman of the world, dressed to show her taste, her superior reserve, her brilliance.

If you are supremely sure of yourself and always know your mind, if you can simulate perfect proportions of figure whether you actually have them or not, if you can carry yourself with distinction and poise, you can show the sophistication and the worldly wisdom that is yours.

If you want to seem really smart, really discriminating, use nothing to excess. Perfection, moderation and smart simplicity should be your by-words. From the close-fitting dashing hats you wear, to your handmade shoes, every line of your costume should mean just what it says, and say just what you mean it to say. You may choose novelty textures in materials for your clothes because they are different and because you want the tailored, long diagonals of your dresses and suits to need no extra ornament. The beauty of materials you select for your costumes must be sufficient. Even your lingerie should be quite tailored, beautifully made, it must not be too romantic nor yet too severe. Sheer hose and handmade shoes aid your type. Black and white is the favored color combination. When you desire more color in your clothes, the color schemes should be subtle and different. Keep your jewelry in gorgeous settings, and keep the patterns modern. The jewels for you may not be many but they should be the best.

A subtle gardenia, an unrecognizable perfume blended for you alone so it is noticeable on you only at odd moments, will give you an elusive, distant aura. Although you may love flowers, the usual run of corsage would appear blatant and ordinary on you. The very rare green-white orchid will become you at times, but you wear it only when it is supremely right with your costume.

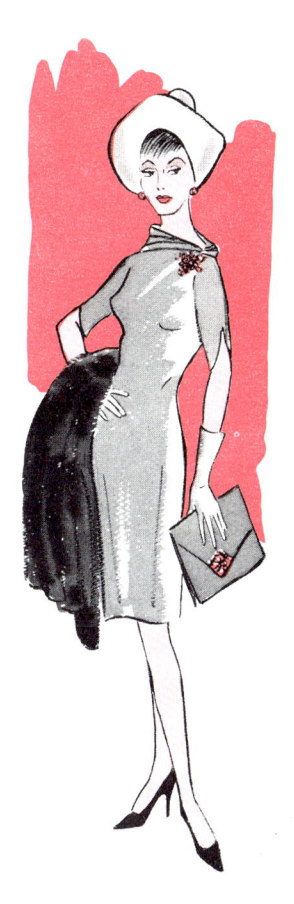

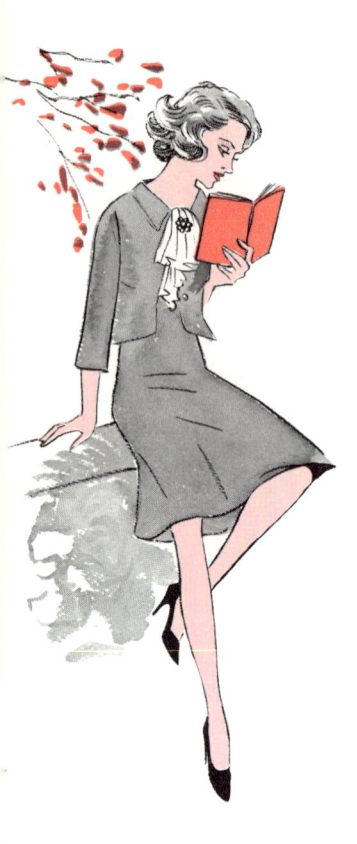

THE INTELLECTUAL TYPE To Sappho, that great poetess of ancient Greece, that intellectual, attractive, famous, individual and distinctive character, goes the honor of immortalizing the intellectual type. Her Greek garments were always beautiful in their fluid line. Simplicity, harmony and moderation were her watchwords.

If you are studious and love the romance of history, if you find happiness in viewing great creations of art, if you enjoy the study of foreign culture, if you are intelligent, critical, appreciative of the creative and very individual, you want your clothes to express your intellect. You will probably love harmony in everything, in music, art, literature, in your clothes, in their line and color scheme. You will like costumes that are artistic, clothes that you feel are personal. Your gowns may have little regard for the latest quirks of fashion. They may not be "stylish," but they should give *you* style, for they should be eminently a part of you.

Choose your costumes because of their beauty of line, because of their becomingness to your personality. They should be timeless, as you are timeless, as art is timeless. Dinner gowns that adapt themselves readily to long straight lines classical in their simple severity, are good for you. Crepes and velvets that fall in gracious folds, in grayed, subtle colors, should be your choice. Your lingerie should be pearly white, simple and aesthetic in its severity. Your hosiery and shoes should be in perfect harmony with your gowns. Your jewelry should be beautifully set, really antique or foreign. The ageless chypre odor is best for your perfume, and your most flattering flower is the classic yellow rose.

THE YOUNG MATRON The Madonna, as painted by any of the old masters, the young mother with a soft expression on her face, a sweet smile on her lips, dressed in the fashionable clothes of her period, is the best example of this type. If you are young and interesting, but a little more gentle, a little more kind than the women of the other types, if you are not too romantic or too much taken up with cultural activities or too dressy; if you are sensible, interested in your home, your husband, and your children, you are the perfect young matron.

You should dress with a *tendency* toward any specific personality type that might be yours, but with a softness that makes your personality less emphatic than that of other straight types. In keeping with the dignity of your position in your home, in keeping with the duties of young motherhood, you must be smart, comfortable, and not "flip."

Becoming hats that suit the occasion, *print dresses* which you can wear all day on shopping trips, to a matinee, to dinner and for an evening at bridge or the theater are especially good for you. Evening clothes and sport clothes you may have, but you will especially enjoy "all-day" dresses. Your lingerie should be slightly lacy and very pretty. Your hose must be right for each occasion and gown. Your shoes should be for the time of day that they are to be worn. You may like seasonal clothes, darker for the cold months and lighter for the warm, and you should wear shades that suit your personal coloring. Usually women of this type like warm colors. You will like costume jewelry, necklaces and bracelets to go with each costume. Your perfume should be sweet and just a little spicy. Your typical flower is the American Beauty rose for you resemble it.

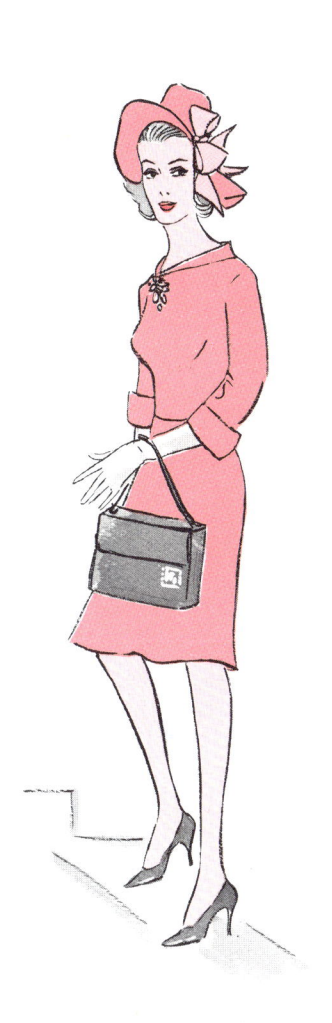

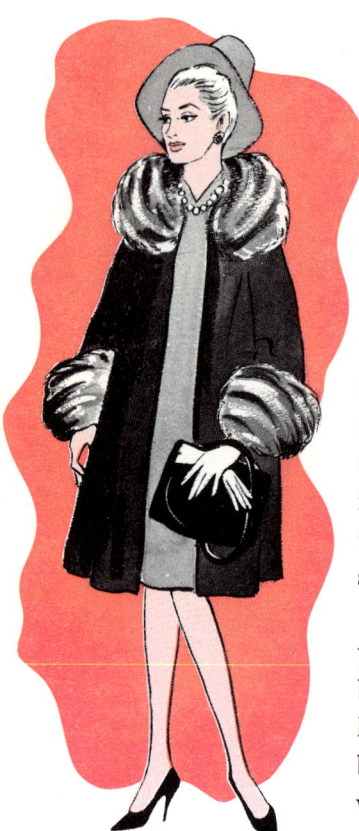

THE MATRON—THE QUEENLY WOMAN Picture Queen Victoria in her prime, dignified, proper, maternal and wifely, the head of her household, beloved of her people, and you have pictured an ideal matron.

The older woman who is charming and beautiful in her proper clothing, no matter what her figure or her age, has style and distinction beyond that of the youthful smartness of the very young. All through history, age has been woman's bugaboo. How she hates to grow old! Yet each age has its beauties. Every stage of life, from childhood to old age, has special advantages that the others lack. If you realize that the added years are making you more charming with experience, more perceptive and more gracious, you will never feel passé, you will never fear growing older. You will wear the clothes that show your poise, your queenly grace and superior understanding.

If you are over 50, you can no longer wear the very youthful and extreme fashions you may have indulged in before, no matter how good your figure. You must choose hats that are not too extreme, hats that flatter the face and bring it smooth, unworried dignity. Your smart, well-cut, well-fitted dresses must be made of quiet, dignified materials which will stand wear. They will not be dresses to be worn a time or two and then discarded. Wastefulness and changeableness should not be for you. Your dress lines, mixed diagonals and straight, will add elegance to your figure, which is no doubt topped by gray or silver hair. Your lingerie, hose and shoes should be fitted for comfort, and pleasure. They should not be varied to follow fashion whims. Old-fashioned, personal jewelry which brings pleasant memories as you don each piece is best for you. Your clean, sweet lavender or floral perfumes tell of the gentle understanding you have learned through the years. *Your* flowers, the violets, are royal purple, the color of the queen; it is *your* color, too, for you reign in the hearts of all who know you.

THE TWELVE PERSONALITY TYPES IN DRESS

THE AMERICAN GIRL TYPE Eve, Adam's companion, sweetheart, wife and the mother of his children, unabashed, unafraid, curious and feminine, equally at home dressed in a fig leaf or in dresses spun, woven and fitted by her own hands, not very tall nor very short, not very thin nor very stout, Eve, the mother of us all, typifies the personality of this type. The American girl type is not *extra*-ordinarily exotic or voluptuous, but she is a mixture of all the other types.

If you are of medium height and build, if you lay no claims to being terribly strong in any of the other types mentioned, if you like business, romance, athletics, intellectual pursuits and motherhood all equally well, you are of this type. You probably enjoy your life immensely and live it gaily. You know that if you want to get a position and hold it, you must dress well. You know the importance of clothes. You know what apparel suits you best and you make every effort to get it.

Your clothes should be smart and useful. You should be able to wear your daytime frock out to dinner and to bridge by changing your hat and shoes. You should be able to wear your formal gown to a dinner party by wearing a jacket over it, and then go on to a dance where you take the jacket off. Your hats must be of smart colors that will go with *several* outfits. Your clothes may be of any color, but you should think of ensembles when you get them and stick to colors that are harmonious together. You don't need very many shoes. Instead, you should select street, sports and evening shoes which will go with several ensembles. Your dresses must be seasonal. The materials you use for them should be warm and wooly for winter, cool and crisp for summer. Your clothes should be styled for the occasions on which you will wear them. And you must have working clothes, sport clothes and evening clothes. Your lingerie, for ordinary use, should be easily washable, for you must *like* to be immaculate. You may have some lacy and extravagant pieces for evening wear, but you probably will not wear very many underthings.

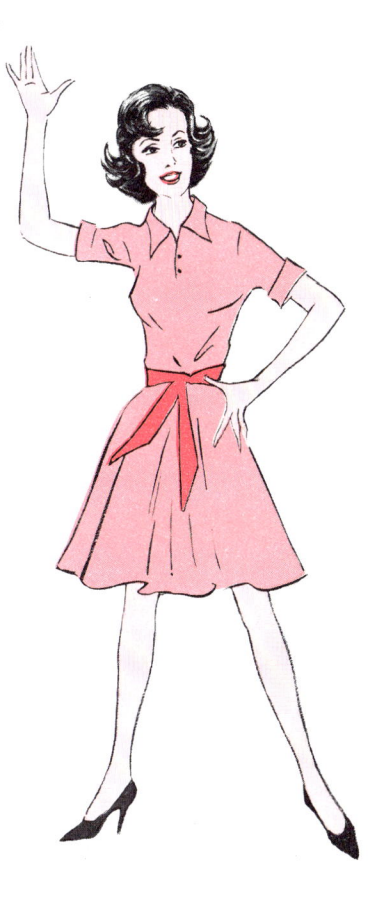

You may wear any kind of jewelry, just as you may wear any type of dress that is not too extreme. Your hose should be suitable for the occasion. They should not be too sheer, for you must get service from them. You will like rare perfumes, and will often select those which are really a little too exotic for you. But they will give you the sense of worldly sophistication that you sometimes desire. Your sweethearts will probably send you gardenias when you go to a dance. They symbolize romance to you, and as such, they will suit you perfectly.

You, the American girl type, set the fashions in America. It is for your comments that the manufacturers have their ears to the ground. The clothes you like and will buy are the clothes they wish to make.

CHAPTER 19

FRAGRANCE

Introduction

Perfume has a magic way of completing your personality and adding the final dainty touch to your grooming. What perfume to choose? That's easy. Select only those that you really like. Experiment by trying the samples at the toilet-goods counters. Put them on your skin so that you will know how they react with your body chemistry. A first love in the bottle might turn out to be a lu-lu on your skin. Buy small bottles and then use them. Don't save your perfume for some vague, special occasion.

WHERE TO APPLY

Rub it on your shoulders, in the bend of your elbows, in the deep V of your blouse. The warmth of your skin will cause the aura of your perfume to float about you—oh, so subtly. Keep a vial in your bag so that you can renew its witchery away from home.

There are three concentrations of perfume and you should learn to use them all. *Lightest is cologne*—wonderful as an all-over body rub. It can be sprayed on, or rubbed on in the form of a "stick." These cooling fragrances are wonderful for warm weather. *Toilet water is stronger.* Spray it on your lingerie or use it as a refresher on your throat and palms. Finally, there is the enchanting concentrate, *perfume,* most potent and lasting of all.

Christian Dior has said, "Femininity is inconceivable without the association of fragrance. When I recall a charming woman, her fragrance is an inseparable part of the memory."

WHICH IS YOUR TYPE?

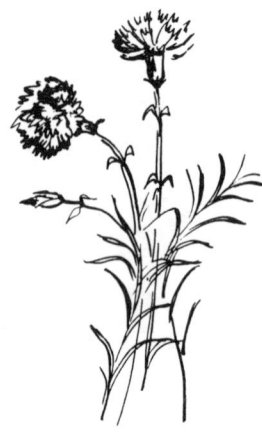

FLOWER FRAGRANCE This is the scent of one flower only. It is charming and appropriate in the spring and summertime. Seems best suited to the "feminine" personality.

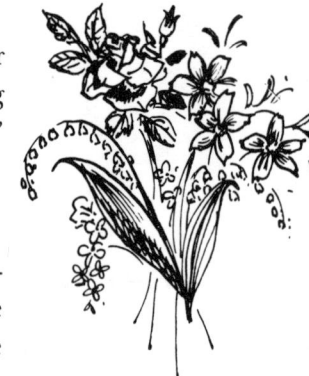

BOUQUET FRAGRANCE The flower bouquets in general have a wearability that's hard to equal. They are year-rounders, never-failers, like pearls. There's one blended, undoubtedly, just for you.

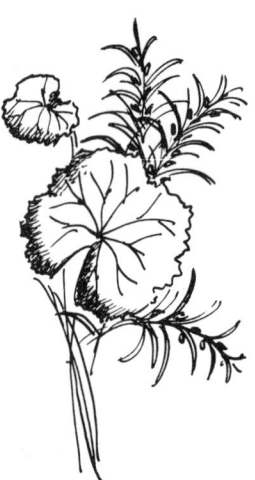

WOODSY FRAGRANCE Some of the most well-liked, best-selling perfumes in America are woods, leaves, grass blends. Wonderful for the out-door, all-around good sport type.

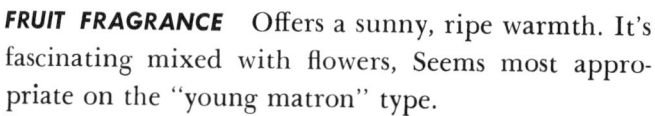

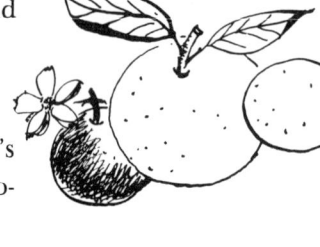

FRUIT FRAGRANCE Offers a sunny, ripe warmth. It's fascinating mixed with flowers, Seems most appropriate on the "young matron" type.

SPICE FRAGRANCE Is intended to awaken the senses. It is sharp and clean-cut. Probably a favorite of several personality types for daytime wear. If anything it seems youthful and alive.

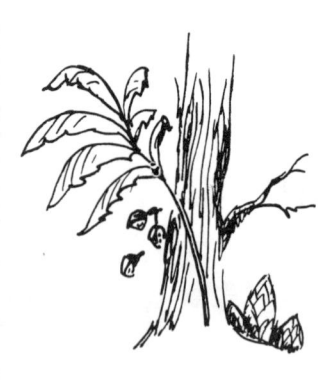

ORIENTAL FRAGRANCE Not for children. It is sultry and clinging. Wonderful for after-five wear on the sophisticated, voluptuous and exotic types.

MODERN FRAGRANCE Is concocted of just the right ingredients to give it a special brand of "chic." Obviously, intended for the busy "modern" woman.

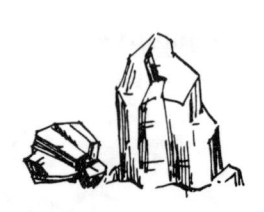

HAVE YOUR SCENTS MAKE SENSE

You are now aware that some perfumes should not be worn to work. Just as you change from day dress to date dress when the evening shadows fall, so should you change your perfume. In fact, the best sense perfume can make is that it be worn when, where and on whom it will be appropriate and enchanting. Here are five suggestions:

1. Take lots of time in selecting the proper scent. Put it on your skin and wait a few minutes to give your own skin chemistry a chance to react with the perfume, then you'll be able to honestly judge.
2. Wear a single scent and carry it through from bath oil to cologne.
3. Change your perfume from daytime to date time. Some scents are too cloying for business wear.
4. Collect a wardrobe of scents to fit the mood, the season and the "types" you want to be.
5. Perfume evaporates, so once you have opened the bottle, use it or re-seal with paraffin.

UNIT FOUR

PERSONALITY DEVELOPMENT

Introduction

Acquiring the knack of getting along with people with ease and assurance is a valuable asset for anyone. For you who are studying for a career, it is a must. Your very livelihood is dependent upon the good human relations you can develop with your co-workers and boss.

It is encouraging to know that all of the traits of personality that make for good human relations can be developed. You simply have to know what they are and apply them in your contacts. Applying the personality traits that don't ruffle others will open the doors of opportunity both socially and vocationally.

The goal of this unit of study is to acquaint you with the personality characteristics that are essential to success. It is designed to give you an insight into your own personality shortcomings so that you can work toward overcoming any traits that might stand as a barrier to your success.

Although everyone does have a personality, it may not be the positive, pleasant variety that arouses love, gathers friends and writes contracts. It may be a negative, ineffectual personality that actually hinders the individual's progress toward his chosen goals. Personality can best be measured by its ability to influence others, and by its ability to open the doors of opportunity.

It is encouraging to know that all of us are striving for the satisfaction of certain basic needs and no matter how far we may have missed the goal of acquiring friends, of finding love, of being happy, we are not alone. Struggling with us are countless others who have not recognized, acquired, and used the keys of personality that open the lid to the Treasure Chest of Golden Opportunity.

You can use the keys to gain: More friends
Enthusiasm for Life
Peace of Mind
Business Success
Greater Accomplishments

CHAPTER 20

PERSONALITY IS PREFERRED

Introduction

Human beings are social animals. They must feel needed, wanted, accepted. They are miserable when they feel rejected and unloved. This applies to you, to me, to your neighbor next door, to the man you wish to have for a boss. You are living in a world populated with people who desire the warmth of your friendship, the gladness of your smile, the strength of your approval. How simple it is to get along with others when you apply a twist to the Golden Rule. Not, "Do unto others as you would have them do unto you," but "Do unto others as they would like you to do."

This calls for a policy of live and let live. It requires a quality of "empathy"—the ability for you to put yourself in the other fellows shoes and to feel as he feels so that you can act and react in a manner that will fill his basic need for being approved, loved and recognized.

THE SCIENTIFIC APPROACH TO PERSONALITY

It was not until recently that Man turned the search-light of the scientific method upon his own behavior. He has come up with a great deal of helpful material on what people like, want and need. He has been able to devise tests that assist in showing you how you appear to others, how you respond to them, what your abilities, aptitudes and attitudes are. These tests can be useful in pointing out personality traits, a knowledge, which when applied, will guide you along the road to your personal Shangri-La.

It is essential that you take heart in the fact that your attitudes can be changed, that your abilities can be developed.

MAKING FRIENDS

Psychologists have made a complete scientific study of nearly one hundred traits and habits that will cause others to like or dislike you. Only those traits that could be changed by will-power were included. During the study, it was discovered that there were certain traits that had definite importance in determining the favorable or unfavorable attitude of people toward us.

It was found that clothes can be flashy or conservative, it makes no difference to your friends, but they would like to see you neat and clean. Forty-eight traits that at first seemed to be really important were found to have little value. On the other hand, there were approximately forty-one traits or actions that did affect how people react to you. Some of these were more important than others so they were divided into three separate groups with a *high, medium* and *low rating*.

THE THREE MAJOR TRAIT AREAS

How to reduce your friction with others to a minimum and how to increase your popularity to a maximum, is here set forth in a set of Do's and Don'ts. The first group of nine has been given a rating of *"high,"* the second group of twelve a rating of *"medium,"* and the third group of twenty a rating of *"low."*

THE TOP NINE TRAITS

(Do's and Don'ts)

A kindly, helpful attitude is a great asset. This trait has been listed as one of the nine most important.

ONE—GO OUT OF YOUR WAY TO HELP OTHER PEOPLE

As one gentleman in a position of prominence advised, "Be kind, friendly and helpful to everyone, even the seemingly unimportant. You never know when your own destiny may lay in his hands."

Until you build the habit of helpfulness, it may be a motivation to remind yourself of the many fortunes that have been left to those who were helpful. You might make a game of wondering and dreaming of all the wonderful things that could happen if you would just take a moment to help that old lady across the street. But far beyond all your dreams, you are actually transforming your personality into a powerful force for the realization of the best within you. So, "Any good that I can do, let me do it now for I will not pass this way again."

TWO—BE DEPENDABLE IN DOING WHAT YOU SAY YOU WILL DO

How your friends love to feel that you are an extension of themselves and that if they ask you to do something you will do it. They also want to feel that if you say that you will do this or that it is as good as done.

No matter how unimportant a promise may seem to you, it is your sacred trust. Besides, the carrying out of the promise will build a mental and moral fiber that will bridge the gap between you and success. It pays to be reliable.

THREE—BE TOLERANT, DO NOT CRITICIZE PEOPLE FOR DOING THINGS YOU DISLIKE

Everyone seems to find criticism hard to take. You will win more friends and make less enemies if you will try to accept others as you find them.

It's true that some people do things of which you disapprove. Fortunately, we do not all like the same things. It has been said that, *"prejudice is being down on what you're not up on."*

FOUR—DO NOT ATTEMPT TO DOMINATE PEOPLE

No one likes to feel that his judgment is so poor and his ability so nil that he must always be told what to do and how to do it. If you attempt to dominate another's actions without regard to his wishes, your attitude is one of dictatorship. It will cause friction in the home and failure in business.

There are always two sides to every disagreement. The pleasure of maturity is the challenge of shaping environment whenever possible and adjusting whenever necessary.

One man divided women into three categories: those who wouldn't say it (the dominated type); those who do say it, and how! (the domineering type); and those who say it and then ask your opinion (the cooperative type).

If your aggressive tendencies sometimes place you in the position of wanting to manage people, fine. It's an important executive trait when used with tact and discretion.

FIVE—DON'T SHOW OFF YOUR KNOWLEDGE

Speaking of tact, people will love you if you will make them seem important. They may admire you for your education and erudition, but they will not love you. It is better to be loved than admired.

Important people are called upon to instruct and this requires superior knowledge, but this knowledge can be conveyed without snobbery. The person who makes much to-do about his education and knowledge is probably using it to cover up a deep-seated feeling of inferiority in other fields. He needs your sympathy.

SIX—DO NOT ACT AND FEEL AS IF YOU ARE SUPERIOR TO YOUR ASSOCIATES

And what about the person who is a personification of perfection in her grooming, speech, and habits? The one who never lets you forget how superior she really is? Is she too hiding behind this facade of perfection with strong feelings of failure? The facts would indicate that she is. She is seeking the approval of her perfection rather than of herself and unfortunately her attitude will lead to a lonely isle. *It's hard on the neck to always be looking "up" at someone. Frankly, they give a pain in the neck.*

If God blessed you with superior abilities, the integration of your personality requires a constructive use of these abilities. They will be as apparent as the first robin of spring. You won't have to broadcast them.

SEVEN—BE HONEST, DO NOT EXAGGERATE IN YOUR STATEMENTS

You have probably heard the parable of the young boy who was tending the sheep and cried, "Wolf, wolf," at which the townsmen ran to help him, but there were no wolves? He did it so many times that finally when the wolves really did come and he called for help, no one came to his aid. This is just about what happens to people who continually exaggerate.

Be careful, you too may call, "Wolf," and no one will come to your aid.

EIGHT—DO NOT BE SARCASTIC

Your personal relationships will have much smoother sailing if you will develop the ability to sense the moods of people around you. There are times when a witty answer will bring gales of laughter, just be sure you can take it as well as dish it out, for sarcasm is resented.

Webster's definition: "to tear flesh like dogs, bite the lips in rage, speak bitterly; a keen or bitter taunt; a cutting gibe or rebuke. Criticism, attack, or reproach of an ironical nature." Not a pleasant word, sarcasm.

NINE—DO NOT MAKE FUN OF PEOPLE

To err is human but the human ego resents being ridiculed. Maybe because it is already painfully aware of its shortcomings. There is nothing that will demoralize us quicker than being laughed at. It makes us feel inferior. It makes us so humiliated and angry that we are sometimes slow to forgive our tormentor.

If you laugh at people behind their backs, you have used a two-edged sword to cut off your friends and make enemies. Put your words through a sieve, are they kind, are they true, are they necessary.

DEVELOP A POSITIVE SLANT

You have just finished reading the nine most important traits. You undoubtedly noticed that most of them are Don'ts rather than Do's. To give a more positive slant to what you have just learned, sit down right now and write up a list of things you can do to gain more friends. For examples:

1. Tell a friend how much you like her new dress.
2. Ask a neighbor about his summer vacation.
3. Ask a member of the family if you can help with something specific, such as washing the dishes.
4. Always leave others with a pleasant word.
5. Keep the promises you have made.

You can think of many more to add to the list. Go over the nine traits again, ask your friends which traits they think you need to develop, what habits you need to overcome. Your instructor may be able to help you see yourself objectively too.

Don't be embarrassed by constructive criticism, if anyone was perfect she'd probably sprout wings and fly out the window.

THE MIDDLE TWELVE

1. Keep your clothing neat and clean.
2. Do not laugh at the mistakes of others.
3. Do not be bold and nervy.
4. Do not pry into other people's business.
5. Do not take a vulgar attitude toward the opposite sex.
6. Do not tell a joke at the expense of those listening.
7. Do not find fault with people.
8. Do not try to have your own way.
9. Do not talk continually.
10. Do not lose your temper.
11. Do not start an argument.
12. Smile pleasantly.

People who are mature and who have good mental health have a good relationship with themselves, with other people and with the demands of life. They have an easy-going attitude towards themselves as well as others. They expect to like and trust others, and take it for granted that others will like and trust them. They feel a sense of responsibility to their neighbors and fellow men. They are able to consider the interests of others. They respect the many differences they find in people. They do not push people around, nor do they allow themselves to be pushed around. They get satisfaction from the simple, everyday pleasures.

THE LOW TWENTY

These are less important.
1. Do not keep up your end of the conversation by asking questions.
2. Do not ask favors of others.
3. Do not be out of patience with modern ideas.
4. Do not be a flatterer.
5. Do not talk about your personal troubles.
6. Do not spread gossip.
7. Do not be dignified.
8. Be cheerful.
9. Be enthusiastic.
10. Do not mispronounce words.
11. Do not be suspicious that people are trying to put something over on you.
12. Do not be lazy.
13. Do not borrow things.
14. Do not tell people what their moral duty is.
15. Do not correct the mistakes of others.
16. Do not tell people what is right and wrong.
17. Do not try to get people to believe as you do.
18. Do not be a political radical.
19. Do not talk rapidly.
20. Do not laugh loudly.

KEEP THE COMMANDMENTS OF FRIEND-MAKING

This is the end of the Do's and Don'ts for personality development in this particular lesson. You might think of them as a sort of set of commandments for social and business success. For you to break these commandments, the result is the loss of friends, popularity and income. For you to keep the commandments for friend-making, the result is increased social and business success.

Cultivation of the habits of behavior that will enrich our own lives and increase the happiness of others is a worthwhile goal. It has been the beginning of success for many. It can be for you!

How wonderful it is to know it is possible to overcome negative traits and to improve positive ones. This knowledge alone should help you to determine to radiate cheer, charm, consideration and cooperativeness.

HERE IS AN OVERALL TEST OF YOUR FRIEND-MAKING SKILL

Most persons realize that their ability to make and hold friends has a great deal to do with their success.

Now and then, therefore, it is good to check up to see how you rate in your friend-making skill, and this simple test will tell you.

Place check mark in the proper column, A, B, or C, according to your honest answer to the questions. "A" stands for "seldom or never"; "B" for "occasionally"; "C" for "frequently or always." Rate yourself, then consult the scoring key that follows.

	A	B	C
1. Do you remember anniversaries or special days on which others like to be remembered?	....	....	....
2. Do you avoid the use of sarcasm or anything which will rub others the wrong way?	....	....	....
3. Do you avoid saying things about others which you wouldn't say in their presence?	....	....	....
4. When you make a promise, are you careful about living up to it?	....	....	....
5. Even in an argument, do you keep your temper under control?	....	....	....
6. If you like your friend's possessions, do you tell him about it?	....	....	....
7. Do you pick out the good points in people and generally advertise them to others?	....	....	....
8. Are you patient and tolerant with people who do not agree with your point of view?	....	....	....
9. Do you avoid arguments if possible?	....	....	....
10. Would you grant a favor, even if in so doing you would be slightly inconvenienced?	....	....	....

KEY If you have at least 5 check marks in the "C" column, you are safe; if 5 or more in the "A" column you had better get busy and start working seriously at the job of making friends.

INCREASING YOUR FRIEND-MAKING SKILL

Most of the good work in the world is done by people who have discovered themselves and their own unique abilities. You may not be able to offer your friends sumptuous suppers or "mink vests" but you can offer them the best of what you have.

In just being yourself you will draw others to you by the strength of your magnetism which has been set free from the shackles of pretence. You will have others return time and time again to drink from your fountain of wisdom and wit and to dine at your table of sincere interest. You don't have to wait until tomorrow when you can buy a new dress or get a larger apartment. The time is now! Check this list to see what you can do in the next five minutes to increase your friend-making skill.

1. Call a friend you haven't seen for "ages."
2. Call a person you know has been disappointed or bereaved recently.
3. Get that "thank you," "get well," "birthday," "remembrance" card in the mail.
4. Ask a friend to help you with a project you know he will enjoy.
5. Tell that acquaintance how much you appreciate her thoughtfulness—any thoughtfulness.
6. Make a three by five file of cards listing your friend's:
    a) Birthday
    b) Anniversary
    c) Favorite Food
    d) Preference in Entertainment
    e) Hobbies
    f) Things that you have done together, that might be conversational material the next time you meet.
7. Try to make amends for any hard feelings that exist between yourself and someone else.

Your friendliness may not always meet with a positive response, and it is not important that everyone should always like you. It is important, however, that you cultivate the social habits that will put you in good stead upon every occasion. The following seven keys to popularity will serve as an excellent guide.

SEVEN KEYS TO POPULARITY FOR WOMEN

1. SMILE! SMILE! SMILE!

Encourage others with your friendliness. They may need encouragement too.

2. BE NATURAL

You can be loved and admired for your weaknesses as well as for your strength. Let others know how superbly human you really are.

3. BE FEMININE

Be the woman you were meant to be. Let your words and actions proclaim your ability to complement all that is masculine. Men will adore and women will emulate.

4. MAKE THE MOST OF ALL THAT WAS GIVEN YOU

Poise is the possession of the woman who achieves it by concentrating on others. She is devoid of self-consciousness because she knows she looks her best, she has made certain she feels her best and she has taken time to fill her mental cupboard with delectable tidbits to share with others.

5. BE INTERESTING BY BEING INTERESTED

The world is so full of new and exciting things that if you are in a rut of boredom you have only yourself to blame. If your days have become a round of routine it is probably your fate to be thought of as a dull and routine person. Adding new interests will multiply your enthusiasm, subtract your dissatisfaction, and divide your drudgery.

6. BE ENTHUSIASTIC

Life attracts life. Your enthusiasm will go out from you in ever widening circles to enchant those who come within its seductive power. Enliven your relationships by bringing fresh fuel to the fire. If your social contacts have grown stale, introduce new and fascinating subjects. Plan new activities. Create an atmosphere of merriment. The unexpected can be amusing. Dress your days with gaiety so that later when you take them out of the closet of memories you can say, "This one was fun to wear."

7. BE OPTIMISTIC

You only have to look at a small lichen clinging to a precipice to realize that life goes on under the most difficult circumstances. Everywhere you can see the marvelous manifestations of life's goodness and abundance. There is enough love, beauty, harmony, for everyone. If you cut your finger, immediately all the forces of your body are brought into action to heal your finger and make it well again. Mother Nature has given you many defenses against the onslaughts of outrageous fortune. She is not discouraged. She never says, "What's the use." She obeys the laws of her being and is ever optimistic. We should not be less. To abandon ourselves to hopelessness is going against all the rules of Life.

SEVEN KEYS TO POPULARITY FOR MEN

1. BE FRIENDLY

Encourage others with your friendliness. They need a lift too and will return your warmth.

2. BE NATURAL, BE YOURSELF

Don't try to affect someone else's personality. Be yourself, in this way you will be different and admired for your strength and forgiven for most weaknesses. No one is infallible.

3. MAKE THE MOST OF YOUR GOD-GIVEN QUALITIES

Take care of your body. Watch your grooming. Strive to become a qualified person. Be aware of what's going on in the world. Achieve self-confidence by knowing what to do, how to do it and then doing it.

4. BE ENTHUSIASTIC

Let people know that you like your work. Let them know that you enjoy working and dealing with them. Enthusiasm is magnetic, it attracts life. It will enhance your social contacts as well as your business dealings.

5. BE INTERESTING AND BE INTERESTED

Let people hear something of what you know and have experienced. Ask about what you don't know. Investigate new activities to eliminate boredom and routine. Rearrange your daily routine now and then by eating in a new restaurant or buying a new brand of shaving cream.

6. BE SINCERE

Let your handshake say "I like you." Smile only if you mean it, but learn to mean it more often. Say "Thank you" because you mean it, not just to be polite.

7. BE OPTIMISTIC

Life in its most basic form never gives up. It overcomes every conceivable obstacle to strive for more and better things, for a better way. Don't anticipate adversity, the world is your oyster if you look at the good side. The time to be concerned is when things go wrong.

THE CORNERSTONES OF SUCCESS

There are four cornerstones upon which a man may build his pyramid of success. These are:

1. *Good manners* as shown in his consideration for everyone, especially for women.
2. *Good grooming* as displayed in the cleanliness of his person and his clothes.
3. *Good speech* as demonstrated by correct grammar and an adequate vocabulary.
4. *Good work* as achieved through industriousness and knowledge.

CHAPTER 21

THE ART OF GRACIOUSNESS

Introduction

There are many ways of doing, of believing, of seeing. The person who is gracious is able to respect the many differences that she finds in people. She is able to admit that the new way may be a better way than the old. She knows that if she closes her eyes to the viewpoint of others she may be limiting her vision.

A STORY TO ILLUSTRATE LIMITED VISION

Four people were in a barn and each one had a knothole to look through. One looked to the east, one to the west, one to the south, and one to the north. The person looking to the east saw the sun come up and said, *"The whole world is nothing but sunrises."*

The person looking to the west said, *"You are wrong, the whole world is nothing but sunsets."*

The person to the north who could see nothing but a haystack said, *"You are both wrong, the entire world is nothing but hay."*

The fourth person looking to the south said, *"I can't understand how all of you can be so stupid. The world is nothing but bales of straw."*

From his own viewpoint, each was right. But, obviously, each one's viewpoint was limited by the size of the knothole through which he was looking.

Get on top of the barn, look in all directions, learn to know that your ideas may be right, but this does not necessarily make the other fellow's wrong. He may be seeing the same wide, wonderful world through a different knothole.

BE PERSUASIVE

The person who is able to get along well with others is the one who has discovered that his way of looking at things is *only one way*.

Those who go through life happily, with success opening new doors for them, are persuasive. Rather than argue with others, the persuasive man or woman leads others to his way of thinking. How persuasive are you? Check now.

HOW PERSUASIVE ARE YOU?

Circle the number found in the appropriate column for each of the following questions.

	Always	Sometimes	Never
1. Do you ask the opinion of others before stating your own?	10	5	0
2. When a member of a group, do you listen more than talk?	10	5	0
3. Do you accompany your speech with pleasant facial expressions?	10	5	0
4. Do you express a contrary opinion with the feelings of the other person uppermost in your mind?	10	5	0
5. Are you more interested in a wholesome compromise than in forcing your point of view?	10	5	0
6. Do you enjoy arguments?	0	5	10
7. Do you use a simple vocabulary so that your listeners understand you easily?	10	5	0
8. Do you become so excited that you interrupt others when they are in the midst of explaining an idea?	0	5	10
9. Is your voice persuasively modulated?	10	5	0
10. Do you use the "you" attitude in putting your ideas across rather than emphasizing "I"?	10	5	0
11. Do you drop ideas in conversation when you see they discomfort others?	10	5	0
12. Are you called upon to smooth out different points of view that arise at home or work?	10	5	0
Total			

Total the circled figures in each column and then add up your totals from all three columns; 60 is an excellent score; 45 is average.

Perhaps the foregoing test has shown you to be a pacifist, or, on the other hand, it may have shown you to be too argumentative. The affable person is one who is able to see the other fellow's viewpoint.

Don't put faith in others liking you, put your faith in your liking them. Your relationship with others will be more likely to succeed if your manner and words speak of your acceptance of them no matter how different their religion, political views or opinions.

GRACIOUSNESS AND MANNERS

Graciousness is the mark of the relaxed personality. It is the quality that invites others to share in our equanimity. Psychologists have proven that there is a technique for getting along with others that can be learned and perfected. Consequently, we should strive to make this technique an integral part of our personality.

It is important to learn the techniques of social custom so that you will be welcomed at home, in the office, in society generally. All of us want to be liked and accepted. It is as natural for us to want to please others as it is for us to want shelter. Moreover, we must develop satisfying social relationships in order to develop a well integrated personality.

You cannot look at someone and tell whether he is honest, considerate, or cooperative. Such characteristics are observable only through prolonged contact. A person's knowledge of social usage or lack of it is readily apparent. A casual meeting may condition your attitude toward him and in like manner his attitude toward you. Surface evidences of culture are not lightly regarded.

We are aware that our knowledge of how to act in social situations is one of the determining factors in people's reactions to us. We must decide now to make our "manners" an automatic part of our social repertoire so that they become an unconscious ally in our design to win friends.

It is not to be assumed that knowing the rules of etiquette is the most important characteristic of a man or a woman. Qualities of considerateness, integrity, fair play, and willingness to cooperate are valued characteristics. It should not be forgotten, however, that the rules of social usage are built upon these foundations. A truly well-bred person would never hesitate to break a rule of etiquette rather than hurt another.

INTRODUCTIONS

The following suggestions are designed to put you at your ease when called upon to introduce one person to another. Simply reading about it will not help, however. You should practice until the accepted forms come automatically when needed.

Introducing people to one another places social intercourse upon a more friendly basis. There are, principally, three kinds of introductions: introductions between two people of the same sex, introductions between two people of the opposite sex, and introductions of an individual to a group.

1. INTRODUCING TWO PEOPLE OF THE SAME SEX

When introducing two people of the same sex, you use the older or more prominent person's name first. (Mention the name of the person to whom deference is being shown.)

Example: *"Mrs. Smith, may I introduce Miss Jones?"*
or *"Mrs. Fifty-seven, may I introduce Mrs. Twenty-five?"*
"Mother, I'd like you to meet my roommate, Sally Brown."

When two people are of approximately the same age, rank, and degree of distinction, the order of introductions is a matter of choice. A great many women would probably prefer that you ignore their extra years and put them on the same level with the younger women.

2. INTRODUCING TWO PEOPLE OF THE OPPOSITE SEX

When introducing two people of the opposite sex, you use the woman's name first, except in the case of a person of distinction.

Example: *"Mrs. Brown, may I introduce Mr. Gregory?"*
or for very informal occasions, you might say:

"Joan, this is Bob Hackett who is a senior at the U this year. (Turning to Bob.) This is Joan Black, Bob."

If you wished to honor a man because of his age, rank, or distinction, you might choose to say:

"Mr. Distinction, may I introduce Betty Roberts?"

This would be a rare exception.

3. INTRODUCING AN INDIVIDUAL TO A GROUP

When introducing a person to a group, do so in the order in which they are sitting or standing, and for the sake of simplicity mention the newcomer's name first.

Example: *"Mr. Brown, I should like you to meet Miss Smith, Miss Burgess, Mr. Brewster, Miss Grey, Mrs. Grey."*

All the men will stand and shake hands as they are introduced. The women may remain seated. Each will say, "How do you do?" as his name is mentioned.

A woman rises for an introduction when the introduction is made by or to an older woman. This matter of an "older" woman is a rather delicate one and should be handled with tact. A hostess does, of course, rise to greet her guests. She should also shake hands with each guest, both men and women.

THE HANDSHAKE

A handshake is an expression of friendliness, it tells the other person that you are really glad to see him. Strive for a happy medium between a vise-like grip and a dead-fish grip. Your handshake is as expressive of your personality as your clothes and your speech.

THE ART OF GRACIOUSNESS

And, if you are wearing gloves, my lady, would you remove them before shaking hands? *No, a woman may shake hands with her glove on.* However, because gloves are for street wear, they are removed as soon as you come indoors.

These are other occasions when handshaking is necessary:

1. Whenever anyone extends his hand to you. If you are a young woman, you would wait for an older woman to extend her hand to you.
2. When men are introduced to one another. Even in a group a man will shake hands with each man to whom he is introduced unless it is most awkward for him to do so.
3. A woman may shake hands with a woman her own age, with a man to whom she is introduced as she chooses. It is the woman who takes the initiative in handshaking when men and women are introduced.

DESIGNATING RELATIONSHIPS

It is necessary to designate your relative's relationship to you by stating it in the introduction, such as; mother, brother, father, sister, aunt, uncle, cousin, etc. However, a gentleman is not a "boy friend" and is not considered a special person with a special name until he becomes a "fiance." This word is used by the boy and the girl and is pronounced the same way for both. The only difference is that "fiancee" has two E's for the feminine gender.

ACKNOWLEDGING AN INTRODUCTION

There is only one accepted way to acknowledge an introduction and that is, "How do you do?" Because it might help to remember the name if you repeat it, you might say, "How do you do, Miss New Acquaintance?"

Exception: Very informal occasion, you might say, "Hi."

FORMALITY AND INFORMALITY

The formality of the occasion would have some bearing on the type of introduction you choose.

Most formal: May I present? "Madam President, may I present the new Chairman, Miss Newcomer?"

Usual form: May I introduce? "Mary Jones, may I introduce Sally Smith?"

Informal: This is. Such as, "May Goodman, this is Jane Lake."

Informal: Just the names with a pause between. "May Goodman, Jane Lake."

WHEN TO MAKE INTRODUCTIONS

When are introductions necessary? A well-bred person would rather make unnecessary introductions than offend someone by not introducing him. The principal point is that everyone should be made to feel a welcome part of the group. Therefore, you should always introduce:

1. Members of any small group.
2. All guests to the guest of honor.
3. All guests at a house party.
4. Friends at a dance who come up to speak to you.
5. All players in a game involving a few players.
6. Dinner partners.
7. Your partner to the host and hostess who have included him on your invitation.
8. Any guest whom you bring into your home, to all other members of the family.

It is not necessary to make introductions on the street. If a person knows your companion and comes up to talk with her, you should walk on a few steps and wait. However, if the third person is invited to join you, then your companion should introduce her to you.

What would you do if you were not introduced? You have no doubt experienced the embarrassment of not knowing a person in your group. The logical thing to do is ask your partner or someone else whom you know to introduce you. If, by any chance, you find yourself with a stranger with no one to introduce you, it is proper for you to introduce yourself: "I'm Jane Doe. I don't believe we have met."

REMEMBERING NAMES

It is not necessary for you to meet everyone at a large private gathering. In fact, you would never be able to remember everyone's name. Which brings us to the question, "What do you do when you forget the name of someone?" If there is no time to ask a third person the name, you will just have to say, "I'm sorry, but I just can't remember your name at the moment." An experienced person will supply his name without having to be asked when he sees your hesitation.

REMEMBERING NAMES THROUGH USE AND ASSOCIATION It has been said that one good way to remember names is to associate the name with something. There is no magical formula for remembering names, but because it is important, you should have a genuine desire and the willingness to try. It may help to:

1. Repeat the person's name in your acknowledgement.
2. Ask him to spell it if it is unusual.
3. Get some facts about the person so that when you see him again, he is a personality as well as a name.

You will want to compliment others by being certain that you are pronouncing their name correctly. If it is a difficult name you might go over it several times until you are sure.

THE ART OF GRACIOUSNESS

ADDITIONAL HINTS ON GOOD MANNERS

1. An invitation in the third person is answered in the third person.
   Invitation: "Mr. and Mrs. Albert J. Smith request—"
   Response: "Miss Sally Smith is happy to accept—"
2. Special kindnesses require a "thank you" note. Thank you notes should be sent to those who:
   1. Send wedding presents.
   2. Send flowers or other "get-well" gifts.
   3. Send cards or flowers in time of bereavement.
   4. Do special favors for you.
3. Acceptance of a weekend invitation demands acceptance of the living pattern of your hostess. She will think you most gracious if you bring her some small, well chosen gift.
4. As a guest you have the responsibility for your own good time and for the good time of the other guests also. It is imperative that you fit in.
5. When making introductions, it is helpful to give a conversation lead, so that the persons being introduced will have a common meeting ground.
   "Mr. Smith, May I introduce Mr. Blank who also works in radio?"
6. When asked to go out on a "date" it is perfectly proper for you to ask the time, the place and the clothing appropriate to wear.
7. You may ask a gentleman whom you have just met to share some activity with you even though he has never asked you for a date. For instance, you might say, "We are having a group in for coffee after church next Sunday. I'd love to have you come. I'd like your opinion of my apple pie."
8. When answering the telephone use your best telephonic manner. Let the other person know who you are—in the beginning, it will save a lot of embarrassment. *Example:*

   John: "Hello, is Mary there?"
   Mary: "Yes, this is she."
   John: "Oh, hello, this is John Smith calling."
   Mary: "Hello, John."
   John: "I'd like to invite you to go with me to the football game next Saturday."
   Mary: "It sounds like fun. Let's see, is the kick-off at one o'clock?"
   John: "That's right. I'll pick you up at 11:30 and then we'll have plenty of time to get parked and in our seats before the game starts. Will that be all right with you?"
   Mary: "That will be fine. I'll bring a blanket if you like."
   John: "O.K., that's swell. See you Saturday at 11:30. Goodbye."
   Mary: "Goodbye."

GOOD MANNERS QUIZ

With a piece of paper, cover the True or False answer and explanation at the end of each statement. Don't refer to it until you have encircled either the "T" or "F" at the right-hand side of the page.

INTRODUCTIONS Circle One

1. A much older person's name is usually used first in introduction.   T   F

   TRUE. To use the older person's name first shows respect.

2. When two women are introduced to one another, the married woman's name is used first.   T   F

   TRUE. Women might resent having age as the determining factor. It is proper to use the married woman's name first even though she may be somewhat younger than the single woman.

3. Women always remain seated for introductions.   T   F

   FALSE. Women usually remain seated for introductions, but they would stand in the presence of a much older woman or when being introduced to a guest of honor.

4. A woman must remove her right glove before shaking hands.   T   F

   FALSE. A woman may shake hands with her glove on.

5. In a private gathering, it is considered bad manners for a woman to speak with a man without an introduction.   T   F

   FALSE. A private roof over the heads of those present allows a woman to speak with anyone present. A man, on the other hand, would be wise to have a third person introduce him before attempting to carry on a conversation.

6. A person's title is always used in an introduction.   T   F

   TRUE. Not only is a person's title always used in an introduction, but a person's relationship to you is also mentioned. Thus, Doctor Brown, your father is introduced, "Father, I'd like you to meet Jim Cook. Jim, this is my father, Doctor Brown."

7. When standing in line to buy tickets at a theater, social courtesy demands that you introduce your partner to friends of yours who happen to be standing near you.   T   F

   FALSE. We do not make introductions in a public place. The lucky girl can keep the fellow all to herself or vice versa.

THE ART OF GRACIOUSNESS

8. If you ask an acquaintance whom you just happen to meet to join your party, then you must make introductions.   T   F

   TRUE. All members of any small gathering are introduced to one another.

9. In a place of business, a customer is either a "lady" or a "gentleman."   T   F

   TRUE. The customer is referred to in this way. For instance, "The lady (or gentleman) who called is here to see you now."
   When speaking directly to the customer, the receptionist would say, "Madam (or Sir), you may come in now."

10. If you have been introduced to someone but have momentarily forgotten their name, you may ask them to repeat it for you again.   T   F

    TRUE. You would say something like, "I seem to have forgotten your name, would you mind spelling it for me?"

INVITATIONS

11. A written invitation must be answered even if there is no RSVP on it.   T   F

    FALSE. If a reply is necessary, the invitation will have RSVP.

12. A written invitation demands a written response, not a telephoned one.   T   F

    TRUE. Unless, of course, the invitation gives a telephone number and requests that you call in your reply.

13. You should wait until three days before the event before sending your reply.   T   F

    FALSE. You should respond almost immediately so that preparations can be made for the number of people who will attend.

14. The reply to an invitation in the third person is made in the third person.   T   F

    TRUE. An invitation in the third person should be answered in the third person; however, formality in these matters is becoming a part of the past. If in doubt, refer to a good etiquette book or do what your heart dictates.

15. Don't issue an invitation to anyone and then let him pay the check.   T   F

    TRUE. It is assumed that if you issue an invitation, it will be at your expense.

16. Women are considered forward when they issue an invitation to a man by telephone.   T   F

    FALSE. A woman may invite a man to any special event. She should, of course, pay his way. By keeping in mind that she is robbing the male of his customary role, she will do everything possible to avoid embarrassing him. She should, if possible, arrange to take care of the financial obligation in advance.

    Girls who occasionally arrange parties, get-togethers, tickets for two or an evening at home with the family are going to be involved in more activities with the opposite sex than those who don't.

WEEKEND GUESTS

17. Etiquette demands that you give your weekend hostess a gift.   T   F

    TRUE. You may either bring a small, inexpensive gift or send it after you leave. It may be something personal for the hostess if you know her very well or it may be a gift for the household to use and enjoy. Potted plants, candy, note paper, large ash trays, cocktail napkins, monogrammed match books, a memo pad for the telephone are all welcome gifts.

18. If you are having a good time, it is proper for you to stay longer than you were invited.   T   F

    FALSE. As soon as the time comes when you should depart, do so.

19. You must fit in with the routine of the family no matter how much it may displease you.   T   F

    TRUE. It is up to guests to adjust to the routine of the family with whom they are staying.

20. If you are the hostess, plan something for your guests to do every minute.   T   F

    FALSE. Although a hostess will plan a number of interesting activities for her guests, she will leave them time to do what they would like to do, even if it is just to sleep late.

21. If you are a guest, expect to be entertained all through your stay.   T   F

    FALSE. It is a guest's reponsibility to entertain as well as be entertained.

THE ART OF GRACIOUSNESS

22. If your hostess has no maid, don't embarrass her by offering to help.   T F

    FALSE. An extra person is always more work, do your share by keeping your bedroom and bathroom neat and clean and by offering to help wherever you can.

23. Use your host's telephone to call home long-distance so your family won't worry.   T F

    FALSE. If possible go to a pay telephone or, if you must call on your host's telephone, call collect. Tell him in advance what you are going to do.

PARTIES

24. Take off your wraps before joining the other guests.   T F

    TRUE. Remove your wraps as soon as you possibly can.

25. Greet your hostess before you greet other guests.   T F
    TRUE. She is the one you seek out first thing.

26. An hour is usually long enough to stay at a tea or reception.   T F

    TRUE. Pay your respects, have refreshments and leave.

27. It is considered good manners to arrive twenty minutes late.   T F

    FALSE. Arrive on time, or better yet, a few minutes early.

28. Show a talented guest you appreciate him by asking him to perform.   T F

    FALSE. He will undoubtedly volunteer to perform if he wishes to do so.

29. If there is a celebrity present, treat him with special courtesy.   T F

    FALSE. Everyone should be treated with courtesy, a celebrity no more so than others.

30. If you are dressed informally at a formal party, go home and change.   T F

    FALSE. Make the best of the situation and for the future, learn to ask what type of clothes would be appropriate.

31. Plan to make a few new friends.   T F

    TRUE. It is a guest's responsibility to mingle and have a good time, not to crouch in a corner and wait to be noticed.

32. Talk only to the people you know or who have been introduced.   T F

   FALSE. At a private party, try to talk with everyone if the gathering is small, and with a few new people if the gathering is large.

33. You will be considered shy if you don't interrupt the conversation of the group you join.   T F

   FALSE. Don't interrupt the conversation. Wait for a break and then join.

DINING OUT

34. On a double date, the girls sit on the same side of the booth.   T F

   FALSE. On a double date, the girls sit on the inside and the boys on the outside of the booth.

35. You should help the waitress by stacking your own dishes when you have finished eating.   T F

   FALSE. The less you move the dishes and silverware, the better.

36. An exclusive restaurant demands better than usual good manners.   T F

   FALSE. Good manners are advocated wherever you may be.

37. A male escort precedes his date to the table.   T F

   FALSE. He does so only if there is no head waiter to lead the way and if the room is crowded.

38. Women should take their coats off after they are seated, not before.   T F

   FALSE. A woman should remove her coat before being seated even though she does not check it.

39. When lunching with a group of girls it is better to ask for individual checks.   T F

   TRUE. Then there will be no mix-up about who owes what.

40. If you don't know what a foreign dish is, ask the waitress.   T F

   TRUE. No one is so widely traveled and so well-read that they know everything.

41. "Table hopping" is taboo.   T F

   TRUE. All the gentlemen will have to stand and their food will get cold.

THE ART OF GRACIOUSNESS

42. If you sneeze or must blow your nose at the table, you apologize.   T   F

    TRUE. You would do this only in an emergency; otherwise, you would leave the table.

43. If you spill something on the person sitting next to you, you must help clean it off.   T   F

    FALSE. A lady would offer her napkin and apologize. A gentleman would ask for a waitress to help and would, of course, apologize.

44. It is permissible to put one's elbows on the table while eating.   T   F

    FALSE. It is permissible, however, to put one's elbows on the table before and after eating and between courses if so doing facilitates conversation.

45. It is permissible to ask your escort to indicate approximately how much you should spend for dinner.   T   F

    TRUE. A woman tries to spend only as much as her escort has planned to spend and she will carry on a conversation with him about what his suggestions are, how hungry he is and this sort of thing to get a hint about how much to spend.

46. If you get up from the table during the meal, you should refold your napkin and place it on the table.   T   F

    FALSE. You may place it on the table, but you do not refold it. There are two rules concerning leaving the table before the meal is finished. One says to place the napkin on the table, the other says, "Do not place a soiled napkin on the table until everyone has finished eating and is ready to leave, place it on your chair."

47. If you are not sure how to eat a particular food, you should ask.   T   F

    TRUE. You may ask or you may observe those around you to see how they are eating. Strange foods can be interesting if you don't panic at the sight of them.

48. Ice cream may be licked off the spoon.   T   F

    FALSE. All food, including ice cream, should be removed from the spoon each time it is brought to the mouth. This means that you have only enough for one mouthful (bite-size) each time.

TIPPING

49. It is not necessary to tip the maid in a powder room unless she performs a special service for you.   T F

    TRUE. Some exclusive clubs may have a powder room attendant who will expect a tip no matter what, but on the whole, you tip for service.

50. In a restaurant where the tables are covered with a table cloth, the minimum tip per person would be about 25¢.   T F

    TRUE. The usual tip is about 15% of the bill, but if the bill is small, the tip will be proportionally larger.

51. Railroads have tipping laws. You tip the redcap about 25¢ per piece of luggage.   T F

    TRUE. Redcaps are tipped according to the amounts posted in the station.

52. A 10¢ tip to a cab driver is never acceptable.   T F

    FALSE. In some communities cab drivers do not expect a tip, in most large cities, they do. A ten cent tip is enough for a 35¢ ride.

53. You must tip a bellboy for carrying your bags to your room.   T F

    TRUE. About 25¢ for medium and small bags and more if they are large and heavy.

54. You tip a doorman who gets you a cab on a rainy day.   T F

    TRUE. You would tip from 25¢ to 50¢ and if you have to think twice about parting with this money, what are you doing where there is a doorman?

55. Usually chambermaids do not expect to be tipped for their services.   T F

    TRUE. Although again it will depend upon where you are staying. Some hotels expect you to tip and leave a dish on the dresser for this purpose.

56. You tip an airline hostess.   T F

    FALSE. You do not tip airline hostesses.

57. A checkroom attendant receives a tip when you pick up wraps.   T F

    TRUE. Usually 25¢ per person.

58. You must tip a bellboy who performs a special service.   T F

    TRUE. You would tip a bellboy for bringing a telegram to your room or for performing other services.

THE ART OF GRACIOUSNESS

FOR GENTLEMEN ONLY

59. A man always removes his hat in an elevator.   T   F

    FALSE. It might take up too much room in a crowded elevator. He would tip his hat to ladies he knows however.

60. A gentleman gets off a bus before his lady companion.   T   F

    TRUE. Whenever there is danger the man goes first. He would get off the bus in order to hold her hand to assist her.

61. A gentleman doesn't speak to a woman on the street with whom he is not acquainted.   T   F

    TRUE. He would not embarrass her by doing so.

62. On the street, a gentleman allows a woman to recognize him first.   T   F

    TRUE. A man waits for a woman to say hello or otherwise show recognition.

63. A gentleman does not go "dutch" treat.   T   F

    FALSE. "Dutch" treats are becoming more common now that women are earning money.

64. To show respect, a gentleman rises when an older person or a woman enters the room.   T   F

    TRUE. And he does not sit again until the other person is seated.

65. A man leads a woman across a crowded room.   T   F

    TRUE. He makes way for her.

66. A man returns his dance partner to the side of the floor or to her escort, he doesn't leave her "stranded."   T   F

    TRUE. He needn't feel embarrassed by leaving her once he has fulfilled this obligation.

67. A man should never ask his "date" if she wants to go to the powder room.   T   F

    FALSE. A gentleman should make sure that his lady companion knows where the powder room is and should make it easy for her by saying something like, "Would you like to powder your nose?"

68. A man says "thank you" after a date.   T   F

    TRUE. A man should say thank you and a woman should say how lovely the evening has been or make some remark about how much she has enjoyed herself.

69. A man allows all women waiting to precede him into an elevator. T F

    FALSE. In a business elevator, first come first served. If he is accompanied by a woman, he would allow her to enter first and would follow.

FOR LADIES ONLY

70. A lady never smokes on the street. T F

    TRUE. She never does.

71. In the business world, a woman should not expect all the usual male courtesies. T F

    TRUE. She should not expect *all* the usual courtesies but neither should she shed her femininity like a snake sheds its outgrown skin.

72. Don't offer to do something for someone unless you know it will be graciously received. T F

    FALSE. Do the nice things because you want to do them not because they may or may not be graciously received.

73. On a date, ask to be taken several places so you'll be "seen." T F

    FALSE. Let your escort plan the evening for you. If he asks for suggestions, try to think of something both of you will enjoy that will not deplete his pocketbook.

74. A lady never offers to pay for a man to go anywhere. T F

    FALSE. A lady may invite a man out for an evening, but she must handle the money situation with tact and diplomacy.

75. A lady is pleasant to everyone, even those who displease her. T F

    TRUE. A truly charming woman tries to smooth troubled waters, not aggravate them.

76. A lady never breaks a rule of etiquette even if it means offending someone. T F

    FALSE. Rules of etiquette are made to be broken if they are out-of-place.

77. A woman should be the first to recognize someone on the street. T F

    TRUE. She may speak with whomever she pleases and may acknowledge those she knows at her own discretion. No wonder some girls who act aloof never get asked out on a date.

78. Answer compliments with a simple, "Thank you."   T F

    TRUE. Do not be embarrassed by a compliment, a simple "Thank you" is all that is necessary.

79. Because you are a woman, you may silently accept little courtesies.   T F

    FALSE. Because you are a woman you may be shown little courtesies, but you should be grateful and say thank you.

80. In a public place, a lady avoids drawing attention to herself.   T F

    TRUE. She is appropriately clothed, she behaves with decorum and speaks in modulated tones.

CHAPTER 22

SOCIABILITY AND PERSONALITY MEASUREMENTS

Introduction

You must keep in mind that ten years from now some of the material discussed in this lesson may have been replaced by results from a more recent scientific study on personality.

The best psychological measuring today is being done in three broad kinds of dimensions or characteristics:
1. *Intelligence*
2. *Personality*
3. *Interests*

This lesson will encompass the last two, personality and interests. These are the two areas in which a person may, by effort, make striking advances.

On the other hand, psychologists have discovered that intelligence is largely innate. Consequently, this lesson will concentrate on personality traits and interests. These characteristics of personality are subject to change through environment, experience and motivation.

Part of the problem the psychologists confronted was just *what* to measure. You have measured your physical dimensions. You have driven past road signs that tell the measured distance to the next town. You have watched a butcher measuring the weight of a steak. But how many inches are there in your courage? How many miles is it to your secret hatred?

PERSONALITY MEASUREMENT

Personality characteristics have been harder to measure than intelligence. A search through a large dictionary will result in finding more than 4000 words in our language that are used to describe personality characteristics. It does not seem likely that there are this many *different* personality dimensions to be measured. Some of these must surely be getting at the same characteristic only in slightly different words.

In the pages to follow, we have listed seven (this is a coincidence, not a magic number) personality dimensions that the social scientists agree on most often in their research. Many months of work (especially during World War II and since), have gone into the job of boiling down the many possibilities, eliminating the duplication, and finding the most measurable of these. If you think of other personality traits that seem to be missing from this brief list, remember that either there may not be a reliable way to measure them yet or that these seven may well account for the other traits you have in mind.

SEVEN PERSONALITY DIMENSIONS

1. AGREEABLENESS—OBSTRUCTIVENESS

Personality traits are usually named by a hyphenated title like this in order to show both extremes of the characteristic. In this personality dimension we have at one end the characteristic of being agreeable, cooperative with others, participating with others in a good-natured and cheerful manner. At the other extreme we find the characteristic of being obstructive, critical of the work of others, spiteful, or "hard" in our dealings with others. Most people fall along the line somewhere between one extreme and the other. Which end are you closest to?

In evaluating or measuring yourself on this characteristic, think back over your past experience. Think of situations like this one:

You are at a meeting or a party and someone makes a suggestion about what the group should do. You think the suggestion needs some improvement. Do you agree to try the idea—or do you point out its weaknesses? Or do you do something in between these two choices?

2. DOMINANCE—SUBMISSION

Do you ever try to argue or bluff your way past a doorman? If someone borrows money from you and doesn't pay it back right way, do you ever ask them for it?

Do you ever complain to the waiter about bad food served you in a restaurant?

If you are more apt to answer yes to such questions, then you are toward the dominant end of this dimension. That is, you tend to publicly put yourself in a superior position to others. At the other end of the characteristic, of course, is the opposite behavior—being more apt to assume a modest, self-critical position, yielding to other persons publicly. As with all these personality characteristics, we are not attempting to say that one end is automatically better than the other. We are asking that you measure yourself as accurately as you can and consider your psychological measurements in terms of what you want to be successful.

3. PERSISTENCE—CHANGEABLENESS

You are close to the "persistent" end of this characteristic if you find that you are usually a determined person, stable and responsible, not often abandoning a task in the face of obstacles. You are closer to the other end if you are more changeable, impulsive and carefree, sometimes frivolous, and preferring to change tasks quite often.

4. SOCIABILITY—SHYNESS

This title just about describes itself. If you are not much of a "joiner," generally keep quiet and stay in the background at parties, then you are more toward the shy end of this trait. If you make new friends easily, join in the party, or can address large groups of people, then you are closer to the sociability side.

5. CALMNESS—EMOTIONALITY

Which list of descriptions below best fits you most of the time?

a) calm	b) emotional
placid	anxious
emotionally mature	childish
stable	worrying
not hysterical	touchy
not jumpy	lose head in excitement

Chances are that you would not claim all of the adjectives in either one list or the other, but you probably know which of these lists comes closest to describing this characteristic of your personality.

6. MASCULINITY—FEMININITY

Do you know some women who are more feminine than others—and some who are really quite masculine? And do you know some men who are rather feminine, yet others who are very masculine? In other words, it is possible for members of either sex to measure some distance from their own end on this personality dimension. Typical characteristics of people who are toward the masculine end are (1) likes to sell things, (2) very interested in athletics, (3) and having mechanical interests or hobbies. More characteristic of the feminine end are such habits as keeping (or kept) a diary, being frequently rather absent-minded, and enjoying music and literature.

7. ENTHUSIASM—SLOWNESS

This dimension has to do with how much energy you usually have and how quickly you spend it. Persons at the enthusiastic end of this are very energetic and are physically active. They have a lot of drive, push, and oomph. At the other extreme are those whose movements are more deliberate, slow, and even languid. This characteristic is not merely a matter of how much sleep you got the night before, but seems to be rather directly related to your physical structure.

A study of how body builds relate to the amount of energy or drive a person has reveals three distinct body types. These are:

Ectomorph—tall, slender, with a narrow chest. This person's energy might be compared with a race horse. He's fine for short spurts of work that require a quick expenditure of energy. He needs "refueling" often and doesn't gain weight easily. He is usually:

Soft spoken	A lover of privacy
Secretive	Sensitive
Self-conscious	Tense
Quick reacting	More likely to be introverted

Mesomorph—muscular, barrel chested, well-coordinated. This person might be compared with a work horse that can expend energy for a long period of time without tiring. He's good for the "long" haul and is often going strong when everyone around him is ready to take a rest. He is:

Competitive	Athletic—loves exercise and physical fitness
Aggressive	
Energetic	Daring—takes chances
Bold and adventurous	More likely to be extroverted

Endomorph—stocky, inclined to look rotund and is often overweight. This is the Shetland pony person. He is:

A lover of physical comfort
Sociable and amiable
Emotionally stable or seems to be
Slow to react
Even-tempered
Complacent and tolerant

You have been aware of your enthusiasm—slowness characteristic for about as long as you can remember. Now you have a reason.

It might be interesting for you to have your instructor and your friends help you decide into which category you fall. However, keep in mind that most persons are a mixture of two types. Very few are a "pure" type.

SOCIABILITY AND PERSONALITY MEASUREMENTS

CHART YOUR PERSONALITY DIMENSIONS

Did you notice that these seven personality dimensions did not overlap much with each other? They were rather independent of each other. To be high on one end of one of these characteristics did not automatically make you high or low on one of the others. Yet your particular *pattern* of combination of highs, lows, and mediums on these seven is of importance to your overall personality. In order to get a better picture of this pattern, psychologists often plot a person's measurements on a psychograph. You might try this yourself. Look at the following chart:

Agreeableness	_____ Obstructiveness
Dominance	_____ Submission
Persistence	_____ Changeableness
Sociability	_____ Shyness
Calmness	_____ Emotionality
Masculinity	_____ Femininity
Enthusiasm	_____ Slowness

INSTRUCTIONS:

Here are the seven characteristics represented as lines—as a measure of distance. Decide where you are along each line and put a small x on the line at the spot. If you then draw a line down across the chart from x to x, connecting them, then you have a rough idea of what psychologists would call your personality "profile." It shows your personality "strong points."

WHAT ARE YOUR INTERESTS

Your interests indicate the *direction* in which you would like to use your mental abilities and your personality characteristics. Most youngsters and adolescents have very changeable interests. It usually isn't until a person reaches the late teens or early twenties that he or she becomes more stable or set in their interests. By now you probably are interested in certain sorts of things and activities, and have settled on these as being most interesting to you. Some of the interests you had in childhood are gone, while other things have become more interesting to you. The interests you have now will probably stay with you for many years.

FIELDS OF INTEREST

Here again, of course, there are literally thousands of jobs, things, situations, etc., which a person could be interested in—just as there are thousands of words that describe personality traits. So there has been a scientific effort to reduce these many items of interests into certain areas or broad fields of interest. If we now take a look at the names of some of these fields, it may help you to see where *your* interests are in comparison to what other choices of interests are available. Dr. John French, a psychologist, has recently reported the collected results of all the scientific work being done on the measurement of interests, so it's his list that we shall examine.

1. **INTEREST IN ATHLETICS** which includes either liking to participate or liking to watch.

2. **INTEREST IN AESTHETICS** liking to do art work, music, poetry, etc., and/or appreciating the aesthetic work of others.

3. **INTEREST IN BUSINESS** preferring the world of finance and practical affairs. People who are strong in business interests are usually lacking in aesthetic interests, and vice versa.

4. **INTEREST IN CLERICAL WORK** liking for office work and the working conditions in offices.

5. **INTEREST IN FAMILY** liking the job of keeping one's family together and contented.

6. **INTEREST IN LINGUISTIC ACTIVITIES** liking to write and talk, and making a living at it.

7. **INTEREST IN PHILOSOPHY AND RELIGION** which includes being interested in, speculating on, the "why's" of life.

8. **INTEREST IN SCIENCE** liking the life of research and the study of the physical world.

9. **INTEREST IN SOCIAL WELFARE** wanting to do things to improve the happiness of others.

APPLY YOUR INTERESTS TO THE WORLD OF WORK

You can undoubtedly see how certain individuals have incorporated their interests into their vocation. For instance:

Interest in Athletics: professional athletes; physical education instructors; dancers; furniture movers.

Interest in Aesthetics: interior decorators; artists; dress designers; window display men; advertising executives.

Interest in Business: production managers; salesmen; corporation executives.

Interest in Clerical Work: secretaries; accountants; bookkeepers; office managers.

Interest in Family: housewives; home managers; servants.

Interest in Linguistic Activities: writers, public speakers; preachers, magazine and newspaper editors; English teachers.

Interest in Philosophy and Religion: clergymen; philosophy professors, missionaries; philosophical writers.

Interest in Science: engineers, science teachers; physicists; chemists; scientific research men; appliance repairmen.

Interest in Social Welfare: doctors; psychiatrists; welfare workers; nurses; hospital administrators.

DEVELOP YOUR INTERESTS

We have already mentioned that *interests* do not generally settle down to a steady pattern until a youngster reaches adulthood. Apparently they are greatly influenced by experience. Therefore, it is possible that new experiences can change them if a person really desires to.

This lesson should have been interesting to you. It is an exciting experience to better "know thyself"—even if what we discover does not always please us.

OVERCOMING HARMFUL PERSONALITY TRAITS

Benjamin Franklin conscientiously worked at improving his personality. He made up a weekly chart on which he would write the traits he wanted to overcome. Whenever he would fall back into his old, bad habit, he would put a check mark beside that trait on the day it happened. As he eliminated a harmful habit or attitude, he would write another in its place. In this way, he made himself into one of our greatest Americans.

His chart method might help you overcome your harmful personality traits. Right now, write down five traits or habits that you feel are holding you back from becoming the kind of person you want to be. Surely you can think of that many.

Traits to be overcome	Monday	Tuesday	Wednesday	Thursday	Friday	Saturday	Sunday

Now, just so you won't be discouraged. Underline ten of the following assets. Be sure to do this so that your picture of yourself will be a balanced one. So often we are willing to admit our weaknesses but not gracious enough to acknowledge our assets.

Dependable	Determined	Sense of humor	Good memory
Ambitious	Talk well	Imaginative	Forgiving
Kind	Thoughtful	Meet people easily	Well mannered
Initiative	Tactful	Sunny disposition	Sing
Generous	Punctual	Slow to anger	Dance
Cooperative	Tolerant	Well groomed	Play a musical instrument
			Good at sports

If you can't think of ten good traits from among the ones listed, ask your instructor, your friends and family to add to the list.

Your personality characteristics have probably been influenced quite a bit by the way in which you were brought up. Since they were learned, these personality traits can still be modified by learning. It was slow work learning what you now know and behaving the way you now behave. It will be slow work re-learning, changing your personality measurements. But you can do it by yourself if you are willing to devote the time to it. Make it a matter of problem solving by the direct approach. Decide what personality traits you need to succeed and then acquire them.

UNIT FIVE

YOUR VOICE AND YOU

Introduction

"How wonderful is the human voice. It is indeed the organ of the soul. The intellect of man sits enthroned, visibly, on his forehead and in his eye, and the heart of man is written on his countenance, but the soul reveals itself in the voice only."

So wrote the poet, Longfellow, whose opinion is substantiated by learned men past and present. One modern husband was asked to list, "What I like about my wife." He said that he would list the ideas as they occurred to him. First on his list was, of course, his wife's lovely, soft speaking voice.

If you are the one who, when in heaven, thought they said "roses" when they said "noses" and ordered a big red one; and when they said "ears," you thought they said "beers," and ordered two immense ones, take heart. Your voice can irresistibly draw others to you. It is your one feature that need never grow old. It is the part of your personality that can be developed beyond your wildest dreams.

With patience and practice you can develop the attractive voice quality, the good speech habits and the art of conversation that will put you in good stead on every social and business occasion.

Beyond this, voice confidence will open up a whole new world to you. How many times have you wanted to speak, to voice your opinion, to add your viewpoint but have been held back by fear? Perhaps there have been many occasions. If so, read through to Public Speaking and how to overcome stage fright. The world is your oyster when you speak well.

CHAPTER 23

VOICE IMPROVEMENT

Introduction

If you are a person with normal voice equipment, your voice can be trained and improved. The main essential in so doing, is to understand clearly the goals toward which you need to work and then to apply your energies toward reaching these goals by following an organized plan of study and to practice regularly and with enthusiasm. Developing the speaking voice is a gradual process involving the mastery of one phase of the subject at a time. If you attempt to correct every deficiency of voice in a short period of time, it will become so frustrating that success will be doubtful.

Obviously, the first essential in voice improvement is a rather objective evaluation of your voice as it now is. Remember that evaluation is not self-criticism, but a sensible cognizance of both the positive and the negative qualities of the voice. It is entirely possible that you do not know what kind of a voice you possess. If you have a recording machine available, it can be used to great advantage in making your personal analysis. A recording is revealing in that we do not generally recognize as our voice the sounds that come out of the mouth. We make sounds within the body cavities and these are sent directly to our auditory mechanism and these are "heard" by the speaker before the sounds actually reach the ears of the listener. Because of this, we are sometimes surprised at what we actually sound like to others. We generally imagine that our voices are lower and more resonant than they are. Such a recording will give you an accurate idea of how your voice sounds to other people.

ACHIEVING A SATISFACTORY SPEAKING VOICE

Most people want a satisfactory speaking voice. Because of this, they usually approach the problem with great enthusiasm. But you should keep in mind that the few weeks or months usually devoted to a beginning course in voice are all too short a time for you to realize your aims fully. Habits are difficult things to change and unfortunate voice habits that have been built up over a period of eighteen or twenty years cannot be replaced by better ones in a few short weeks. Such a course as is here proposed should give you a good start in the right direction and, with the knowledge and skill gained, your own interest and ambition should stimulate you to continue your personal development.

SETTING GOALS FOR VOICE IMPROVEMENT

1. Flexibility — By this we mean meeting any voice need readily and easily.
2. Vitality — This suggests a reserve strength under all situations.
3. Expressiveness — A voice capable of immediate response to all intellectual and emotional meanings.
4. Sincerity — A voice which reveals inner meanings without affectation or showiness.
5. Pleasantness — A voice that has a quality which attracts rather than repels the listener.
6. Intelligibility — A well-articulated voice having clear and acceptable diction.

YOUR VOICE IS YOU

What does *your* voice sound like? Does it radiate beauty from within you? Is your voice complementary to your physical beauty, good grooming and proper choice of clothing? Does your speech convey the real you?

There is very little that one can tell about a book by examining the cover. No matter how interesting a book may be, most of us never bother to open it unless the cover is eye-catching and attractive. Yet, even with an attractive cover, if the story and contents do not live up to our expectations, we cast the book aside. To make an analogy, we, like the book, must present an attractive exterior. We must be prepared to follow up this first impression with inward qualities that will create continued interest. We must always remember that there is no truer index of individual personality than the voice.

Speech communicates to everyone we meet what we really are. Every tone of a person's voice and every word she utters is a living comment on her personality and individual effectiveness. Try as she may, a woman cannot separate what she says from what she is. We have all heard the old saying,

"I cannot hear what you *say*, because what you *are* is ringing so loudly in my ears." So let us not imagine that what we are can be hidden from others. The minute we open our mouths to speak, the truth will be discovered.

Exactly what does our voice tell about our personalities? First of all, it tells the state of health. If a person is sickly and weak, the voice, too, will be frail and lacking in resonance and beauty. We can readily tell how one is feeling merely by the sound of her voice. We use a great deal of energy in good speech. When we do not feel well, we do not have sufficient energy to give to alive, attractive speech. Thus, the weak, thin quality is produced.

How about our philosophy of life? Have you ever tried to keep from expressing a deep conviction about some aspect of life or belief? It is difficult to convince anyone of something you do not believe yourself, and this lack of conviction shines through like a beacon piercing the darkness of a mountain peak.

What about emotions? Have you tried to keep anger out of your voice? You may deny that you are angry and publicly state that it really doesn't matter, but beware, your voice is giving you away. Observe someone who is fairly bursting with the joy of an occasion and you will readily detect that pleasant rapture of the voice. Greed, hate, envy, jealousy—name any you wish, and then try to conceal an emotion that you feel. The task is nearly impossible.

Have you ever seen a person who is to speak before a group of people? He approaches the podium with an air of utter confidence and poise. He stands relaxed and pleasant before the audience. But wait! As he starts to speak, he cannot hide the insecurity he is feeling inside. His voice comes in rasping, short phrases. He is experiencing stage fright and everyone is aware of it.

When you hear a gruff, rasping voice, don't you judge that person to be unsympathetic and perhaps even unkind? He might not be at all, but you have judged him so. You see, you have judged him by his voice.

DEVELOP YOUR MOST ATTRACTIVE VOICE

Just how important a role does a female's voice play in her success as a career woman. Although there may be some jobs that do not require the use of the voice very much, it's difficult to imagine a successful secretary, nurse or receptionist without an attractive voice and good speech habits. Certainly the supervisory and executive-type promotions will go to those who are prepared to use their voices effectively.

You may well ask what type of voice you should try to develop if you are going to perform more effectively as a person and as a career woman. There are several qualities that you should attempt to develop to be more effective in your habits of speech.

VOICE IMPROVEMENT

QUALITIES TO DEVELOP

1. A NATURAL, ATTRACTIVE PITCH

Above all, we must learn to be natural. We must be ourselves in the pitch of the voice. We can do no more to change the *basic* pitch of the voice than we could do to change the color of the eyes or the length of the fingers. It is determined anatomically, and we should avoid forcing it lower to "sound more sexy" or to strain it to be higher because we may feel we would sound more feminine. Lest there be some misunderstanding, it should be stated that we must not be content with the pitch of the voice, if it should be unattractive. We can do much to enhance the beauty of the basic pitch by correct breath control, resonance, and production of harmonic quality. But to abuse the voice by forcing and tension will eventually result in permanent damage to the vocal folds which cause the voice to break down in later life. So be yourself, be natural. The pitch most generally is very flattering to you without your doing anything to create unnatural conditions and make unreasonable demands upon it.

2. A MUSICAL QUALITY

Music in the voice is made with only eight (8) sounds. These are m, n, ing, and the vowel sounds. These sounds are the sustained sounds of the English language. They are, therefore, the ones which allow melody and song to be heard in speech. It is impossible to achieve music when saying the sound of "b" or "t" or "g" or any of the consonants for that matter. So become accustomed to giving the musical sounds a little greater emphasis and watch the gratifying results. You, too, will have a voice that is a delight to hear. You might use these sentences for practice:

The light is on.   The rug is brown.
The walls are gray.   The day is dark.

3. A FRIENDLY VOICE

Friendliness is achieved primarily through the medium of inflection of pitch. This variation conveys a feeling of well-being and wholesome interest on the part of the speaker. Note the difference in Good Morning and . . . Good Morning. We are too prone to speak along on the same old line of monotony, without variation of pitch and rate of speech. This renders friendliness practically impossible. Don't be afraid to let the voice become flexible and expressive. Change it as you speak and note, with satisfaction, the enthusiastic response it invokes from others. Then too, friendliness is catching, and the world becomes a nicer place when this attractive quality is spread to others.

4. A STRONG VOICE

By strength we do not mean volume. Strength is an inner reserve or vitality that can be brought into play if needed. It is a basic fiber which is capable of suggesting reserve strength under all situations. Proper volume will result from controlled strength. But volume by itself, and in and for itself, should be avoided. Speak up as if what you are to say is important. This strength will give you confidence that what you speak will be accepted as having been spoken with authority. For practice, repeat with authority, "move aside, please."

5. THE QUALITY OF SOFTNESS

This may seem, at first, to mean the opposite of strength. Nothing could be more erroneous. In softness, we do not sacrifice vitality, but we trim down the rough edges and the harshness to create a light, airy quality to voice. When we say, "I saw a lovely, white, fluffy cloud," make it sound white and fluffy. This is achieved by reducing the volume and letting the words flow out of the mouth, gently and softly. Try this one, "now is the time for us to go." Keep it up, it's fun.

6. A CLEAR, UNDERSTANDABLE VOICE

Nothing is so unnerving as to be forced to listen to a "mush-mouth" quality to speech. If it is worth saying at all, it is worth saying well. Make certain that the sounds are made properly and well. Let the tongue wag, the lips open and close freely, and the jaw move with freedom and ease. Attempt to remove any strain from the parts of the body which produce words and a clear, attractive voice will result. It is suggested that some of the tongue-twisters we said as children will assist us in speaking clearly and correctly. They give good practice in moving the articulators and "spitting out" the words. Remember that good voice is in vain, if the words cannot be understood. Watch how you say that word!

Here are some tongue-twisters for better articulation to make the voice more Clear and Understandable.

Rubber baby buggy bumpers.
Fuzzy wuzzy was a bear, fuzzy wuzzy had no hair,
    fuzzy wuzzy wasn't fuzzy, was he?
A big black bug bit a big black bear.
Many a wit is not a whit wittier than Whittier.

7. A FLOWING QUALITY

Don't speak in short sentences or phrases of mere words. Get into the habit of taking a deep breath and allowing the ideas to flow together to make attractive and complete thoughts. Just as a brook runs downward toward the river, so should speech flow from one phrase to another, with ease and beauty. Short, disjointed speech is unpleasant to hear, but the effect of flowing sentences and ideas is most gratifying.

A Flowing Quality comes from controlling the breath. Practice saying the longer and longer sentences of the story, "This is the House that Jack Built" until you can get through the eighth one without taking a breath.

This is the house that Jack built.

This is the malt that lay in the house that Jack built.

This is the rat that ate the malt that lay in the house that Jack built.

This is the cat that killed the rat that ate the malt that lay in the house that Jack built.

This is the dog that worried that cat that killed the rat that ate the malt that lay in the house that Jack built.

This is the cow with the crumpled horn that tossed the dog that worried the cat that killed the rat that ate the malt that lay in the house that Jack built.

This is the man all tattered and torn that kissed the maiden all forlorn that milked the cow with the crumpled horn that tossed the dog that worried the cat that killed the rat that ate the malt that lay in the house that Jack built.

This is the farmer who sowed the corn that fed the cock that crowed in the morn that waked the priest all shaven and shorn that married the man all tattered and torn that kissed the maiden all forlorn that milked the cow with the crumpled horn that tossed the dog that worried the cat that killed the rat that ate the malt that lay in the house that Jack built.

Remember that the voice is, in reality, a wind instrument. And just as there is a difference in Benny Goodman's clarinet playing and the noise of the little boy next door as he toots on his instrument, so is there a difference in effective speech and just plain, "devil-may-care" talking. The voice is a lovely thing to hear when it is played well. Master the techniques for so doing, and open the door to a more interesting, more gratifying life. Reveal to the world the person you know yourself to be. And remember always, *your voice is you!*

EXPRESSIONS TO BE AVOIDED

There are some types of expression which are to be avoided if we are to be accepted by people with whom we associate. There is no uniform classification of these objectionable terms, but most of them will be included in one of the following categories:

ARCHAIC WORDS Archaic words are those which are old-fashioned. They are not used in the language of our own time. You will still see them written in some forms of writing, but they are not now used.

Examples: Forsooth for indeed, thee for you, quoth for said.

PROVINCIALISMS OR LOCALISMS Provincialisms or localisms are words and expressions which are peculiar to a given locality. They are frequently not understood by people residing in other sections. These words, which you have frequently heard from your childhood and now use without thinking, are the most difficult to detect in your own language and generally very hard to correct. They may sometimes be used in speech, but they must be avoided in formal speech and in writing.

Examples: Plumb for entirely, chuck for throw, pack or tote for carry, carry for accompany, and reckon for think.

IDIOMATIC EXPRESSIONS Idiomatic expressions are those which are peculiar to a language, and often they are not governed by the rules of grammar. Because of this, it is difficult to translate them into another language. In spite of the fact that idioms defy the laws of grammar, they have, through long and tried usage, become firmly established as standard in the English language. There are still many "authorities" who would have us abandon our use of idiomatic expressions. We should not become so dependent upon them that we cannot speak correctly when called upon to do so. Nevertheless, many of our very best writers and speakers make frequent use of the idiom. It adds color and variety to our language.

Examples: Put up with, with a grain of salt, get rid of, in the long run, get into hot water.

VULGARISMS OR ILLITERACIES Vulgarisms or illiteracies are words and expressions which are characteristic of uneducated people. They are the most serious violations of good English. They are never correct in either formal or informal expression and should be carefully avoided at all times.

Examples: The use of the wrong case of personal pronouns, (Me and him went, Between you and I, A group of we neighbors), the confusion of the parts of the verb, (He begun, I have drank, He come early, I'll lay down soon, ask, busted, brung, etc.). Many common expressions, (them there, hain't, nowheres, borned, irregardless, ain't, you was).

IMPROPRIETIES Improprieties are good words that are used inappropriately in an incorrect meaning or in an incorrect function.

Examples: set for sit, leave for let, bad for sick, accept for except, most for almost, affect for effect.

COLLOQUIALISMS Colloquialisms are expressions which are correctly used in informal conversation and writing, but which are not generally acceptable in formal, literary style. Colloquial words are more homely and less dignified than proper English.

Examples: The contractions, (can't, don't, isn't, etc.) Abbreviations, (Jap, taxi, phone, auto, chum, O.K., spunk, newsy).

VOICE IMPROVEMENT

SLANG Slang is a most controversial form of speech. You will find that many of the best writers condemn it in formal use, yet they readily admit that it has a place in informal writing and conversation. Greenough and Kittredge have defined slang as "a peculiar kind of vagabond language always hanging on the outskirts of legitimate speech." Much slang was originally the secret speech of tramps, thieves and others of similar reputation. Today, it is at best a cheap substitute for good English. It conveys both laziness in thought and great poverty in vocabulary. Slang weakens one's ability to think clearly and express one's thoughts in concise, attractive language. If you value the power, charm and vigor of good language, you should avoid this weakening element in English.
Examples: swell, lousy, wow, flunk, hot stuff, washout, I guess.

HACKNEYED OR TRITE EXPRESSIONS Hackneyed or trite expressions are those which have been so overworked that they have lost their effectiveness. It is by no means easy to avoid such expressions and to substitute fresh and exciting new words. We are, however, tempted to use them too frequently and we become unimaginative and dull.
Examples: strong as a lion, pearls before swine, busy as a bee, green as grass, cold as ice, a bolt from the blue, crazy as a loon, fat as a pig, nick of time and many hundreds more. Many of them, right or wrong, are in common use today.

WORDS FREQUENTLY MISUSED

The use of the word *get* is frequently misunderstood. In a strict sense, it means to obtain. It might be better, therefore, to substitute another word when we mean "to become" such as, "If she doesn't come in out of the storm she will get sick." This is not, technically, a correct usage.

There are certain words which take the objective case *at all times.* Two of them are "except and between." Therefore, it is not correct to say, "No one listens to her except I," or "It's a matter between she and I."

The old question of "Who" and "Whom." There seems to be a movement underway to completely eliminate the use of "Whom." It will undoubtedly be much better for our language when this happens. In spite of this, we must live with "Whom" until this transition takes place. So when you need an object for a preposition, the proper form is still "Whom."
Example: "Whom are you going with"? or "By whom do you live"?

Remember that the word "neither" is singular and must take a singular verb. An expression such as "Neither of the girls are pretty," is incorrect. The singular verb "is" would be necessary.

A picture is hung, but a man is hanged. So let us never say "He was hung at dawn."

The use of "It is me" has now become accepted by many of the world's best speakers. It is still considered to be a gross violation of grammatical law, however. It is colloquial in nature, and must not, as yet, be used in formal use. The correct is still, "It is I."

In conclusion, since usage is constantly changing and it varies considerably among educated people according to age, locality and extent of their experience, there is still no *one* and only one correct set of rules for grammar.

PRONUNCIATION

There are some standards by which a person may govern his pronunciation:
1. Know the sounds in English, and learn to think of them in terms of their sound, and not by their spelling.
2. Attempt to avoid eccentricity and affectation in your pronunciation. Pronunciation varies a little with each individual. People, however, expect a familiar pattern from you.
3. Be consistent with your own practice of pronunciation. If you are in the habit of saying "deta" at one time and "data" at another, it will be confusing to those with whom you associate.

Become conscious of the manner in which you pronounce words. Eliminate habits of sloppiness in this essential part of speech. Do not run words together. Try not to use new words until you know what the accepted forms of pronunciation are. This will eliminate embarrassment on your part.

The pronunciations used by cultivated speakers are doubtless the best guide. This coupled with the use of a good dictionary should allow you to strike a happy medium for good pronunciation.

You, as a student, will find it both interesting and valuable to consult several books and journals in an effort to satisfy your own thinking on the rules of good grammar and pronunciation. There is no sure guide to correct English. Be alert to the changes and do not be dogmatic in your point of view. Work toward better and more effective usage and you will find yourself to be as acceptable as the next person.

VOICE IMPROVEMENT

HOW ARE THESE WORDS PRONOUNCED?

address	drama	Italian
agile	err	mischievous
bouquet	facet	municipal
chic	gala	often
corps	forbade	forehead
debut	grimace	perspiration
divan	harass	reputable
docile	idea	route

Look them up in the dictionary so you will be sure yourself. Add others to the list.

CHAPTER 24

CONVERSATIONAL CHARM

Introduction

One of the occasions when it is vital that we use good speech is in the art of conversation. It is also important to know something about what makes a conversation sparkle.

During your career, you will be called upon to carry on conversations every day both in your social activities and in your business life. It is imperative that you learn to do so with great skill and ease. Confidence and poise can be established only through the practice that makes conversational topics come automatically.

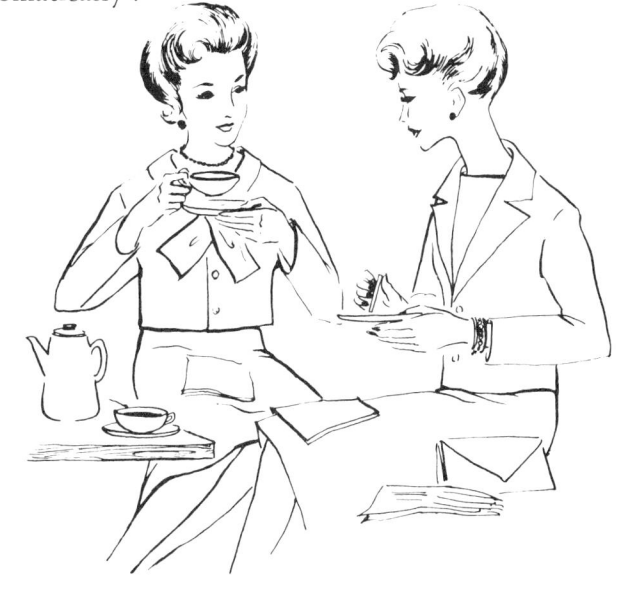

THE TEN COMMANDMENTS FOR CONVERSATIONAL CHARM

Sometimes it's most difficult to be charming, especially when others irritate us to the "nth" degree. What can we do about the other person's hostility? What can we do about his rebuffs and negative attitude? Well, it's not always possible to change another person, but it is possible for us to adjust so that the irritation and discord is lessened. You might even begin to enjoy someone whom you had formerly disliked if you understand his reasons for acting the way he does.

Many people unconsciously throw up barriers that irritate and annoy. Conversationally they unmeaningly hurt and offend. This is due to a lack of imagination. For one thing, they cannot put themselves in the place of their victim to see how what they say, sounds.

A young man said to an older gentleman, "Are you going to come with us?" And when the man replied that he was, the younger one stated, "Boy, we'll sure be crowded with seven in the car."

To the young man this was a statement of fact, but to the older man it implied that he was unwanted and would be in the way. Needless to say, it resulted in a rather unpleasant scene.

It would have been much better for the younger fellow who was driving the car to have said, "Fine, the more the merrier. I hope you won't be too uncomfortable with seven in the car." On the other hand, why should the older man have assumed that he was unwanted? They both lacked imagination. Our first commandment then is going to be:

ONE—TRY TO UNDERSTAND THE OTHER FELLOW'S VIEWPOINT

As Jack Webb says, "Get the facts. That's all I'm interested in is the facts."

Just a few of the barriers that people throw up include:

POSITIVENESS They are afraid that if they are not assertive what they say will not hold weight. This type of person will respond to your show of sympathy and respect. He will no longer need to be positive in his statements when you display esteem for his opinions.

VERBOSITY Some talk too much because they have been repressed. A sympathetic ear is so welcome that they just don't know when to stop. If you allow them to unwind a little they can be led to share the conversation rather than to monopolize it.

NERVOUS HABITS Annoying physical mannerisms can make you forget what the person is saying and close out the good that you might get from the conversation. Your making the person feel at home will diminish his nervousness and make him a more pleasant companion.

CONVERSATIONAL CHARM

ARGUMENTATIVENESS A person who has a chip on his shoulder and believes the world is against him has probably had experiences in his life that caused him to feel this way. You can successfully counteract his attacks by passive nonresistance. It is practically impossible to fight without an opponent.

"I" ATTITUDES Funny thing that this is only annoying when we find it in another person! It might be interesting to see how guilty we are ourselves. The conversationalist who has only her small, personal interests from which to draw conversation is bound to be boring. She needs to be encouraged to discuss events and ideas outside her own realm of experience.

You can have a gay time, if not listening to the conversation, figuring out what you can add that will give spice and zest. With a little pre-flight training, a few hours of practice and some solo flights, you will be able to soar through any evening with the greatest of ease. Keep conversation light, airy and effervescent.

TWO—FIT YOUR MOOD
TO THE MOOD OF THE OCCASION

The seasons change and so do people's moods. It would be a mistake to put the solemnity of a church in the raucousness of a circus tent. However, some people mistake seriousness for dignity. They are afraid to let their hair down and fit in.

A young woman was invited to meet her fiance's family and, wanting to make a good impression, she wore her best clothes, high heels and all, only to discover that the family was at a canyon picnic. What did she do? She took off her shoes and hose and joined in the baseball game. She made a hit too. If not with the ball, then with her young man's family. Today they are happily married. She knew how to fit in.

THREE—LEARN TO GUIDE THE CONVERSATION

You don't want to overestimate your importance to the conversation, neither do you want to underestimate it. It is quite possible with tact and discretion to change the conversation when it becomes sidetracked onto a subject that is depressing. Under no circumstance should you change the topic under discussion simply because it is of no interest to you. Gossip should be outlawed although human interest stories have their place in good conversation. Let us imagine that we are with a group of fuddy-duddies who insist on talking about their operations. How are we going to get them away from this subject and onto something more entertaining, educational and uplifting? You could, of course, simply say that you didn't want to hear about the operations; but this would bring a precipitation of wrath and silence. How much better to introduce a new subject in such a way that the others would come with you on your conversational train of thought and be glad to do so. You might say, "I have been waiting to tell you how well you look in that color, Grace. Is it a new dress?" Or, "All this talk reminds me of an article I read on emotional stress causing disease. Stress is something we can control. What do you think?"

Best of all, you can sincerely ask for their help. It may be that you need a new cake recipe or something of the kind. Many cosy evenings have been spent with a group, each one contributing his unique slant to one particular subject of interest to everyone present.

FOUR—DON'T BE SILENT

Social courtesy demands that if others are giving their opinions that you do also. If you do not join in, you will be thought stupid or stuck-up. Neither of these impressions will add to your popularity.

After one housewife had completed a charm course, her husband took her out for the evening with a group of friends they had known for a long time. This apt pupil had learned how to join in the conversation, for when the husband later met one of the men in the group, he said, "How come your wife has gotten so smart all of a sudden?" It really wasn't all of a sudden of course. She had simply uncovered opinions and let others see that here was a woman who was aware of the world around her.

FIVE—DON'T MONOPOLIZE THE CONVERSATION

Conversation means to talk with. It is never a monologue nor a lecture. It is a give and take of ideas where everyone benefits. If you are going to play the game well then you need the proper equipment.

1. *Ideas*—varied and interesting.
2. *A vocabulary*—with which to express your ideas.
3. *A modulated voice*—that colors your words to make them interesting.
4. *Diction*—that is clear and distinctive.

If you have the ball, toss it back to someone by asking a question. In this way even the very shy can be drawn out. They ofttimes have much to contribute if you can just get them to express themselves. You will learn only when you're listening.

SIX—USE SIMPLE LANGUAGE THAT ALL CAN UNDERSTAND

As has been said, conversation is to entertain, not to instruct. Your communication lines in conversation will be only as strong as your ability to make others understand what you say. Not that we mean to discourage the development of a large and adequate vocabulary. No, indeed, for only after you have many words at your disposal can you pick and choose to get just the proper shade and meaning. It is helpful to think of having not just one vocabulary, but four:

1. *For speaking.*   This one has the short, one syllable words.

2. *For writing.*   This one has descriptive words that will color experiences.
3. *For listening.*   A person must be able to understand what words someone is using or remain alone.
4. *For reading.*   This should include all the words in the English language so that an individual can gather to himself the wisdom of the ages.

SEVEN—FIND OUT HOW PEOPLE SPEND THEIR LEISURE

Leisure time is spent doing the things we like to do. We like to do these things because they interest us. We might compare conversation with a game of darts. The bull's eye is the center of the other person's interest. The closer we can come to this center, the more response we are going to get. We throw our dart in the form of a question and trust that it strikes home.

It is an advantage then for us to know some of the things people like to do with their leisure time. They like to:

Participate in sports	Belong to clubs
Have a cultural interest	Travel
Keep scrapbooks	Have a hobby
Go to plays and movies	Read books
Attend concerts and musical events	Collect stamps or other objects

By observation and questions you will be able to learn the burning interests of a conversational partner. Just as soon as you can get him talking about his favorite subject you can become the charming listener of whom it has so often been said, "My, she is the most interesting woman," or "He is the most interesting man." And all because you encouraged him to talk.

EIGHT—DON'T BECOME PERSONAL

People resent our prying into their private affairs. The questioning that you must do to draw out a person and find topics of conversation that will be interesting to both of you must be done on an impersonal basis. Rather than saying, "Where did you get that suit?" It would be better to say, "That's a lovely new suit. Don't you think the new fall Y line is better than Dior's H line?" Or, "I see you are wearing a new suit, I can recognize the Y line influence."

Rather than, "Where did you get that tan?" You might say, "It seems to me that the only way you could get such a tan this time of year would be for you to go skiing, did you?"

You will find an assignment at the end of the lesson asking you to reword a question three ways. It will pay you to do this with several questions so that you recognize the most tactful phrasing.

NINE—TALK ABOUT IDEAS RATHER THAN PEOPLE

There are three levels of conversation. One is ideas and it is the best one. It is the safest too unless you insist on talking about religion or politics. The second level is personalities. If you don't have something nice to say it will be better for you to remain silent. The third level is gossip and is small talk for small people. It should have no place in your conversations. It will act as a boomerang and will return to you the ill will that you send out.

What are some of the good topics involving ideas? You might discuss:

Science: What man has discovered and invented.
Literature: What man has written.
Philosophy: What man has been able to discern.
Art: What man has been able to create.

TEN—SELECT ENTERTAINING RATHER THAN ARGUMENTATIVE SUBJECTS

It has been said that every time a person wins an argument he loses. He loses his charm in his stubborn pride of being right. It is mentally rude to insist upon only one point of view. The error of arguing is worse than the error of judgment or belief that the other fellow holds. Besides, "Convince a man against his will and the man is of the same opinion still." How much better to learn the art of compromise. It affords a cultured individual the opportunity to show wisdom in meeting difficult situations with the good taste that smooths troubled waters.

AVOIDING AN ARGUMENT In order to avoid an argument, you do not have to capitulate or be wishy-washy in your convictions. You can enlarge your reservoir of knowledge by discussing topics with those who hold a view different from your own.

For example:

You like Chinese modern furniture well enough to defend it and someone says, "I just can't see putting money into anything but conventional furniture." What are you going to reply? Are you going to tell her that she lacks intelligence and good taste if she doesn't like your Chinese-modern? (You might be thinking it.) Or are you going to respond with interest to her ideas and perhaps ask her the reasons for preferring conventional furniture? You might say, "Well, that is interesting. What one thing do you like especially well about this type?" She replies, "I won't get tired of it." To which you might add, "Do you think you would get tired of comfortable furniture even though it is modern?" "No, I guess not, who gets tired of comfort?" Now might be the time to ask her taste in color and line. You have already won her over to your way of thinking, about comfort in furniture, by using the persuasion by discussion method. In the meantime, she may give you some valuable ideas that will broaden your knowledge.

LEADERSHIP THROUGH CONVERSATION

A discussion is not an argument until one or the other loses his perspective and forgets that conversation was intended to be a bridge upon which we cross to meet our fellowman.

Let your conversation be light and gay so that to bask in it will be like standing in a ray of sunlight. Be sure that you let others know how appreciative you are of just being alive. They will seek you out as the leaves of plants seek out the light.

It is healthy to be gay. It is wise to be optimistic. It is fun to live! Your enthusiasm will attract people to you, and, inasmuch as you would like to increase your sphere of influence and become a leader, you might check the following list to see if you are ready.

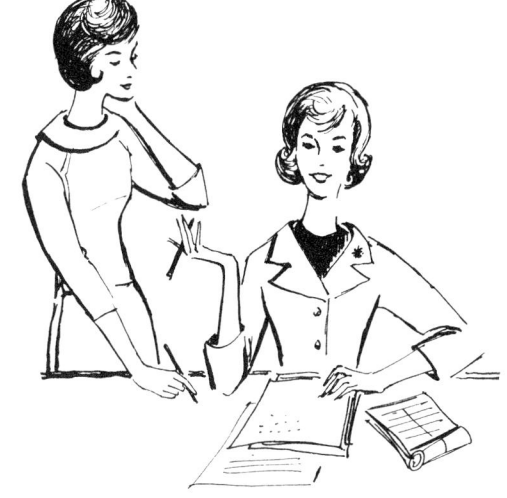

do you	*L*—love
do you have	*E*—enthusiasm
do you develop	*A*—ability
are you noted for	*D*—dependability
do you strive for	*E*—efficiency
will you accept	*R*—responsibility

ASSIGNMENT FOR REWORDING QUESTIONS

Here is a list of questions that are to be reworded three ways. These are the type of questions that might be used to open a conversation with a new acquaintance. But they should be asked more tactfully.

1. I understand the price of compact cars is going to be less this year than last. Have you heard this?
   Example of rewording: Did you read in the newspaper yesterday that the price of the compact cars is going to be less than last year?
2. Who do you think will win the World Series this year?
3. Did you take your vacation at the seashore this year?
4. Did you read about the peasant in Mexico who won $300,000 in a lottery?
5. Where did you get those lovely shoes?
6. Have you been in this community long?
7. Don't you hate living in an apartment?
8. Do you own a car?
9. What do you think the hairstyle trend will be this coming year?
10. Don't you think Jane Powers will make a good president of our Co-Ed Society?

CHAPTER 25

PUBLIC SPEAKING— PLATFORM TECHNIQUES

Introduction

This section is devoted to learning how to talk well before a group. You may be tempted, at this very moment, to say, "This is not for me." But just take a minute to reflect back over the personalities who have been successful in various walks of life and you will quickly realize that a part of their success can be attributed to their ability to use "word power." They are able to communicate their ideas to others and, ofttimes, to move them to action.

Whatever the future holds in store for you, you will find a knowledge of public speaking valuable. The same techniques are employed whether you are trying to convince your son of the necessity for going to college or whether you are collecting money for a church drive. Even the telling of a joke utilizes all the arts of public speaking.

Within your family circle and with your friends, you will be better able to avoid misunderstandings if you can express yourself adequately. Within your community, you will be prepared to advance civic endeavors if you can speak convincingly.

Your professional life will be enhanced by the ability to speak "on the platform." The lesson material is intended to facilitate the organization of your ideas into consecutive order so that you will be able to tell your story convincingly.

As a rule, most of us have no real difficulty when we are talking with our friends or even with chance acquaintances. It seems to be almost universal in scope though, that as soon as we are called upon to talk to strangers we always start experiencing "butterflies" in the stomach. More difficult than this however, is the task of speaking before even a small group. The butterflies suddenly become magnified into something the size of elephants. This is an understandable feeling, and it is not reserved for only those who are not accustomed to speaking in public. *Even seasoned troupers confess to a feeling of uneasiness and some small degree of stage fright.* But there are many things which, when practiced, will assist us to feel more at home on the platform in front of a group of people.

STAGE FRIGHT

There are several reasons for this mental confusion and the accompanying physical evidence of fear and insecurity. The one which is most common is a lack of preparation in the subject which we are to discuss. If we feel secure in our preparation, we have overcome the most frustrating aspect of public speaking. Another reason is that we are thinking of ourselves and not of the material we are to present. This form of self-consciousness can be readily overcome by transferring our thoughts from ourselves and the insecurity we feel, and concentrating on the material which we are to present. Believe it or not, very few audiences are hostile, and generally speaking, they are pulling for you one-hundred percent. If you will give them an opportunity to show their friendliness and support, they will indicate that you have no need to fear them.

HOW TO OVERCOME STAGE FRIGHT

The answer to what we must do to overcome insecurity and stage fright is: Learn the techniques which are necessary to build an effective speech. A speech will "make or break the speaker," but if it is well organized and familiar to the speaker it is almost certain to be accepted by any audience. A good rule to remember in any speaking situation is that a deep, sustained breath tends to relax you and gives just a moment before you must begin to actually speak. Use this device to collect your thoughts.

COMPONENT PARTS OF A SPEECH

Any speech is composed of three parts: the Introduction, the Subject Matter or the Body of the speech, and the Conclusion. One of the best outlines for effective speech making is to tell the audience what you are going to say (The Introduction), then say it (The Body), and then tell them what you have said (The Conclusion). There are several well tested means of developing these three main divisions of a speech.

INTRODUCTION:
1. A story
2. A startling statement (something to attract attention)
3. Poetry
4. An applicable quotation
5. A stimulating question

THE BODY OR SUBJECT MATTER:
1. Draw mental pictures
2. Vivid, descriptive words and phrases
3. Examples and illustrations

4. Stories, everyone likes a good story
5. A logical sequence of detail
6. Definitions
7. Contrasts and comparisons, very effective
8. Statistics
9. Repetition, reiteration is our most effective means of making a point.

THE CONCLUSION:
1. A direct appeal
2. A definite conclusion—"and in conclusion . . ."
3. A story
4. An illustration
5. A short quotation
6. A logical summary of what you've said.

THE IMPORTANCE OF PLANNING

Remember that all art has a plan to go by. We cannot overstress the great significance of having some means of effective organization as a key to success in public speaking. Strive to include unity, proportion, arrangement and sequence in what you do. Every speech plan should answer the three questions: What? Why? And What for?

GATHERING AND ARRANGING MATERIAL Before you can begin to be concerned about delivery in a speech you must gather material which will be useful in putting a speech together. The following suggestion will be helpful in doing this.

After you have chosen your subject, write the title on the top of a piece of paper. Then, begin to think out loud and make notes on this page. Do not try to put these ideas in order. Just jot them down as they come into your head. You will find that one idea gives rise to another and then another. Soon you will be writing furiously and before you know it, the page will be filled with information. Now you should begin adding other materials to your own thoughts. Have you a good quotation or interesting illustration that you think will be appropriate?

Then you can begin grouping ideas. This one will fit in the Introduction, that one is the Conclusion, etc. A good idea is to number the notes and put them in natural order. In this new order, put them on a clean sheet of paper, and see if that is the way you wish them to be in developing main ideas for your speech. Now break this sequence into the Introduction, The Body, and the Conclusion, and fill in with illustrations and stories. Just keep filling in until you have all the material you need. When you become familiar with the order and the subject matter, you can easily reduce this information to small note cards and there is your speech all ready for an audience.

SELECTING AND DEVELOPING THE SUBJECT

Whatever subject you may select to speak about must become a highly personal matter. It is literally a part of yourself. The primary source for speech subjects and materials is within—in the field of your own interests, experiences, convictions, desires and ambitions. This is true even about those who have lead quiet, sheltered lives and often have not been out of the city and state where they were born.

Have you a hobby that literally fascinates you? If so, you can make it equally interesting to others. Your school life has provided you with intensely personal experiences that might be of interest to others. Perhaps you have learned and understand some new and exciting game which is not generally understood. Any of the familiar things about you, many times which you take for granted, will give you your most effective background for good public speaking.

In choosing a subject, remember:
1. It must be of interest to your audience.
2. It must be of interest to yourself.
3. It must fit the time alloted and the occasion.
4. It must not be so broad in scope that it becomes too complicated to follow through to a logical conclusion.

HAVE SOMETHING WORTHWHILE TO SAY

The very first requisite for good speaking is to have something worthwhile to say. Generally the beginning speaker's most common error is failure to develop his ideas. He is content to merely state the idea, and let it go at that. He may wonder what more can be done with it. There is actually a seven-fold plan of development of an idea for speech making.

1. MAKE IT CLEAR Be certain that your idea is clear to yourself first; next, phrase it clearly for your audience. The use of an illustration or two is invaluable in clarification. Whenever an audience is uncertain as to a speaker's meaning, a "for instance" will always bring expressions of relief and understanding to their faces.

2. MAKE IT INTERESTING AND ARRESTING This is a task of the utmost importance. If you do not catch the interest and attention of your audience, it is essentially useless to continue with your speech. This point can be easily illustrated by observing your television and radio programs. We readily "tune out" speakers who do not seize and command our attention. The first thing we must do to be certain we are not "tuned out" is to make our ideas striking and unusual. You can easily shock an audience into attentiveness. Secondly, be sure to make your idea personal. Call attention to the fact that what you are about to say is of utmost concern to everyone within listening distance. Aim your speech directly at your audience and you will generally hit it. Thirdly, make your ideas concrete. Abstractness in speaking means sudden death. Concreteness is the breath of life in speaking. Make certain that what you have to say bears directly upon the subject at hand.

3. **MAKE YOUR IDEAS SIGNIFICANT** You must convince your audience that it is worth its while to listen attentively. One means of doing this is to stress the importance of the theme.

4. **MAKE YOUR IDEAS CONVINCING** You must be in a position to substantiate your words to be truly convincing. Therefore, you must use all the resources of logic, facts, examples and opinions of authorities. Your chief task should be to demonstrate the *truth* of your ideas.

5. **MAKE YOUR IDEAS FAMILIAR** To do this, you must associate them with what your audience already knows and is interested in. You begin with what is known, and go from there to what is unknown and unfamiliar. How often in describing something do we say, "It is about as large as our car." Or, "She is about the size of Dorothy Green." By using this method in form, you may make an entrance into your audience's minds by giving facts that are well-known and at the same time arouse their interest and curiosity by promising to give this familiar idea a new and startling significance.

6. **MAKE YOUR IDEAS ATTRACTIVE** You must make your audience wish to accept what you are telling them. People desire things which are to their advantage. Thus, you will find your audience eager to accept your ideas if you can show that it will be to their advantage to do so. This does not mean that the speaker should present only the attractive ideas. People sometimes have to be urged to do things which are not always to their advantage. In such cases, the speaker's task is to find the attractive features of his proposal and elaborate upon them.

7. **MAKE YOUR IDEAS APPEALING** Show what positive good will be accomplished by what you are saying. One element in human nature is the desire to do what is decent and proper, even though this might involve some sacrifice. Capitalize on this trait and you will be more effective. The speaker who shows his audience the moral significance of his ideas is using one more method of securing support from them.

The speaker makes his chief contribution to a subject on which he is to speak by the manner in which he develops it. The above suggestions will enable you to expand and develop your ideas so that you need never fear about having too little to say, but your main problem will become how you may limit what you wish to say about a subject.

APPLYING THE "SEVEN-FOLD PLAN"

Let's take the subject "Letter Styles" and see what devices we can incorporate into a short talk to make this subject interesting.

As you read the lesson material, you learned that every speech plan should answer these three questions: What? Why? What for?

WHAT is a letter style or format? It is the "frame" of your letter and just as the wrong frame can detract from the appearance of a lovely picture, a poor layout can spoil the appearance of a well-phrased letter.

WHY should you be concerned with the style of your letters? Because no letter can have an inviting, easy-to-read appearance without careful attention to its "grooming" or margins.

THE WHAT FOR is answered by remembering that first appearances make lasting impressions and that properly spaced letters are easier to read.

GIVING YOUR SUBJECT LIFE

For you to put the importance of letter styles across to your audience, remember the seven-fold plan suggested to give your subject "life" and make it seem worthwhile. You must make it:

1. Clear
2. Interesting or Arresting
3. Significant
4. Convincing
5. Familiar
6. Attractive
7. Appealing

PUBLIC SPEAKING—PLATFORM TECHNIQUES

A SAMPLE OUTLINE

Introduction to your talk

1. **CLARITY** To make the importance of your subject of "letter styles" clear, you might say,

    "Our company wants the letters that go out from this office to be a credit to both the company and the typist. Our letters are our personal representatives to hundreds of customers." (This is a statement.)

Body of talk

2. **ADD INTEREST** Hold up two letters, one clean, neat and with a good format; and the other with erasures, poor spacing and sloppy margins. (This utilizes visual comparisons.)

3. **MAKE IT SIGNIFICANT** Ask, "Which letter would you give attention and consideration?" (This question requires audience participation.)

4. **BE CONVINCING** Use a blackboard or large scratch pad to explain how each typist can judge where to start typing and how to judge her margins. "With a little experience you will know that a letter of approximately 200 words will start about three inches from the top of the page. You will also realize that the proper place for the complimentary close and signature will be about three and a half inches from the bottom of the sheet. Set up your work so that all margins form a balanced arrangement." Show various letter formats.

5. **FAMILIARIZE** Continue to talk about the accepted forms for business letters. Show a sample of each as you discuss it.

6. **MAKE IT ATTRACTIVE** Hold up the well-spaced letter and tell the group what pride they will experience when they know that their letters are well groomed and inviting.

Conclusion of talk

7. **MAKE AN APPEAL** Inform the group that the company has decided to use the Full Block Style on all letters. They have selected this particular style because all structural parts of the letter are flush with the left-hand margin which eliminates indentation and tabulation. Therefore, it is a simplified form and will make their work easier. Are there any questions? Thank them for their interest. You will look forward to any communication from them—in Full Block Style. (A direct appeal.) *End.*

BODILY ACTION

Bodily action means speaking with the whole body. Speech is a product of movement. That action is a natural part of normal speaking, which can be readily recognized by watching people in conversation. It is sometimes difficult to get into the habit of using gestures before a group of people because we have the mistaken idea that it is unnatural to do so. It is *not* unnatural; rather it is the most natural thing we do. Cicero of old, praised action as a kind of physical eloquence. Demosthenes when he was asked for the first requisite of good speaking replied, "Action." And when he was further questioned for the second and third requisites, he said, "Action!" From this we may conclude that effective speaking is speaking with the whole body. The meaning of a speaker is determined as much by the eye as by the ear. We must always be certain that the action is suited to the word and the word to the action.

For the purpose of our study, we will concentrate on three important types of body action. They are: *Movement, Gestures and Facial Expression*.

MOVEMENT

Movement refers to the change of position on the platform. It is the pacing back and forth, the shuffle from side to side, or the leaning on the podium. Movement is achieved with the entire body.

GESTURES

On the other hand, *Gesture* is a significant use of hand or arm, or of both hands and both arms. It is also common to speak of a head gesture. Gestures help us to relax the body when we become too tense, especially in the beginning of speeches. The best way to relax the muscles of the body and help to overcome stage fright is by gesturing. Many speakers release this energy by movements or by toying with a pencil, glasses, watch-chain, ring or other object. This distracts the audience while it is relieving the speaker; whereas, a gesture well made will accomplish the same result while it is enhancing the effectiveness of the words. A goal in learning proper use of bodily action is to learn to retain the *value* of action while making those same actions serve as aids, rather than hindrances, to the audience. An effective speaker plans to use enough *purposeful action* so that he will not need to indulge in any other action solely for the purpose of draining off excess nervous energy.

ADDITIONAL USES FOR GESTURES

Gestures have three additional uses:

1. ***TO HELP CLARIFY THE SPEAKER'S MEANING*** This is used when indicating the size, shape or position of any object. In enumerating a series of points, the fingers may be extended as the points are mentioned or clarified. In many ways actions do indeed speak louder than words in revealing the meaning of the speaker to his audience.

2. ***TO HELP REVEAL THE SPEAKER'S ATTITUDES*** If he feels a close, intimate relationship to his audience, he steps toward it, and leans a bit toward it. If he is denouncing something, he can do it by pushing his hand away from him, with palm down. To suggest doubt or indecision, the hands

PUBLIC SPEAKING—PLATFORM TECHNIQUES

may be raised waist high at the same time the shoulders are slightly shrugged. Other gestures reveal other attitudes. It is not intended to offer a complete listing of them. Gesturing is both an individual and a social thing. We must be constantly alert to it, however, so that we avoid artificiality. Each speaker must use the type of gestures and the kind that have grown out of his own personality and experience. One way to develop effective gestures is to acquire the habit of observing conversationalists who are completely unconscious of any attempt to observe "rules and regulations" of body action. Then seek to use these movements in public speaking just as naturally as they were used in conversation. Also, practice before a full length mirror, this is very helpful. Many of the nation's best orators practice for many long and useful hours before a mirror. The rewards are great and recognizable.

3. **TO LEND EMPHASIS** The attention of an audience is certain to lag at times during a speech. When a speaker comes to points of chief importance he wants to be sure that his audience is alert and paying strict attention. An effective means to achieve this is to use suitable gestures. They may take the form of pounding on the table with a clenched fist, slapping the two hands together, pointing a finger at the audience or a number of other effective devices. The chief point to be aware of is that the emphatic gesture actually suggests forcefulness. Weakness used as force is laughable or to be pitied, but never is it impressive. Gestures must not become habitual or they will lose any value in emphasis. Emphatic gesture has the disadvantage of attracting attention to itself instead of the speech and must be used with a great deal of skill and care.

FACIAL EXPRESSION

The third type of body action, *Facial Expressiveness,* is effective only in an intimate speaking situation. It would be useless to use this type of movement if we're to be understood and seen by people sitting say one-hundred feet from the platform. Yet it is still indispensible in conveying emotional responses to spoken words. Use it well!

TWELVE STEPS TO SUCCESS IN PUBLIC SPEAKING

1. Be sure of what you are going to say.
2. Do not memorize your speech word for word. First make many notes and become familiar with them. Then throw them away and use only a short outline on small, easily handled cards.
3. Practice, and then practice, and then practice again until you are saturated with the material of the introduction of the speech.
4. Practice before a full length mirror and see how the audience will see you. Check all aspects of your appearance and facial expression.

5. Practice your introduction aloud so that you can hear your voice saying the things you intend it to say.
6. Check your pronunciations and diction to see that they are as they should be.
7. Study your audience. If possible, arrive early enough to size them up beforehand. When you finally get up to speak, look at them for a moment until they settle down. Then take a good, deep breath and let them have it. This will give you composure and it will give the audience more confidence in you.
8. Keep your posture easy and relaxed; move around occasionally. It is great for relieving tension.
9. Use gestures, but use them to complement what you are saying, not to detract from the speech. Also, gestures give freedom from platform jitters and tend to relax you.
10. Look at your audience at all times. Do not let your eyes wander out the window or at the pictures on the walls. Keep someone's eyes as your focus at all times. Let your glance go to all sections of your audience from time to time. You will keep better control of your audience.
11. Lose yourself in your subject. Really be interested and you will be interesting. Enthusiasm is catching. If you are interested and enthusiastic, your audience will be too.
12. Use as much variety as possible with your voice. Change the inflection and pitch level, as the content dictates. We all become lulled by a monotonous voice. Don't let it happen to you. A change of volume and rate of speaking lend drama and interest to your speech.

UNIT SIX

BEING SUCCESSFUL ON THE JOB

Introduction

Are you successful? That is, are you getting what you want out of life? Chances are that you are like most people—you have experienced the very pleasant feeling that comes with success. There have been and still are times when you are successful in getting what you want for yourself and for others. Probably, however, you would like to increase the *number* of times that success comes to you. And most of us would like to be successful at those times and places that really count—the times and places that are important to us.

CHAPTER 26

THE PSYCHOLOGY OF SUCCESS

Introduction

Let's pause for a moment and consider the sorts of things that made up some of the successful occasions in your life. In the first place you must have wanted or needed something. That is, you must have been *motivated* or moved toward getting something—toward reaching some goal. Secondly, there was undoubtedly something or someone that had to be taken care of before you could satisfy this want or motive. There is almost always some sort of *obstacle* in the way of the goals we seek—this is partly why we still seek them. Finally you must have figured out some way to handle the problems between you and your goal. You did satisfy your need. You did get what you wanted. You must have reached some sort of *goal. So, you were successful.*

In considering the psychology of success, then, let's look at each of these parts and see how much psychological information we can gather to help us understand the nature of our successes.

WHAT DO YOU WANT?

Part of your success depends on what you want. How realistic are your wants? Why are some of our wants or motives stronger than other wants? As psychologists look at us individuals they see that we have many different motives, but they also find that we all have some motives in common. Some of these, called the inborn or biogenic motives, are so vital to life that our society has pretty well worked out ways for us to successfully satisfy them. For instance, it is *not* very likely that as you read this lesson you are completely at a loss as to where your next bite of food is coming from or where you are going to sleep tonight. These biogenic wants, such as hunger, thirst, sleep, need for oxygen, and elimination are satisfied with a fair degree of success every day by most people in our society. This doesn't mean that they are not important. It means that they are not as apt to be the kind of success problems that bother us.

MOTIVES

The motives or wants that are particularly related to success in our society are the motives that we have been learning ever since childhood. For instance, having been brought up with people (instead of birds and animals, like the fictional Tarzan) we now as adults want very much to belong to groups of people. If here you stand, while there goes a group of persons who didn't invite you to go along with them, it may well be that you don't feel very successful.

EGO MOTIVES Most of these learned motives can be called "ego" motives, meaning that they are concerned with things you want in order to satisfy your "self" or ego. *You* are about the most important person you know and you certainly know more about yourself then you do about anyone else. So psychologists see in us such learned motives as belongingness, self-respect, recognition and respect by other people, and self-expression.

It is natural to have this kind of selfishness. It is quite understandable that we feel especially unsuccessful when we cannot overcome the barriers that get in the way of satisfying these ego motives. So—

WHAT IS BLOCKING YOUR PATH

Believe me, you are certainly not alone if you find your life frustrating at times. Does it sometimes seem that life is just one thing after another? Do you sometimes feel down in the dumps, or irritated for no particular reason at all? This happens to most all people at some time or another. The reasons are many—and some people's reasons are so complicated and difficult that they need the professional help of their medical doctor, a psychologist or a religious advisor.

There are some things that any normal person can do, however, to have more success in handling her or his life. One big step is taken when we track down just what it is that is blocking the path to the satisfaction of our motives. Just knowing what the barrier is can be a big help in overcoming it.

You may reply, "Oh, I know only too well what is frustrating me—but it would take a miracle to do anything about getting rid of it." You may be right, and we'll discuss that possibility later. But first make sure that you *do* know what the barrier or barriers are.

A FEW OF THE MORE COMMON SUCCESS BARRIERS Let's look at some of the possibilities. Some of the barriers to our success are inside of us. Lack of ambition, personality characteristics that aggravate other people, insufficient knowledge or simply not enough of the right kind of intelligence, physical illness, prejudice, fear, one motive interfering with another motive—these are some of the barriers that exist within us. Until they are recognized by us we don't know where to begin the battle for overcoming or handling them.

Equally close to us are the possible barriers that result from our outward appearance. Check your posture, facial expression, your grammar, your clothes, your manner. Many people are potentially handicapped by the results of crippling illness or accident.

Then there are the host of things around us that get in the way. For instance, other people who want the same thing we do, other people who discourage us, other people who demand our time, and just plain other people—also, economic conditions, the town in which you live, international tension, etc.

LIST YOUR BARRIERS This begins to paint a pretty black picture. No wonder we seem to fail so often and succeed so rarely. And yet you know you have succeeded at times. You know people who succeed quite often in the things they undertake. The idea here is that you can get a better picture of *how* you can succeed and *where* you can succeed when you first make a list of the things and situations that are blocking your path.

Now having made such a list, or having recognized obstacles many times before, the crucial question is. . . .

HOW DO YOU USUALLY MEET SUCH BARRIERS

There are a variety of ways that everyday, normal persons such as you and I meet their obstacles. Some of these ways have proved to lead to success more surely than others. Some of them only get us into deeper trouble.

THE PERSONALITY INFLUENCE The particular ways that a person has developed, that is the habitual ways that you and I use to adjust to the barriers between our motives and goals, can be referred to as our *personality*. Psychologists have found it convenient to catalogue or classify these typical methods of adjustment or approach to barriers. Here are the methods we most often use. When you recognize some of the less satisfactory methods in your own behavior, don't think this means you are abnormal—remember, these are used to some degree by all of us.

METHODS OF ADJUSTMENT:
1. The direct approach.
2. Substitute action that sometimes helps.
3. Substitute action that usually doesn't help as much as it hurts.

In order to better understand each of these adjustment methods, let us take the case of Jane and see how she could have used each approach.

JANE'S PROBLEM

Jane is a successful graduate from a business college. It was a struggle for her to get the tuition together, not because her family lacked the means, but because they wanted her to marry rather than start a career. After several years of success, Jane wants to own her own business but, the lack of money is a barrier. How does she solve her problem?

1. THE DIRECT APPROACH Jane may not have known that she was using the direct approach when she applied to the bank for a loan. But her action is a good example of this method. It requires that we analyze the barrier, then decide how to reduce or remove it. This is known as problem-solving behavior. The direct approach has to lead to success, since we have defined success as the act of reaching our goal—getting what we want.

Of course it is entirely possible that our first try at a solution will not be the one that leads to success. We have to be flexible and try a number of possible solutions.

It would be nice if we could handle all our barriers by this direct approach method, but we don't.

2. SUBSTITUTE ACTION THAT SOMETIMES HELPS There are some things that we do, even if they don't directly approach or handle the barrier, that nevertheless may satisfy our wants and motives.

(a) *Aggression*

Jane got mad at her father and told him if he didn't let her have the money to open her business, she would go to the bank for it. He decided that if she really was this determined, he would see what he could do about it.

(b) *Compensation*

Jane decided that inasmuch as she didn't have the money she would become a manager in someone else's business.

To compensate means to let this motive or goal go and satisfy another one instead. Or, to find another goal that will also satisfy the frustrated motive or goal. That is, success sometimes comes only when we realize that we are just beating our head against a stone wall in trying to overcome a certain barrier. So we compensate by taking another path whose barrier we can handle more easily.

(c) *Resignation*

Jane decided that if she couldn't own her business now, she'd give up being a career girl and get married.

Closely related to compensation is resignation or giving up. In using this method the barrier is not really handled and the motive is not satisfied by reaching the goal on the other side of the barrier. But at least the person stops beating against too tough an obstacle. It may well be that certain barriers are nearly impossible to overcome. Perhaps the energy wasted on such barriers is better spent in other ways. If this method is used, the person just has to learn to live with the barrier, to live short of success in this pursuit.

3. SUBSTITUTE ACTION THAT USUALLY DOESN'T HELP AS MUCH AS IT HURTS

(a) *Aggression*

Jane got mad at her father and told him that if he didn't let her have the money to open a business of her own, she would get it somewhere else. He told her to get out of the house.

Although aggression might work some of the time, there is a certain amount of risk that it will make the obstacle even bigger. Think twice before you use aggression and fight back.

(b) *Resignation*

Jane gave up wanting a business of her own. She gave up the idea of marriage too. It seemed easy to resign herself to a world that was against giving her what she wanted.

Although resignation is sometimes the best way to handle certain barriers, we have to be careful about forming a habit of giving up.

(c) *Regression*

Jane asked her dad for the money and when he turned her down she cried, ran into her room and slammed the door.

Regression means *to back up to an earlier age,* to act childish. Since most people expect adults to act like adults, childish behavior usually leads further away from success.

(d) *Projection*

Jane didn't go to the bank, she didn't ask her father for the money. After all, he hadn't given her the money for school, had he? So she simply told people that she could have owned her own business but her dad was too selfish.

Projection, as the word sounds, means the act of projecting or putting the blame on someone else. This often includes seeing in someone else the bad things or weaknesses that we wouldn't dare admit about ourselves.

We have now reviewed some of the main ways that people use every day to meet the obstacles that stand in their path. We have also followed the case of Jane to see how each of these methods would have worked in this rather simple case. Some of them are very helpful in adjusting our life to our failures, only a few of them can lead to success in reaching our goals.

Did any of the above methods of adjustment seem familiar? They should have. The psychology of normal people is based on the study of you and me by the scientific tools of psychologists. Did you see in all this, any suggestions for improving your chances for success?

PRACTICE THE DIRECT APPROACH

People who get practice in using the direct approach whenever it is possible tend to make a habit of it. You can just about say that they make a habit of success. With this habit there comes a feeling of confidence. You can develop a belief in your ability to adjust directly to the obstacles in your life. Such a positive attitude can actually *help* you have success more often. This is not magic. This is not a rash promise that you can smile bravely and the world will obey your every wish. Instead this is a scientific postulate. As a famous psychologist, said, *"Our belief at the beginning of a doubtful undertaking is the one thing that insures the successful outcome of our venture."*

THE POSITIVE ATTITUDE

Psychologists have evidence to show that our attitudes and beliefs effect us and the people who look at us quite strongly. If you get in the habit of looking at your life situations as interesting (even if sorrowful or aggravating) problems to be handled as you have successfully handled other problems in your life, then you tend to act in a positive way toward analyzing your wants, your goals, and the barriers that often stand in the way. This habit of tending to act as if the problems can be handled is exactly what we mean by a positive attitude. That this attitude can change the outcome of the situation has been seen time and again. A very popular writer on this subject today is Dr. Norman Vincent Peale. There have been other such writers in the past and there will be more in the future. This is because what they say has always had some supporting evidence and it is gaining more all the time.

THE CYNICAL ATTITUDE Some people feel that such a positive attitude of being able to work out many of your problems is an unrealistic attitude. Many people, and some very intelligent ones at that, seem to prefer a cynical attitude. It is as if they would prefer to bet that they will fail. This way if they do fail they can point to how right they were in their prediction. If they succeed, then they can forget their pessimistic prediction and enjoy the success. However, it would appear that they are stacking the odds in favor of being "correct failures." With an attitude that failure is the most likely outcome, this very tendency to act as a failure is incompatible with the behavior needed to analyze and handle the situation.

So this positive attitude that success *can* be worked out is actually a realistic assessment of yourself and your surrounding. It means that you must know your strengths and weaknesses. It asks you to consider in which endeavors you are most apt to succeed.

SUMMARY

Have you made an assessment of your assets and liabilities lately? In the earlier chapters or lessons you had a good chance to measure your outward appearance. The work at hand is to get the most out of this present lesson. It is the groundwork and the blueprint for success. As you well know, this lesson is not a ticket to success. It is instead a psychological viewpoint of what you yourself can do to get the success you want. What did it say?

1. *Consider your wants and motives.* Know why you feel restless or dissatisfied. Recognize just which motives are not being satisfied. Weigh the importance of these motives. Compare them to your other motives and the similar motives in other people. Take a good look at the goals or objects or events that you feel will satisfy this hungry motive. Are there any other goals that might also fill the bill?
2. *Get a good picture of the obstacle or obstacles* that are blocking the hungry motive. Is it as tough as it looked to be at first, or is it even tougher after close analysis? Consider how much effort you want to devote to handle the obstacle in terms of how strong your motive is and how satisfying the goal is to the motive.
3. *Consider carefully the various ways you can adjust* to this situation. Be flexible—remember there is usually more than one way, and there is usually more than one direct approach that can be made.

Finally consider the proposition that confidence can come from success and that success can come from confidence.

CHAPTER 27

PERSONALITY POTENTIAL

Introduction

One of the greatest sources of waste in business today is people's failure to live up to their potential. Most modern business executives climbed up the ladder of success because they understood the value of good personality traits in getting ahead. Oh, yes, they did not ignore education or physical fitness, they needed these assets to work their way above the crowd. But neither did they leave the development of their personalities to chance. They spent time on personal improvement. They acquired a winning personality by climbing the:

TWELVE STEPS TO A WINNING PERSONALITY

1. **CHARACTER** is a combination of qualities, traits and virtues that distinguish an individual. For success, he must have a reputation for:

honesty	fair dealings
sincerity	integrity
loyalty	tolerance

    Andrew Carnegie said, *"No amount of ability is of the slightest avail without honor."*

2. **ENTHUSIASM** is the magic ingredient that makes tasks lighter. *"Nothing is so contagious as enthusiasm. It moves stones and charms brutes. It is the genius of sincerity, and truth accomplishes no victories without it."* Bulwer

3. **ATTITUDE** is either positive or negative. In this modern world, a constructive, positive, businesslike attitude is a major necessity. No boss can afford to waste time on a careless, negative or indifferent employee.

4. **IMAGINATION** makes it possible for us to anticipate the outcome of our actions. It makes us interesting, helpful and welcome to everyone around us. Turn your daydreams into actualities. *"The soul without imagination is what an observatory would be without a telescope."* Henry Ward Beecher

5. **INITIATIVE** is what makes a person a *self-starter*. It is the personality that has the ability to do things under its own steam rather than waiting for someone to tell it when, where, how and what to do. Employees with this quality are at a premium. They face problems and develop their own methods and techniques for solving them. They have a reputation for getting things done.

6. **AGGRESSIVENESS** is the quality that lights the spark for constructive, bold action. To be acceptable, aggressiveness must be pleasant, not pushy or quarrelsome. Continually strive for a diplomatic, tactful aggressiveness that *makes* the breaks. Create opportunities.

7. **FRIENDLINESS** is the ingredient that pays the biggest dividends. It is the outward evidence of a cheerful willingness that begets a similar friendliness. To have a friend, be a friend. Samuel Johnson said, *"If a man does not make new acquaintances as he advances through life, he will soon find himself left alone. A man, sir, should keep his friendships in constant repair."*

8. **GOOD MANNERS** are the blossom of good sense and good feeling. *"If the law of kindness be written in the heart, it will lead to that desire to oblige, and that attention to the gratification of others, which are the foundation of good manners. A man whose great qualities want the ornament of exterior attractions, is like a naked mountain with mines of gold, which will be frequented only till the treasure is exhausted."* So sayeth Samuel Johnson.

9. **GOOD GROOMING** is a distinct promoter of a winning personality. Appearance is extremely important in this modern world. People generally judge more by appearance than reality. A good first impression is important, you don't always get a second chance to correct a bad first impression.
"Dress is an index of your contents." Johann Kaspar Lavater

10. **PERSONAL HABITS** can sometimes mar an otherwise faultless character. Ear pulling, nose twitching, finger drumming, etc., can prove to be the undoing of otherwise delightful personalities.
"Sow an act, and you reap a habit; sow a habit, and you reap a character; sow a character and you reap a destiny." G. D. Boardman

PERSONALITY POTENTIAL

11. HUMANISM is good business. It involves realizing that the average person appreciates being treated like a human being rather than a number. It is the practicing of the Golden Rule. It is the quality that will bring people around to your way of thinking. Anyone aspiring to leadership should keep in mind the basic needs of the people around him:

1. *Recognition.* People appreciate having their name remembered, along with all the things that are important to them.
2. *Acceptance.* Like them for what they are and try to understand their shortcomings.
3. *Admiration.* If you admire something about a person, don't keep it under a barrel, tell it to him.

12. SPIRITUALITY endows a person with ethics and sound religious, social, intellectual and cultural values. In the words of Maltbie Babcock: *"Spirituality is best manifested on the ground, not in the air. To have bread excite thankfulness and a drink of water send the heart to God is better than sighs for the unattainable. To plow a straight furrow on Monday or dust a room well on Tuesday or kiss a bumped head on Wednesday, is worth more than the most ecstatic thrill under Sunday eloquence. Spirituality is seeing God in common things, and showing God in common tasks."*

These are the twelve personality rungs in the ladder of success. To make them a part of our personality means that we shall know more success than we thought possible.

PROMOTION

Whether or not you want to get a promotion depends partly on your "level of aspiration." By this, psychologists explain, just how high do you want to go? Some people find the work they are doing satisfying enough and the worst thing that could happen to them would be a promotion. But if the goals you seek include a better job at a higher level, then you are undoubtedly interested in the chances for promotion.

RECORD YOUR PROGRESS If you keep your own personnel record and check your own progress, you will be able to see where your weaknesses still are. If you carefully consider what you, the boss, the job and the business all need for success, then you should be able to rate your own merit. You must consider what obstacles still lie in the path of success. If you notice that there have been some successes and improvements, give yourself a pat on the back.

YOUR BOSS IS ALSO HUMAN If you can sincerely see some successful action that the boss has done, you should pat him on the back too. Remember that one of the the strong motives in our society is the need for public recognition of our place or standing. You need it. The boss needs it. If you can give it to your boss, he or she is more secure, less frustrated, and hence more free to give it to you in return.

Here is a list of nine items that should be included on your personnel record so that you can be successful by "filling the bill":

1. What does this business need to be successful?
2. What does my boss need not only to be, but to feel successful?
3. What does my job need to be successful?
4. What do I need to be and feel successful?
5. What weaknesses do I have to overcome to be successful?
6. What obstacles still stand in my way?
7. What are my successes so far? My improvement?
8. What are my boss's successes?
9. What am I doing to improve and to remove the obstacles?

LEAVING THE JOB

When you leave a job, you should try to leave in a business-like manner. Perhaps you are moving on to greener pastures or are getting married and you may not feel that an "exit interview" is nearly so important as the opening interview. Yet the job you are leaving becomes a part of your work references and, as such, will probably be contacted by your next place of employment. Every work reference is a vital part of the information the next employer will want about you.

PLAN YOUR EXIT

You should plan for an "exit interview" and, at the very least, discuss your leaving with your supervisor. How much more courteous than just not showing up one day and then calling to say you have quit.

WINNING CONFIDENCE

Let's be honest. We need things from other people if we are to succeed. We need their goodwill and friendship, their recognition and acceptance. Sometimes we need them to "sponsor" us so that we can get what we want. If we are going to have people's help, then they must have confidence in us.

You must win the confidence of your boss, of your fellow workers and of your friends if you are to succeed. In addition, you must win the confidence of the community. How are you going to do this? By making the Twelve Steps to a Winning Personality a part of yourself you build an image that begets confidence.

You must be careful not to lose this confidence in an unguarded moment when you might think it makes no difference. It is extremely important that you behave socially in a way that will continue to win confidence and not destroy it in one fell swoop. It's almost embarrassing to mention that socially unacceptable behavior such as getting pregnant out of wedlock or getting dead drunk can, like other unacceptable behavior, ruin an otherwise promising career.

It is important that you realize that you must continue to learn about your profession after you finish training. You can do this by attending:

Post-graduate classes
Specialized courses
Seminars for advanced techniques
Institutes of higher learning
Local, State and National Conventions

You can keep up-to-date by subscribing to trade magazines and by reading newspaper articles and news items that are pertinent.

The world of work is an exciting new country, you can become a successful part of it!

CHAPTER 28

CHARM IN THE OFFICE

Introduction

As a female in a man's world, the world of business, you may sometimes find yourself wondering what to do and what to say in certain situations. It may help you to know that in every office there are two sets of rules to which you must adhere.
1. Rules and regulations of the office, such as; tardiness, vacations, lunch hours, etc.
2. Rules of etiquette, such as; showing consideration, deference, thoughtfulness, kindness and loyalty.

It is with the second set of rules, those of etiquette, that this chapter will deal. Usually the office "rules and regulations" are carefully outlined, clear-cut and easy to follow. It is not with these that you might stray and find yourself in a maze wondering which way to go.

RULES OF OFFICE ETIQUETTE

On the other hand, the rules of etiquette in an office are not written. It will take good manners (a considerate attitude) on your part to discover just what they are and to make them work for you and not against you.

Even though rules of etiquette are not written laws and may seem nonessential, they are practical. They make it possible for there to be greater understanding between polite people. A respect for rules of conduct contributes to the general welfare. Ignorance of them may cause you to appear at best, inexperienced, or at worst, rude.

As a woman, it is up to you to contribute "charm" to your office. Not cloying, clinging femininity, but genuine graciousness and consideration.

As you read through the following suggestions, keep in mind that good manners stem from thoughtfulness and are the *spirit* of polite behavior . . . etiquette is the *embodiment* of the rules. If you ever get into a situation where you must make a decision between the two, let your consideration for the feelings of the other fellow be your guide. You can't go far wrong if you, "Do unto others as you would have them do unto you."

ETIQUETTE WITH EXECUTIVES

You have already learned that the most important person in the world of work is "the boss". You have learned that your relationship with him will be more satisfactory if you try to *understand* him, his problems, pressures and responsibilities.

The employer, because of his position, deserves your respect and deference. You can give him these things in a number of ways.

USING TITLES

USE HIS PROPER TITLE Never call him by his first name unless you have been asked to do so. When visitors come to the office, it is more respectful to refer to him by his last name rather than as "he". For instance;

Right	Wrong
Mr. Smith will see you now.	He will see you now.
Mr. Smith is out of his office.	He's out.

VALUE HIS JUDGMENT If he has suggestions as to the way he would like you to do things, do them his way. If he has ideas about how to increase your efficiency, pay him a compliment by adopting his ideas as quickly as possible.

Right	Wrong
Thank you, Mr. Smith, I will do it.	But in school I was taught this way.
I see, I will try it.	I can't do it that way.

CHARM IN THE OFFICE

WHEN INSTRUCTIONS ARE NOT CLEAR

DON'T WASTE HIS TIME Perhaps you will be given orders to finish a particular project and you are baffled about certain details. Before going back to your executive, make sure that you *can't* get the information by:

    a. Looking it up yourself.

    b. Getting a fellow employee or a junior executive to help you.

If you must make a request for information, make it as brief as possible. There is no need to preface your remarks with apologies.

Right	Wrong
Excuse me.	I don't like to interrupt you but . . .
Concerning that report . . .	I'm sorry, but I have a problem.

He knows you have a problem, that's why you have come to him. He will not be displeased by short, direct questions . . . if your voice is pleasant and you maintain a friendly facial expression.

AVOID BEING A PEST

CONSIDER HIS FEELINGS If he is busy and harrassed by a thousand things on his mind, remember that timing is important. Be sure you have selected an appropriate time to discuss problems. You'll make it easier on yourself and your employer if you will "store up" your questions and problems for times when you know he's relaxed. He'll then be happy to help solve your difficulties.

Right Times	Wrong Times
The boss's door is ajar, he's not busy.	He's on the telephone.
The work schedule is light for the day.	He's waiting for an important call.
The boss has placed a priority on the job.	He's asked not to be disturbed.

DO NOT DOMINATE

LET HIM TAKE THE LEAD Your employer takes the initiative in deciding what your routine in the office should be. It is only at his suggestion that you call him by his first name, and just as he takes the lead during working hours so it is up to him to propose any activity outside the office. You do not suggest lunch together, neither do you "invite the boss to dinner".

Right	Wrong
You may invite the boss and his wife to dinner *after* he has first invited you.	You may never invite him to a social function of any kind before he has invited you.
The boss asks you to perform some personal function such as buying his wife's birthday present.	You would never offer to take charge of his personal matters.
He buys you a Christmas present.	You give him a present when he has not arranged to give you one.

Concerning presents, although your boss may wish to remember your birthday or Christmas with a present, you are under no obligation and should not worry about giving him one in return. If you have worked together for some time, and you wish to give him something, you may quite properly do so. It is assumed that you will both exercise discretion in the choice of your presents and *refrain from giving items of an inappropriately personal nature.*

OBSERVE PROTOCOL

RESPECT HIS RANK Your executive may not be the president of the company, but to you, he's "The Boss". Your job is to take care of the work he assigns you, not anyone else's. It would be chaotic, to say the least, if other executives were to give you work assignments without your boss's knowledge. In another way, it's just as improper for you to go over the head of your executive to his superior. If you have a question, problem or complaint, speak to your own "boss" about it.

WHAT WOULD YOU DO?

1. You have been given an assignment by another executive without your boss's knowledge.

Right	Wrong
You would immediately inform your boss.	You would go ahead with the assignment and let your boss's work pile up.

2. You are dissatisfied with the amount of work you have to do.

Right	Wrong
You would discuss it with your boss.	You would go to his superior.

When you side-step proper business channels, you lose the respect of your boss, of your co-workers and of the higher executives. They cannot help but wonder why you can't stand up for your own convictions and conduct yourself according to established procedures.

WHEN THE BOSS IS ANGRY

RESPECT HIS MOODS Although your executive may lose his temper or treat you in a way that seems to be brusk, you should never let his behavior ruffle your feathers. Perhaps he has many vexing problems on his mind of which you are not aware. A truly gentle person exercises tact and patience and realizes that the only actions she is responsible for are her own.

Benjamin Franklin wrote in his Poor Richard's Almanac, "He is not well-bred, that cannot bear ill-breeding in others." If you become angry with another person's bad behavior, you become his "mirror". Better to return good for evil.

CHARM IN THE OFFICE

WHAT WOULD YOU DO?

1. Your boss finds an error in a report, which the typist under you has typed. Angrily, he asks, "How did this happen?"

Right	Wrong
Say, simply, "I'm sorry", without making an issue of it.	To fib, "I don't know." or "Miss Jones did that."

In reality, he doesn't expect you to turn in an elaborate explanation, and give one only if he insists upon it.

2. A slow assistant prevents you from completing a report quickly, your boss impatiently asks, "What's taking that report so long?"

Right	Wrong
You explain that perhaps you should supervise your assistant more closely so you can discover the difficulty.	You put all the blame on your slow assistant.

No one loves a "tattler". Better find out why she's slow and then help her along.

3. Your boss makes a mathematical error in a report, checking the report you find the error.

Right	Wrong
You make the correction without bringing it to his attention if it is minor. Otherwise, you might say, "I seem to get another total, would you check me?"	"Mr. Smith, you have made an error."

None of us like to be shown how stupid we really are and inasmuch as you are hired to "help" your boss, soften any criticism you have of him until it is not criticism but helpful suggestion.

LOYALTY IS IMPORTANT

SHOW HIM LOYALTY Loyalty is part of the nature of the kind and considerate person. With a genuine interest in the welfare of others, you will not have to *try* to be loyal.... It will come naturally. It will include loyalty to your company as well as to your boss. If you are always conscious of his best interests, you will sense the right thing to do.

WHAT WOULD YOU DO?

1. You have had a busy and trying day. You are vexed with your boss's seeming disregard for your efforts in his behalf.

Right	Wrong
You realize that tomorrow is another day and get some relaxation after work.	You unload your annoyances on the ready ears of your fellow employees.

2. An executive asks you for a report that you think is confidential.

Right
You tell him that you will ask your boss, Mr. Smith, to give it to him.

Wrong
You give it to him.
or
You say flatly, "That's confidential."

Note: If the owner of the company or the president asks you for something, your discretion would probably tell you to give it to him immediately.

3. Your boss asks you to tell a certain caller that he isn't in even though he is.

Right
You respect his wishes and say something like, "I'm sorry, but Mr. Smith will not be available today."

Wrong
You decide to tell the stark truth, "Mr. Smith doesn't want to see you." or
"Mr. Smith told me not to tell you he's in."

4. Your boss insists upon every visitor having an appointment, but Mr. Blank doesn't, what would you do?

Right
Tell Mr. Blank that because of the heavy work load Mr. Smith is seeing only those who have made appointments and who have pressing business.

or

Ask Mr. Blank if he might take the matter up with another executive in the company.

or

Ask him if you might be of service.

Wrong
"You can't see Mr. Smith without an appointment."
or
"Mr. Smith is too busy to see you."

As your boss's assistant it is your job to handle every difficult situation with as much tact and consideration as possible. Make friends for him and the company, not enemies.

5. A dissatisfied customer bursts into your office and starts raking you over the coals as though it's all your fault.

Right
You respond with calmness and a genuine concern for his dissatisfaction.

Wrong
You defend your company and the boss and insist that it must be the customer's fault.

CHARM IN THE OFFICE

Right

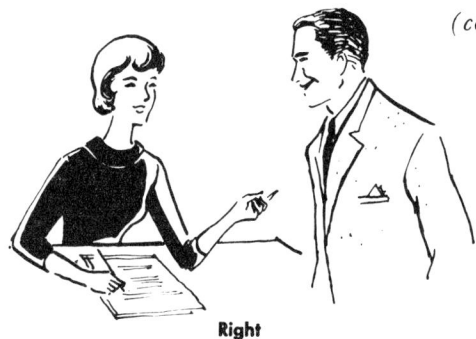

(cont.) You get very angry and tell him you had nothing to do with it. You abruptly tell him you're busy and don't want to hear about it, he'll have to tell your boss.

You assure him that your company and your boss will do everything possible to right the wrong.

You ask him to tell you all about his complaint so that you will thoroughly understand it. Give your boss an idea of the nature of the customer's complaint prior to showing the customer in.

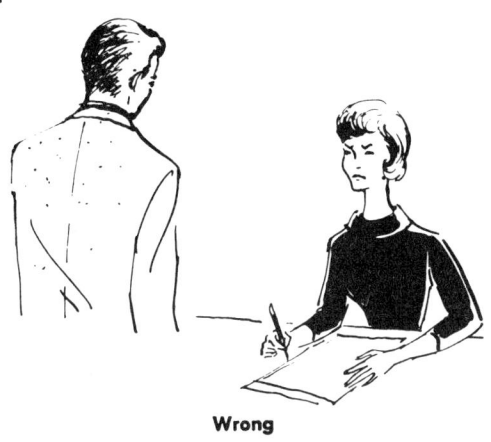

Wrong

THE GOLDEN RULE

Remember, a wise person recognizes the fine line that separates the distance between walking on another's sensibilities and handling difficult situations with decorum . . . that which is the ideal of what is decent. If you value your position in the business world you will practice the Golden Rule upon every occasion. Trying situations give you practice, so think of them as challenges rather than holocausts.

COOPERATING WITH YOUR CO-WORKERS

It pays to be polite, not only to your boss, but to everyone with whom you come in contact. One wise sage said, "Treat everyone as though your life depended on him." This is good advice for maybe your life does depend on him—at least the way you act, habitually, depends upon how you treat others as a matter of course.

THREE WAYS TO PROMOTE OFFICE COURTESY

1. *Respect the property of others.* Don't borrow without asking. Also, nobody enjoys having his desk disarranged, his papers roughly handled and his books carelessly soiled.
2. *Be friendly but not familiar.* For instance, it's awkward for you to break up a routine that you have established with a co-worker, if you suddenly wish to eat lunch with someone else or go home with other friends.
3. *Keep your private life out of the office.* In your business life, your company's interests must come first. What you do with your private life is your business, keep it that way.

Many companies do not allow husbands and wives to work together or even for the same company. Experience has shown that they interfere with each other's ability to handle business hours in a business-like way. This can be true also of attachments you might form with a male co-worker. Move cautiously and wisely in office friendships. Always ask yourself, "If we decide to cut off this relationship, will it prove embarrassing to either of us?"

OTHER WAYS TO PROMOTE COOPERATION AND GOODWILL WITH CO-WORKERS

GIVE ASSISTANCE When asked, give as much help as you can. Don't, on the other hand, give advice that is unasked for and is resented.

There are times when your assistance is required. For instance:
   a. When you are a "sponsor" for a new employee.
   b. When you are the immediate supervisor over other employees.
   c. When you are assigned to help with a special project because of your background and knowledge.
   d. When your boss asks you to give another employee instructions.

Under these circumstances, it will promote good-will if you will word your instructions, suggestions and advice as tactfully as possible.

HOW WOULD YOU SAY IT?

1. You have shown a new employee how to use the postage meter. Now a letter is returned because of insufficient postage.

CHARM IN THE OFFICE

Right
You say, "Mary, somehow this letter was sent out with insufficient postage. Perhaps I didn't explain thoroughly to you how you weigh each letter before you put postage on it. Let's go over the steps again."

Wrong
"Mary, this is a stupid mistake. How could you possibly have sent out this letter without enough postage?"

2. You are the supervisor over a pool of employees who are on a "rush" job.

Right
"We are expected to get this job out as quickly and accurately as possible, do you have any suggestions?"

or

"As you know, our company is depending upon us to get this job done in a minimum amount of time, when shall I tell the president to expect its completion?"

Wrong
"I don't care how you get the work done, just get it done. I'll report anyone who is slow."

or

"I'm here to see that this job gets done by Friday. Go to work. I won't allow any loafing while I'm here."

3. You have been sent to another department to offer your assistance on a project because of your superior background and experience.

Right
"The boss seems to think that I can be of assistance here. If you have any questions, I will be happy to try to answer them."

or

"We anticipate some very special problems on this job, maybe if I tell you about some of my past experiences with jobs that were similar it will help you avoid them. At least I'd like to help."

Wrong
"I've been sent here because I know more than you do."

"I know all about this job, you'll do as I say."

4. You have been asked by your boss to give another executive instructions on how to get out a report.

Right
"Mr. Smith has asked me to show you how we have been doing these reports in our office."

Wrong
"You're to do the report this way."
"I'm here to check on your report and see that it's done right."

or

"Mr. Smith thought it might help you if I showed you how we have been doing these reports."

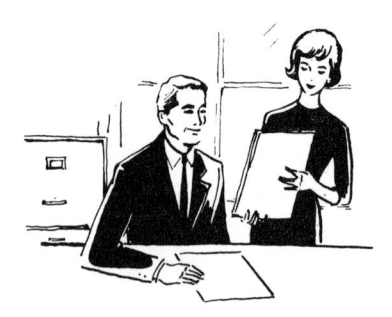

When your boss asks you to pass on instructions or suggestions, do so with a pleasant manner and considerate speech. A thoughtful conversation will avoid antagonism to your employer and you.

OBSERVE COMMON COURTESIES

As a representative of the company for which you work, you should treat repairmen and other service personnel with the same friendly manner you use with your boss and customers. If you have to request their services you do so in a kindly manner realizing that they have other obligations and may not be able to come the moment you want them. You are genuinely grateful for their services and never fail to thank them when they have completed their work.

Right	Wrong
"Joe, my typewriter doesn't seem to be working just right, could you come over and see what's wrong?"	"Joe, my typewriter isn't working, I want you to come right now and see what's the matter."
"Thank you for putting in a new ribbon."	Ignore the service.

SITUATIONS THAT REQUIRE COURTESY

THE PARKING LOT Your parking lot manners are put to the test at closing time. When the driver behind you crowds you out of line, don't hoot and fume. You can set a good example by using as much courtesy behind the wheel as you do at a formal dinner.

THE REST ROOM Here is one place you're not under pressure to keep up appearances for the sake of your job, but, it's important to be considerate for your own sake. Check your restroom manners.

Do you consider those who will use the facilities after you and keep the washroom clean?
Do you avoid marking up the walls with lipstick?
Do you avoid congregating with friends in a small washroom?
Do you avoid loud laughter or talking in the washroom?
Do you ever make that extra thoughtful gesture of cleaning up after a careless person?

THE TIME CLOCK Don't race ahead of others to beat them to the clock. Arrive for work a few minutes earlier and you won't have to worry about being late.

CHARM IN THE OFFICE

THE LUNCH PERIOD Are you willing to uncomplainingly take your place in the cafeteria line? Are you willing to sacrifice the convenience of your own lunch period in emergencies?

THE SUPPLY CABINET You owe it to your co-workers to keep supplies in neat piles and stacks. You owe it to your company not to take more supplies than you reasonably need. You also owe it to the person in charge of procurement to report when certain items are getting low.

WHEN THERE HAS BEEN A MISTAKE You don't point an accusing finger. You should pitch in and do whatever is required to correct it.

WHEN YOU DEAL WITH RUDE PEOPLE What obligation do you have to be polite to those who are rude? It's a test of your good-will if you can maintain a friendly attitude in the face of rude or careless behavior. Be polite, by all means, even to those who: jostle against you; push ahead of you in line; get angry because they have to wait; make unreasonable requests.

Remember, these short phrases were made especially for the civilized, polite person . . . you.

Thank you. *I beg your pardon.*
Excuse me, please? *How do you do?*
I'm sorry. *Let me help you.*

MAKING OFFICE INTRODUCTIONS

More important than the form of introduction you use, is the way you help others become acquainted by being pleasant and friendly. However, there are certain instances in which you will want to follow the rules.

WHEN INTRODUCING A NEW FEMALE EMPLOYEE It is correct to introduce all persons to her. For instance, "Miss Brown, this is Mr. Jones." Also, "Miss Brown, this is Mrs. Lyons."

WHEN INTRODUCING A NEW MALE EMPLOYEE Introduce him to female employees, but let the men handle the male introductions. Such, as, "Mrs. Johnson, I'd like you to meet our new accountant, Mr. Jones." "Mr. Smith, this is Mr. Jones."

KNOW HOW TO WORD YOUR INTRODUCTIONS.

1. When a distinguished person such as a judge calls on your boss and you are required to introduce this person to him, you may say, "Judge Harrison may I introduce Mr. Smith?" A variation of this form is also perfectly correct. If you happened to address Mr. Smith first, you might say, "Mr. Smith, may I introduce *you* to Judge Harrison?"
2. When introducing a *man* to a group, say his name first, such as: "Mr. Dean, this is Mrs. Anderson, Mr. Smith, Mr. Jones, Miss Taylor." When introducing a *woman*, you may say, "Mr. Dean, Mrs. Anderson, Mr. Smith, Mr. Jones . . . Miss Taylor."

3. When introducing a male co-worker to a new female employee, you may say, "Miss Cole, this is Mr. Jones."
4. You may introduce a member of your family to your boss in one of the following ways: "Mr. Smith, may I introduce my husband?" or "Miss Taylor, this is my daughter, Joan," or "Mr. Smith, I'd like you to meet my mother, mother this is Mr. Smith, my boss."
5. When you introduce yourself, say something like this: "I'm Helen Miller, Mr. Smith's assistant. May I help you?"
6. If you are not sure two people have met, you may say, "Mr. Jones, do you know Miss Taylor?"
7. In an informal office, you may wish to use both first and last names and you may properly do so if the people you are introducing are of fairly equal age or position. In this case, "Bob, this is the new accountant, Jay Jones, Jay, this is my boss, Bob Smith."

MAKING SPECIAL REQUESTS

USE A LITTLE SALESMANSHIP Get the person's attention, arouse his interest, fire his desire, get him to act.

WHAT WOULD YOU SAY?

1. You are given the unwelcome job of raising money for a special fund.

Right	Wrong
"We are taking up a collection for Mr. Wilson's widow, if you feel you can contribute, it will be appreciated."	"We expect you to contribute to our Widow Wilson fund."

2. You are asked to tell a fellow employee about B.O.

Right	Wrong
"Mary, sometimes a person has a real problem controlling body odor, even though they take all the normal precautions. Maybe this is your problem. Would you let me make an appointment with the company doctor for you?"	"Mary, you've just got to do something about your B.O."

3. You have to cancel an appointment for your boss.

Right	Wrong
"Mr. Smith is so sorry that he can't see you this afternoon. He has been unexpectedly called out-of-town. May I send you to someone else? Or perhaps you would rather wait for Mr. Smith's return."	"Mr. Smith told me to cancel your appointment."

TURNING DOWN A REQUEST

BE AS KIND AS POSSIBLE It is not always an easy thing to be firm but gentle, but it can be done.

WHAT WOULD YOU SAY?

1. You are asked for information which you consider confidential.

    Right
    "I'm very sorry, but you will have to talk with Mr. Smith about that."

    Wrong
    "I don't know." (A lie.)

2. You are asked to work in another department on a project that doesn't have the sanction of your boss.

    Right
    "I'm sorry, but it looks as though I will have to say no, Mr. Smith wants me here."

    Wrong
    "You know I can't do that."

3. You have been asked by your boss to refuse an interview to a certain individual.

    Right
    Unless your boss has given you specific instructions on what to say, here is a suggestion: "I'm terribly sorry, but Mr. Smith is very busy on a special project and will be so for a number of weeks. He is limiting his interviews only to those directly involved in this activity.

    Wrong
    "Mr. Smith told me to tell you he refuses to see you."

YOUR BUSINESS MANNERS IN ACTION

Etiquette provides a framework for your dealings with people. It helps you show consideration at the appropiate times. And above all, your business manners help you prevent misunderstandings, resentment and chaos.

WATCH TIME LOSERS There are many "honest" employees who wouldn't think of stealing stamps or supplies from the company but who manage, not withstanding, to steal many dollars of *time*. If you are a considerate and appreciative person, you will watch such time stealers as:

1. *Smoking.* Where and when may you smoke? If you don't know, ask.
2. *Applying make-up.* Do you arrive at the office only half-dressed, punch the time clock and then apply your make-up? If so, this seemingly small discourtesy could cost you your job.
3. *Needless conversations.* Do you take up your own time and that of other employees discussing personal matters? If you must tell everyone of your date last Saturday, don't do it on company time.

4. *Personal telephone calls.* Most offices restrict personal telephone calls to emergencies only. If you are in a more permissive office, don't over-do the privilege. It may be here today and gone tomorrow.

5. *Family office visitors.* The office is a part of the business world and should be apart from your homelife. Plan to meet your family and friends elsewhere.

6. *Arriving late and leaving early.* If you expect big dividends from the business world, you won't get them if you are a "minute grabber." Add up those extra minutes you steal by being late, leaving early, over-staying your coffee breaks. Just ten minutes a day in 365 days will rob your employer of over sixty hours that rightfully belong to him. This is much more than a week's work. If you wouldn't actually steal your salary from him, don't be a guilty "minute grabber."

BUSINESS ETIQUETTE AWAY FROM THE OFFICE

LET THE SAME RULES APPLY Business etiquette provides rules of tact, good judgment and thoughtfulness that should be adhered to both in and out of the office.

WHAT WOULD YOU DO IN THE FOLLOWING SITUATION?

1. You have been invited to dine with a male business associate.

Right	**Wrong**
You will expect the social courtesy and deference accorded any "lady."	You will not expect the usual male courtesies such as his helping you with your coat.

2. Your business duties require you to take a male visitor to lunch.

Right	**Wrong**
You will avoid, if possible, the awkward situation of paying for the meal in his presence. You will either arrange to pay in advance or put the meal on the company charge account.	You will fight him for the check when it is presented.

3. You are invited to dine with a group of employees.

Right	**Wrong**
You would expect to pay for your own meal and assume your share of the tip.	You would expect someone in the group to pick up your tab. After all, they invited you, didn't they?

"Dutch treats" are always popular because each person pays for his or her lunch.

4. You are dining in a restaurant and your boss asks to join you, who pays the check?

Right	Wrong
Your boss offers and you let him.	You insist on paying your own way.

5. You are asked to be hostess at an office party.

Right	Wrong
You oversee the party, making sure that all guests are having a good time.	You assume no responsibility for the comfort of the guests.
You help distribute refreshments.	You let "everyone fend for themselves."
You encourage group conversations.	You talk with one of your friends all evening.
You encourage husbands and wives of employees to get acquainted.	You make no attempt to see that all guests are introduced to one another.
You help remove the wraps of older guests.	You let the guests find the cloakroom and the rest rooms by themselves.

Whatever a good hostess does, she encourages the guests to have a pleasant evening. All this is done, of course, in an inconspicuous manner. *She must not appear to be manipulating the activity in any way.*

6. You have been asked to accompany your boss on a business trip.

Right	Wrong
You keep accurate records of any money you spend for expenses.	You insist upon being a "clinging vine" unable to take care of yourself.
You do any necessary work in an appropriate room.	You work in your hotel room.
You wait for your boss to take the lead and invite you to meals, if he wishes.	You expect him to have all his meals with you.
You request that your room be on another floor away from your boss's room.	The hotel has given you an adjoining room. You don't think it looks right but you say nothing.
You dress and act in a manner that is above reproach.	You figure that now you are out of the office you can "cut up" in both conversation and appearance.

APPROPRIATE DRESS AND GROOMING

FOLLOW THE CUSTOM IN YOUR COSTUME Have you noticed the similarity in the two words "manners" and "manner"? It's as much *how* you do it as *what* you do. This is particularly true of the way in which you dress. You may be a most desirable employee, but who will know it if you disguise the fact with inappropriate appearance? Let's assume for a moment that you are going into an office for your first day of work. How should you look? What should you avoid?

GROOMING

Right	Wrong
Make-up that has an essentially daytime look.	No make-up; or a "showgirl," painted doll look.
Hairstyle that is up-to-date but not extreme.	An intricate, hard-to-keep-in-place hairstyle.
Finger nails that are of moderate length.	Long finger nails, some of them broken.
Nailpolish that is neat and subdued in color.	Bright red or "gilted," chipped polish.

DRESS

Right	Wrong
Jewelry that is "dress-down" and that is conservative in appearance.	Rhinestones and jangling jewelry.
Shoes that have a medium heel with closed heel and toe, in a conservative color.	Plastic mules with two inch heels; or flat loafers.
Hosiery that is either seamed or seamless without decoration.	No hosiery; bobby sox; or nylons that are highly decorated.
Underwear that gives adequate support to the breasts and the buttocks. Wear both a bra and a girdle in a color to blend with the dress.	No bra; no girdle; or underclothes in a color that "shows through."
Perfume that has a nice, gentle fragrance.	Perfume that will "knock 'em dead."
Dress or Suit in a conservative color that is essentially "covered up" with a relatively high neckline and sleeves.	A low-cut dress. Splashy prints. Loud colors. Conflicting color combinations. Too tight sweaters; or sloppy joe sweaters.

KEEP IN MIND Your business appearance and wardrobe will be influenced by the type of business for which you work, its locale and the climate. You may find, after the first day, that the other girls are either "fancier" or "plainer" in their appearance than you are. But, you will also find, that your relationships within the office will go more smoothly if you lose no time becoming "one of the group."

DATING AFTER WORK

If you work in a large community where going home before a date presents an insurmountable problem, you can have "basic" dresses that will change from "dress-down" to "dress-up" simply by changing the accessories. These accessories can be carried to the office or kept there for just such occasions.

In fact, it's a good idea to keep a "make-up" case at the office in which you can keep all the items essential to your good grooming. You will not use them, however, at your desk but will take the case to the restroom.

BEING PREPARED

Think what a nice sense of security it will give you to know that you are ready for unexpected pleasures like a luncheon away from the office or a dinner date right after work. You'll be forever grateful for items such as these tucked away in a desk drawer:

A small sewing kit	A clean handkerchief
A tooth brush and paste	A fresh pair of white gloves
An extra stocking	Facial tissues.
An emery board	Cosmetic items for make-up repair
Hand lotion	A small bottle of cologne

PERSONS AND PITFALLS TO AVOID

Just between us girls there seems to be, in every office, the person who does everything to disrupt good human relations. She's the *gossip monger* who can't wait to tell a new employee all about the idiosyncrasies (true and untrue) of each employee. She's a trouble maker. Avoid her like the plague.

Then there's the *unpleasant co-worker* who makes heavy schedules, deadlines and rush projects more difficult by making life miserable for everyone around her. Do you "let off steam" by telling her what you think of her to her face or by waiting until lunch period and then attacking her behind her back? Etiquette says "no" to both these tactics. There's no such thing as justifiable temper tantrums. First of all, examine your own habits to see if you might be partially at fault. Then if you feel the situation justifies attention, go to your supervisor.

A WORD ABOUT SEX APPEAL

What about the girl who hopes to get ahead in business because of her *sex appeal?* A pretty face and a curvaceous figure may be successful in attracting male attention, but they won't get the work done. A company that is concerned about forging ahead can't afford to hire a girl who is prepared to do nothing but look pretty. This type usually dresses inappropriately—an indication of her lack of good taste.

Then there is the *opposite type*, the girl who figures that if she's going to fit into a man's world she may as well act like a man. She's in the center of the group telling questionable stories. She learns to fight like a man and swear like a trooper. She's a real "go-getter," but she'll never get the coveted promotions. They'll be reserved for the career girl who displays femininity without frills.

THIS IS YOUR CHALLENGE AS A CAREER GIRL To roll up your sleeves and pitch in to a man-sized job without even chipping your fingernail polish or fraying your womanliness. This is possible because you will be firm without raising your voice, quick thinking without sounding abrupt or discourteous, cool headed without being hard as nails. You will develop work habits that are tops. And even though you are in a hurry with telephones ringing, the boss heckling and a deadline to meet, you will never sidestep the line of good manners. You will remain what you essentially are, a lady.

CHAPTER 29

THE BUSINESS TELEPHONE

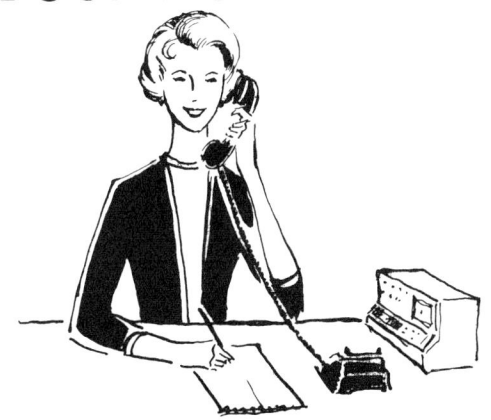

Introduction

Every time you answer a business telephone, your voice and manner of speaking are, in the truest sense, representing your company. Your telephone techniques can increase business or drive it away. It's important that you give the very best impression to all those who call. By speaking with clear pronunciation, correct grammer and a pleasant voice you will build an image of prestige in the public's mind.

ANSWERING THE PHONE

GREETING THE CALLER Most companies agree that it's more efficient to say "Good morning" before introducing yourself. If you say, "Good morning, Mr. Smith's office, Miss ...... speaking," your caller need only say, "May I speak with Mr. Smith, please?"

FIND OUT WHO'S CALLING When a person calls and fails to give his name, it's your job to find out who he is. A curt, "Who's calling?" will never do. Try to say, pleasantly, "May I tell Mr. Smith who's calling?" or, it doesn't take much longer to inquire: "I wonder if you would tell me your name, so that I can tell Mr. Smith who's calling?" The extra seconds it takes, to show consideration for the caller, add immeasurably to good public relations.

When the tables are turned, and you are calling, don't make the other party wait for your name. Announce: "This is Mr. Smith's office calling." By announcing the name of your office first, you do not give the other person a moment to wonder to whom she is speaking.

Keep in mind that these techniques are only suggested. When on the job, you will adopt the procedure used at your place of employment.

BASIC PRINCIPLES OF TELEPHONE ETIQUETTE AND TECHNIQUE

1. **AVOID INTERRUPTIONS AND SIDE REMARKS** It is discourteous to expect a person to wait while you chat with another. Concentrate on the telephone conversation. And you will, when you realize that the person on the other end of the wire has no way of knowing what is going on in your office.

2. **EXPLAIN DELAYS** If a caller must be kept waiting while you call your executive to the wire, let him know there will be a delay. Maybe he would rather call back. In the event that he wishes to wait, don't leave him waiting indefinitely. Courtesy demands that you speak with him about every sixty seconds with, "Sorry to keep you waiting, I believe Mr. Smith will be free in just a moment," or "Sorry, Mr. Smith is still busy, do you mind waiting a moment longer?"

3. **MAKE NOTES AND USE THEM** Keep a telephone message pad and pencil handy. Use it to take messages for your boss or other employees who may be out when the call comes in. Don't delay your callers with, "Just a minute, I can't find a pencil."
When you have several items to go over with a person you are calling, have the list written down before you telephone. Check the items off as you cover them. Jot down important points.

THE BUSINESS TELEPHONE

HANDLING TELEPHONE COMPLAINTS

HANDLING AN UNPLEASANT CALLER It's fairly easy to keep a pleasant voice when the caller on the other end of the line is also courteous, but the handling of an irate or dissatisfied customer can be a difficult task. If you are confronted with a complaint, here are a few ground rules for retaining the customer's goodwill.

1. Don't take the complaint as a personal affront.
2. Keep the tone of your voice sympathetic and reassuring.
3. Make the caller aware of your concern by your manner of speaking and the words you use.
4. Let him tell his whole story. Avoid interrupting.
5. Suggest an adjustment or the firm's willingness to make one.

You have two obligations. One is to follow the rules of the firm in adjusting complaints. The other is to retain your composure. An attitude of resentment will only make matters worse. But a relaxed and courteous tone will induce your caller to adopt an agreeable manner.

TELEPHONE SPEECH HABITS

IMPROVING YOUR TELEPHONE SPEECH HABITS If a tape recorder is available, it will be helpful for you to hear how you sound to others by having your voice taped and played back. If not, you can discover how distinctly you are speaking by standing in front of your class or your family and pretend to answer the telephone. *Ask your "audience" to give you constructive criticism.*

Can they understand each word?
Are your speech habits good? Do you use correct grammar?
Does your voice convey cheerfulness and enthusiasm?

To improve your speech habits over the telephone, it is suggested that you adhere to the following rules:

1. Watch your posture.
2. Breathe deeply.
3. Pronounce all your words distinctly.
4. Speak at a moderate pace.
5. Use a pitch that is neither too high nor too low.
6. Speak with the right amount of volume.
7. Hold the telephone instrument so that it is neither too close nor too far away.

The most effective speech is that which is correct but unaffected. The tone of your voice should convey friendliness, cheerfulness and alertness.

PERSONALITY-PLUS

With personality-plus, the first few words said over the telephone register an attractive personality and give prestige to the firm. It is important to greet every caller with a cordial welcome. It shows your firm is pleased to receive the call and wants to be of service. Here is a list of do's.

DO

Use correct grammar and clear speech.
Sound cheerful and alert.
Show enthusiasm through the tone of your voice.
Observe basic telephone courtesies.
Be prepared to answer questions about products and services.
Take accurate messages.
Book appointments efficiently.
Answer complaints tactfully.
Overcome price objections.
Write out a sales talk.
Identify both yourself and the company.
Be prompt in answering the phone.
Here is a list of don'ts.

DON'T

Speak too loudly or too softly.
Ask blunt questions, such as, "Who's calling?"
Make side remarks.
Allow interruptions.
Keep the other person waiting without an explanation.
Bang the receiver.
Become irritated.
Argue.
Refuse to give requested information.
Trust your memory for messages.
Use slang.
Sound disinterested.

USE LITTLE NICETIES In addition to answering the telephone promptly and giving proper identification, it is necessary to observe other rules of good telephone usage. These include:

1. Displaying an interested, helpful attitude.
2. Supplying requested information with efficiency.
3. Saying, "I'm sorry to keep you waiting," or "May I ask who is calling, please? or "I'll get that information and call you back."

It's amazing how many people do not realize that it is courteous to let the other person know the conversation is finished by saying "goodbye" before hanging up. It is gracious to pause for a moment before setting the receiver in its cradle.

GOOD BUSINESS PRACTICE

The telephone serves many useful purposes in a business when it is used capably and with understanding.

Good business practice requires that the business telephone be freely and prominently displayed on cards, stationary, advertising circulars, newspaper and telephone book ads. It makes it easy for people to call.

Good business practice also requires that a trained person be put in charge of the telephone calls. Should you be given this job, you must have the qualities of personality that have been discussed in previous lessons. But in addition, you should be thoroughly familiar with the workings of the office so that you can:

1. Make or change appointments.
2. Use the telephone for sales promotions.
3. Adjust complaints and satisfy customers.
4. Receive messages.
5. Order equipment and supplies.
6. Give information about products and services.
7. Overcome price objections.

This is a rather large order and a lot to expect of a young person new to the business world. It goes without saying that your job requires so much concentration that you should not be bothered by other members of the staff nor should you engage in unnecessary conversation with customers. You should have a helpful, efficient attitude and an awareness of the importance of your job. You are the customers first contact and create a lasting impression.

THE TOOLS OF THE TELEPHONE

Your job will be made easier if you are given the proper equipment with which to work. This means that your telephone be in a convenient location with a comfortable chair furnished. Readily accessible and close at hand should be:

1. The appointment book.
2. Record cards.
3. Appointment cards (if these are used).
4. Message pad and pencil.
5. Often used telephone numbers in a number finder that is easy to use.
6. A telephone directory.

RATE YOUR TELEPHONE MANNERS

To see if you have "telephone charm," answer yes or no to the following ten questions.

YES__ NO__ 1. Do you make your voice pleasant, your diction clear and speech correct?

YES__ NO__ 2. Do you answer the telephone by identifying the time of day, yourself, and the company or office?

YES__ NO__ 3. Do you answer the telephone promptly?

YES__ NO__ 4. Do you avoid interruptions and side remarks?

YES__ NO__ 5. Do you explain any delays and re-explain every few seconds?

YES__ NO__ 6. Do you keep much-used information conveniently close at hand?

YES__ NO__ 7. Do you write down messages giving adequate information, such as: the date, the name of the person calling, his telephone number, the name of the person for whom the caller asked, and a message that makes sense?

YES__ NO__ 8. Do you courteously handle complaints and thereby create good-will?

YES__ NO__ 9. Do you go out of your way to be helpful to the caller?

YES__ NO__ 10. Do you constantly try to improve your telephone speech habits.

"*Yes*" answers mean that you are creating good-will and adding to the good name of the firm.

"*No*" answers mean that you are not benefitting yourself or your business. Maybe you are benefitting your competitors.

CHAPTER 30

APPLYING FOR A JOB

Introduction

The responsibility for getting the job you want will fall upon your shoulders as the job seeker. The acid test will come at the time of your personal interview with a prospective employer. Because this interpersonal situation is so important to your success, let's devote a few moments to determining what you can do to heighten your chances of hearing, "When will you be ready to go to work?"

The word interpersonal is used in place of personal to stress the mutuality of the situation. The employer needs you or someone who is qualified to fill his job opening and you are interested in the position. Some job applicants take the stand that they want to know as much about the employer as the employer wants to know about them. However, after you have been accepted is time enough to ask for details. You can always turn down an offer, but you can never accept one that is not offered you.

On the other hand, your chances of success in the interview will be enhanced by your knowledge of the firm, the job for which you are being interviewed, and the interviewer himself. This will require some advance preparation which is not always easy, and in some cases is impossible, but you must do what you can.

Unless you are extremely fortunate, you will not have unlimited opportunities for interviews with employers who have jobs you want. Therefore, the interview is not the place to experiment. You will get too few chances to correct your mistakes. Some persons handle their interviews smoothly and effectively, and land the job. What is their key to success? They are prepared; they know what is expected of them. Advance preparation has made them seem confident, natural and at ease. They have the pertinent facts about themselves in logical order and they are ready to present them in clear and concise language, without the need for cross-examination. They are aware that the interviewer is a human being who is seeking evidence of the job hunter's ability to handle the position.

PREPARING FOR A JOB INTERVIEW

To Handle a Job Interview Successfully, You Must:
1. Be prepared by knowing whatever you can about: (a) the firm (b) the job (c) the interviewer.
2. Have the facts about yourself in logical order.
3. Be ready to present them in clear and concise language.
4. Be aware of the interviewer as a human being.

This advance preparation will make you seem confident, natural and at ease.

KNOW YOUR OWN QUALIFICATIONS

The easier you can make it for the interviewer to get a clear picture of your ability to handle the job, the more successful your interview is going to be. How can you acquire competence in handling interviews? By a number of small and large things. You will have a definite advantage if you have a clear idea of the standards you will have to meet when applying for a particular position. You must be prepared to emphasize your education, interests and background that are relevant to the job and pass over those in which the employer may not be interested.

Before going for an interview, be sure you know your qualifications both as an employee and as a person. The time you will spend in an interview is limited. You have only a few minutes in which to sell yourself. The interviewer is going to form opinions before he knows you very well. His quick judgment will be based on a host of small factors.

DRESS CORRECTLY

It may seem elementary to mention personal appearance, but it is sometimes surprising to see how people dress when applying for a business position. You'd think it would not be necessary to mention that no one applies for a responsible position in a cocktail gown or in a sweater, skirt and bobby sox. It is true that modern day living tends toward informality, but a neat well-groomed appearance cannot be over-emphasized.

APPLYING FOR A JOB

FEMALE GRADUATES SHOULD:
1. *Wear a basic dress* (simple style) with a "covered up" look. It should have sleeves and a reasonably high neckline.
2. *Wear conservative jewelry* that doesn't "jangle." No shining baubles.
3. *Wear nylon hosiery* rather than bobby sox or no hose at all. Teenagers wear bobby sox and the world of work is for adults only.
4. *Wear gloves* no matter what the time of year. Ladies always wear gloves on the street.
5. *Wear simple pump shoes* with closed heel and toe. Open shoes are for resort and vacation wear, this is no picnic.
6. *Carry a handbag* that has been cleared of clutter. You should have a pen and note pad for on-the-spot use.
7. *Bring a resume* which will list pertinent data.

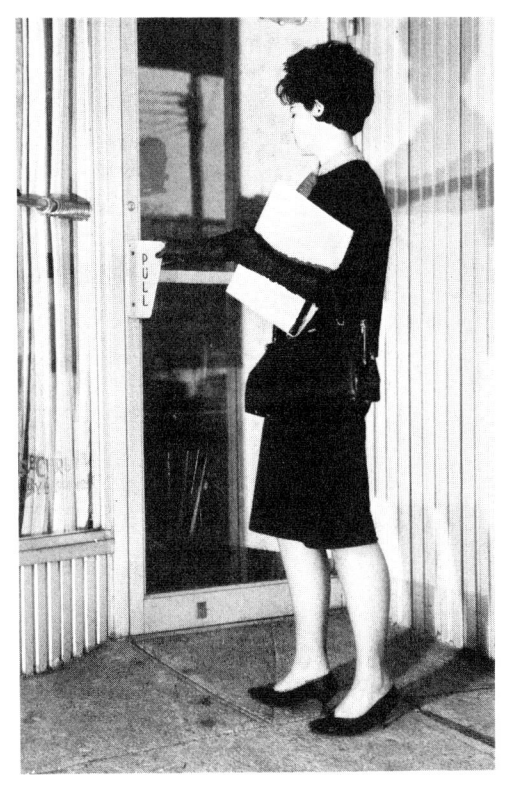

MALE GRADUATES SHOULD:
1. *Wear a suit or conservative sport jacket and slacks.* A suit is preferable.
2. *Wear a white shirt with a necktie.*
3. *Wear business-type shoes, not brogans.*
4. *Sox that are conservative* in color and blend with the pants.
5. *Bring your resume* in some sort of carrying case even if it is only a manila folder. You should not fold the resume.

Your entire appearance should be *conservative*. Not because the interviewer might be an old fuddy duddy, but because you will score a bigger hit if you concentrate on impressing the interviewer with yourself and your abilities rather than with the clothes you are wearing. One well-chosen outfit will serve you for your entire job hunting period.

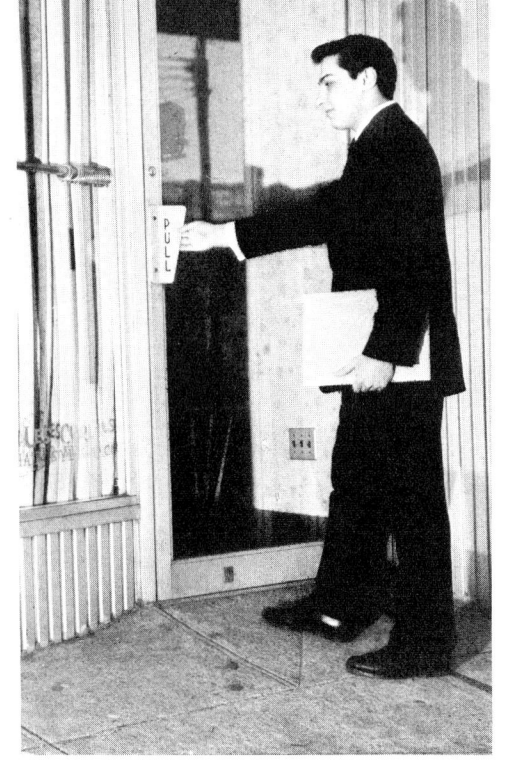

Whether or not girls should wear a hat is debatable. It probably will depend upon your location, the time of year and type of business.

LAST-MINUTE SUGGESTIONS

Here are listed other small, last-minute suggestions:
1. Don't carry any packages. You won't have any place to put them.
2. Have only essentials in your handbag (for girls) pockets (for boys).
3. Be certain your hair and hands are well-groomed and neat.
4. Have two copies of the resume. One you can hand to the interviewer and the other for you to look at while you talk with him.
5. Plan on doing without a cigarette until after the interview.
6. Have your Social Security card with you.

You will certainly be better able to give the impression that you qualify if you *have all the pertinent data on the tip of your tongue.* This data is the center of the interviewer's interest. He wants to know how well you qualify. How well you can do the job.

Constantly keep in mind that the *interviewer is more interested in what you can do for him rather than what he can do for you.* He is not particularly interested in your dwindling financial reserve or social position except as these factors affect your value to him as an employee.

THE RESUME

The resume represents a lifetime of experience condensed onto one page. It should unerringly paint the picture you want of yourself during the interview. It should be prepared after much thought. It is the outline you are going to follow in talking sharply, factually and to the point about your ability to qualify for the job.

The idea of a personal data sheet or resume is a very handy one. It takes the place of an application blank and saves the interviewer's time in finding out what he needs to know about an applicant.

It should include a brief outline of the following items:
1. Your name, address and telephone number.
2. Your educational background.
3. Family information, such as; marital status, number of children, your father's or your husband's occupation, other dependents, if any.
4. Your work experience.
5. Your hobbies, clubs, interests.
6. Your occupational goals.
7. The names and addresses of former employers and responsible persons (other than relatives) to whom the interviewer could write for references about you.

A SAMPLE RESUME

Name: *Brown, Mary* Marital Status: *Single*

Address: *100 Maple Ave. Bayview, Ohio*

Telephone: *PE 1-3700* Age: *20*

Education: *Graduate of the Tip-Top Business School*
One year Ohio State University
Graduate Midway High School

Work Experience: *Part-time receptionist, Tip-Top Business School*
Evening cashier, Loew's Theater
Sales Clerk, Broad's Dept. Store during Holidays

Occupational Goals:

It is my desire to obtain a full-time secretarial position. During my schooling with the Tip-Top Business School, I received an award for accuracy in typing. My typing speed is 70 words per minute. My dictation speed is 120 words per minute.

One of my main interests in high school was bookkeeping and business machine operation. In fact, I worked in the principal's office on a part-time basis.

I have no plans for marriage at the present time and plan on being a career girl.

I would like to be employed by your firm because it is a growing concern and offers me the type of job I would most enjoy, that of being a personal secretary to an executive. If there is no opening in this area at the present time, I would be happy to be a member of your secretarial pool until I have proven myself.

References: *Edna Smith, owner of the Tip-Top Business School*
Mr. John Roper, personnel manager, Broads Dept. Store
Mr. Robert Grover, manager Loew's Theater

THE INTERVIEW

Two questions put by interviewers sound deceptively simple and then turn out to be stumbling blocks. These are:

"Tell me something about yourself."

AND

"Why do you think you best qualify for this job?"

The answers to these questions should be convincing and persuasive. They should be smooth and logical. Rehearsing answers to these and other questions in advance will give you a feeling of confidence.

Other questions should be answered specifically and factually. When asked, "How long did you work at Broad's Department Store?" To answer, "Oh, I left there last year," doesn't really answer the question and gives the impression that you weren't really listening. How much better to say, "I have worked in the cosmetic department during Christmas Holidays for the last three years."

HELP THE INTERVIEWER TO GET INFORMATION

Some interviews are so difficult that an interviewer ends up feeling more like a dentist pulling eye teeth. *A prospect should make it easy for him to get the information he is seeking.* Leading questions can be answered and then followed up with additional important information as well. To the question, "Can you handle cash?" You might answer, "Yes, I was bonded by Loew's Theater to handle their receipts. I also had experience in making change when I worked as a clerk for Broad's Department Store. On both these jobs it was necessary for me to keep books on the sales I made and to balance them at the end of the month." You have told the interviewer of your ability to handle money and you have also indicated that you have had some bookkeeping experience.

A TIME TO SPEAK AND A TIME TO . . . Naturally, if the interviewer interrupts, you will allow him to speak. Otherwise, it is advisable for you to talk for approximately two minutes—no longer. And, remember; the moment you are no longer talking about the qualifications that make you suitable for the job, you are no longer in a job interview; you are simply having a pleasant social chat.

Your interview began the moment you walked through the door. Your appearance has already told something about you. And now he is going to hear your voice and manner of speaking. You will say something like this, "Good morning, my name is Mary Brown. The Tip-Top Business School sent me to apply for the secretarial job that is open." You will notice that you have identified yourself and the position for which you are applying. If you know the interviewer's name, you use it when you first speak. "Good morning, Mr. Jones."

APPLYING FOR A JOB

GOOD MANNERS DURING THE INTERVIEW:
1. You will not sit down unless asked to do so unless it is quite obvious that the interviewer expects you to sit.
2. You will not smoke, especially if you are a girl. A fellow might accept a cigarette if offered one.
3. You will not lean on Mr. Jones' desk or touch anything on it.
4. You will not fidget. If you cannot control your hands, hold the note pad and pen.
5. You will not ask personal questions about salary until you have been hired.

It is permissible to say how much you want if the interviewer asks you, but it is wise to leave some room for bargaining. Don't appear to be choosey, standoffish or hard-to-get. After you have been accepted for the position will be time enough to ask the interviewer for information that will tell you how well you will like the job.

Midway through the interview Mr. Jones has formed his opinion of you. He is interested in your attitudes as well as your qualifications. Watch carefully for his reactions. If he is not sold on your qualifications perhaps he has overlooked some important data. Bring it to his attention.

CLOSING THE INTERVIEW Usually the interviewer will close the interview with some remark, such as, "Well, Miss Brown, we expect to make a decision by Thursday. If you are chosen, we will get in touch with you." If this information is not forthcoming, it is acceptable practice for the applicant to ask how soon her application will be decided upon.

ACKNOWLEDGING AN INTERVIEW

Finally, you should acknowledge every interview that you have been granted and express your appreciation in a brief note. Send it the day after your interview. It needn't say much.

> Dear Mr. Jones:
> This is to express my appreciation for the courtesy you extended by granting me an interview yesterday for the position of secretary. I very much enjoyed talking with you.
> I am very much interested in securing this position and I'm looking forward to the possibility of hearing from you.
> Sincerely,

Happy Job Hunting!

CHAPTER 31

HOW TO CONDUCT A MEETING

Introduction

This lesson is inserted to acquaint you with the obligations, rights and privileges that are inherent in belonging to democratically run organizations. It is to be hoped that you will become and remain active in the various clubs, societies and associations that exist in the business world. Membership in these organizations makes it possible for career girls to expand their knowledge, acquire leadership and gain recognition in their chosen field. A knowledge of parliamentary procedure, terms used and order of business will also be very helpful if you are called upon to act as a recording secretary.

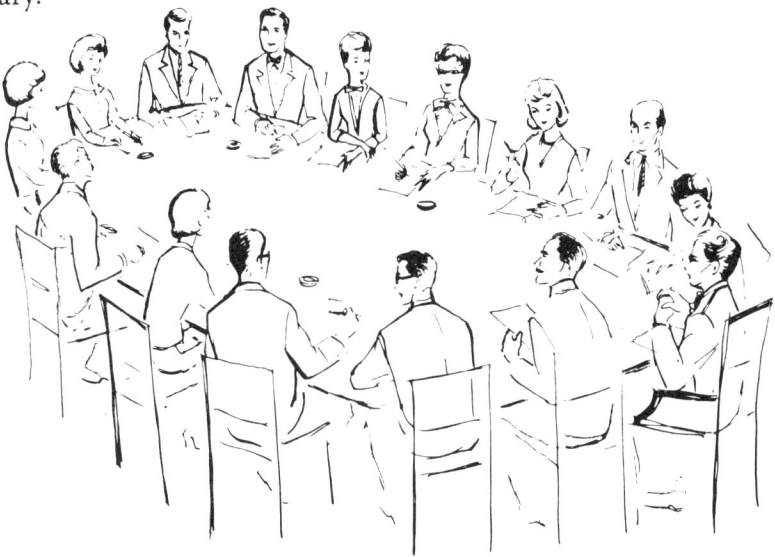

PARLIAMENTARY PROCEDURE

If you have never before belonged to an organization where parliamentary procedure is followed, the terms and methods of running a meeting may seem very foreign and frightening. This lesson will dispel your fears with a few pointers. It will give information so that you will be able to participate with confidence.

It may be that you will aspire, one day, to the elected position of an officer. In this event, you should know what duties are involved so that you will be prepared to devote the time needed to keep the club active and successful.

MEANING OF THE TERM "PARLIAMENTARY PROCEDURE"

In order that you may comprehend the term, "parliamentary procedure," you should have a clear understanding of each word. Webster's dictionary defines them this way:

PARLIAMENTARY

According to the usages of Parliament or of deliberative bodies.

PROCEDURE

Customary method of conducting business in a deliberative body.

The whole term may be defined thus: "Parliamentary procedure is the established system of laws commonly used for transacting business in assemblies."

BASIC PRINCIPLES OF PARLIAMENTARY PROCEDURE

Any system of laws must have a foundation. This foundation is composed of definite principles which are "basic." There are many rules which derive from them, but if one has a reasonably clear knowledge of the principles, it will be comparatively easy to learn the rules.

Some of the very important principles underlying parliamentary procedure include:

1. *The purpose of parliamentary rules is to facilitate action.* If properly applied, the rules are of valuable assistance in expediting business and protecting the rights of members.
2. *The majority rules.* The principal purpose of parliamentary procedure is to ascertain the will of the majority and see that this will is carried out.
3. *The minority must be heard.* The minority has the right to be heard on any question presented for decision. Every member should be vitally concerned in the protection and preservation of the rights of the minority.
4. *Every proposition presented is entitled to full and free discussion.* Members of the assembly have the basic right to express their opinions fully and freely so long as they abide by the rules of debate and observe the proprieties of good conduct.
5. *Only one item at a time.* If several propositions were presented at one time the assembly would be thrown into such confusion that it would be impossible to transact business. It is of greatest importance that the presiding officer and the members of an assembly be ever on the alert to guard against infraction of this principle.
6. *Justice and courtesy for all.* It is the business of the presiding officer to conduct the proceedings of the meeting in a fair and impartial manner to the end that justice will prevail.

DEFINITIONS

To make the lesson understandable, here is a list of definitions for words that are liable to come up even in the most informally run association meeting.

Adjourn — To call the meeting to a close until it assembles again for the next scheduled meeting.

Adopt — To accept formally. A "motion" or "question" is put before the group for a vote and when it has received a favorable number, it is then "carried" or adopted.

Agenda — A list of things to be done during the time of the meeting.

Amend — To change the wording of a "motion."

Articles — The sub-divisions of a constitution or by-laws.

Aye and No — The terms used in voting out loud. "Aye" is pronounced "I," means yes.

Ballot — Any object, sheet or slip of paper, used for secret voting.

Business — All matters of whatever nature that are considered by the meeting.

By-laws — The rules or laws of a society that may be in addition to the constitution.

Chair — "The Chair" is the title applied to the presiding officer who guides and leads the meeting. This is usually the president but may be either the vice-president or someone else appointed to preside.

Chairman — The Chairman is the presiding officer of a committee or temporary gathering. The presiding officer of a permanent organization is the president.

Committee — A group or individual within the organization assigned to do a particular job.

Declare — To announce or affirm as, "The Chair declares the motion carried."

Floor — Was originally meant to be the area on which the speaker stood. Today, "to have the floor" is to have the right to speak without interruption.

Majority — More than half of the votes cast.

Members	The individuals who comprise an organization.
Minority	Any number less than a majority.
Minutes	The minutes of a meeting are the records of the proceedings at a meeting of the organization.
Motion	A proposal that something be done. This is the method of bringing a question before the assembly for consideration. For instance, "I make a motion that . . ."
Nomination	To propose or present the name of a person for appointment or election to office.
Parliamentary	To proceed in a parliamentary fashion is to observe the rules of Parliament. These rules have been derived mainly from the practices of the English Parliament and have been predicated on the theory that the majority can take care of itself, but that the minority has rights that should be protected.
Question	The motion or subject that is before the group to be acted upon.
Quorum	The number of members required to be in attendance to transact business. It may be any number provided for in the rules. Unless there is a rule to the contrary, a quorum is a majority of members.
Recognize	A member is recognized by the Chair by announcing his name, or by a nod.
Second	To support or back up; to express support of a motion as a necessary step to further discussion of it or to vote on it.
Unfinished Business	Any pending business that has not been disposed of.

DUTIES OF THE OFFICERS

THE PRESIDENT Every organization should have at least two officers. Some may have more. The first and most important is the administrative head of the organization and its presiding officer. This is usually the President, but he may be known by one of many other titles. In carrying out his duties, the President of a society will:
1. Preside at meetings of the society.
2. Be responsible for the administration of its affairs.
3. Appoint committees.
4. Sign all papers on behalf of the organization.

VICE-PRESIDENT In the absence of the President, the First Vice-President shall exercise all of the functions of the President and is vested with all his powers.

THE SECRETARY Next to the President, a Secretary is most essential to the welfare of an organization. A Secretary should be competent in keeping the records and handling the correspondence. It is the duty of the Secretary to:
1. Keep the minutes.
2. Read all papers ordered to be read.
3. Call the roll of members when necessary.
4. Keep the books and papers of the organization.
5. Prepare a program of the meetings for the Chair.
6. Keep a list of all committees.
7. Endorse reports and other papers received with the date of their reception and what further action has been taken on same.
8. Sign papers as required and attend to the correspondence, unless there is a corresponding secretary.

THE TREASURER In small societies, the office of Secretary and Treasurer is often combined. The Treasurer acts as banker for the organization, receives funds and makes disbursements when authorized to do so. She should:
1. Keep a record of all receipts and disbursements.
2. Periodically report to the organization, showing the money on hand at the time of the last report, subsequent receipts and expenditures and present balance.

HISTORIAN The duties of the Historian include the keeping of accurate records which clearly explain the month by month activities of the association or group.

ELECTIONS AND VOTING

A nominating committee is usually appointed by the President to decide who should be nominated (named as a candidate) for office. This committee may be appointed or elected, according to the by-laws.

DUTIES OF THE NOMINATING COMMITTEE:
1. To keep a record of the candidates chosen and the alternates to be asked if a candidate declines; to keep an accurate list of all names proposed and comments to be passed on to the next nominating committee.
2. Select a candidate or candidates for each office, according to the by-laws.
3. Decide which member of the committee is to ask each candidate. The chairman of the committee usually asks the candidate for the presidency.
4. Submits the report on nominations. This may be at the time of election or at a time specified in the by-laws.

NOMINATIONS FROM THE FLOOR When an election is to take place, the chairman of the committee reads her report and then hands it to the presiding officer. The Chair again reads the nominations for each office and asks if there are any further nominations. *If there is more than one candidate for each office, it is customary to vote by ballot (secret ballot).*

THE BALLOTS A slip of paper (ballot) is passed by a "teller" (two of them if the assembly is large) to each member. The "tellers" are selected by the presiding officer to handle the election. They pass out the ballots, collect and count them. The Chair announces the new officer just elected by the majority.

PRESENTING NEWLY ELECTED OFFICERS The retiring President, wishing to present the new officers to the group, will probably call for a vote for the office of the treasurer first. As each officer is elected she will come forward until finally the new president is elected. The President will hand over her gavel with some appropriate remarks for the success of the new administration and a pledge of her support.

THE VOICE VOTE In the event that there is only one candidate for each office nominated, then the presiding officer would call for a voice vote. Those in favor would say "Aye." If an individual is not particularly keen on the candidate, she may refrain from voting.

BASIC RIGHTS AND OBLIGATIONS OF "THE CHAIR":
1. To call the members to order at the appointed hour.
2. To announce the order of business.
3. Entertain all motions when properly made and in order, state them properly, submit them to a vote and declare the results.

HOW TO CONDUCT A MEETING

4. Preserve order and maintain decorum in debate.
5. Recognize who, in the judgment of the Chair, is entitled to the floor.
6. Rule on all points of order or submit the question of order to the decision of the assembly.
7. As soon as a motion has been made and seconded, the Chair restates it clearly and accurately, asks for discussion and then calls for a vote.
8. The Chair should rise when asking for a vote, but may restate it while sitting.
9. Under no circumstance should the Chair monopolize the time of the assembly or take part in the debate.
10. Call attention to business that is pending and to matters that require the attention of the assembly.
11. To report on the duties of her office.

BASIC RIGHTS AND OBLIGATIONS OF MEMBERS:

1. To request a copy of the By-laws and to understand its covenants.
2. To receive all notices and to attend all meetings.
3. To be prompt, keeping in mind that business cannot be transacted until a quorum is present.
4. To be thoughtful and not speak until recognized by The Chair once the meeting is in progress.
5. To ask questions concerning proceedings; to participate actively.
6. To present business in the form of a "motion" or "resolution."
7. To nominate, and accept office. To resign if necessary.
8. To inspect the organization's records.
9. To insist upon enforcement of the rules and regulations governing the association.
10. To pay dues and assessments.
11. To accept majority rule on decisions.
12. To accept elected officers whether the member's choice or not and to be loyal.
13. To bring in new members and generally promote the objects and aims of the organization.
14. To be cordial to new members.

THE ORDER OF BUSINESS

Before we can actively participate in any activity, we must know the "rules of the game." The rules that govern the outline of a meeting of an association are called "The Order of Business." Your enjoyment of being either a spectator (member) or a participant (officer) will be heightened by knowing exactly what is taking place.

Although the "Order of Business" which is the sequence of events during meetings, may be altered to meet the demands of the occasion, this is the outline that is generally followed:

1. CALL TO ORDER
The president or The Chair rises, raps the gavel once and says, "The meeting will please come to order."

2. DEVOTIONAL EXERCISES AND ROLL CALL
—if customary, and welcome to new members and guests.

3. READING OF THE MINUTES
The president calls on the secretary to read the minutes taken at the last meeting. These must be approved as correct.

4. CORRESPONDING SECRETARY'S REPORT
The corresponding secretary reads communications relating to the general work of the organization; resignations, acceptance of membership, etc. If the organization has no corresponding secretary, the president or recording secretary may read these communications.

5. TREASURER'S REPORT
There is no motion to accept the treasurer's report because the members have not seen the vouchers or statements. The treasurer's report is made ahead of other reports so that members will be informed of the financial standing of the organization before taking any action.

6. PRESIDENT'S REPORT
The president should report the meetings she has attended or what she has done as official representative of the organization.

7. COMMITTEE REPORTS
Both standing (permanent) and special (temporary) committees report at this time.

8. UNFINISHED BUSINESS
The secretary reminds the president of any unfinished business or of items undecided at the last meeting.

9. NEW BUSINESS
The president, or any member, can introduce new business.

10. PROGRAM—if any.
Introduce speakers and their topics.

11. ANNOUNCEMENTS
The Chair always announces date, time and place of next meeting.

HOW TO CONDUCT A MEETING

12. CHAIR INSPIRES
The Chair leaves some brief inspiration with the members.

13. ADJOURNMENT
If there is no further business, The Chair may adjourn the meeting without requesting a motion to do so.

DUTIES OF A GOOD CHAIRMAN

A good chairman in addition to being familiar with rules of procedure would do well to observe the following "common-sense" principles:

1. Restate a motion before taking a vote.
2. In a debate, recognize, insofar as possible, speakers on opposite sides of the question.
3. In calling for a vote, everyone should be given an opportunity to vote. Thus, even though it appears that the "ayes" have an overwhelming majority, the chairman should still call for a "no" vote.
4. If there is any doubt about the outcome of a voice vote, she should ask for a show of hands or a "rising" (members to stand) vote.
5. She should announce the results of a vote immediately.
6. Speed up proceedings by handling routine affairs with a vote by "general consent" (no opposition).
7. Go along with the wishes of the group for more formality or less.

The chairman does not refer to herself as "I," but rather as "The Chair." If she is president and is giving her report on outside activities then she refers to herself as either "the President" or "your President."

A DRAMATIZED EXERCISE FOR "ORDER OF BUSINESS"

So that our imaginary meeting will have meaning and substance, let's say that it is a meeting of the school alumni. The meeting is being held for the purpose of deciding how to handle an Open House the school is planning for National Business School Week.

1. CALL TO ORDER
It is customary for the officers to sit in front of the group. The secretary sits to the left of the president. The president opens the meeting. She:

1. Rises,
2. Raps the table with the gavel once,
3. Says, *"The meeting will now come to order."*
4. Pauses and says, *"The Secretary will call the roll and read the minutes."*
5. Sits down.

2. DEVOTIONAL EXERCISES AND ROLL CALL—(if customary.)

The secretary will call the roll to see if a quorum is present. (Remember, a quorum is the number of members necessary to conduct business, usually over half.)

3. READING THE MINUTES

The minutes are an accurate record of business transacted at previous meetings. It is a written history of what has transpired that affects the organization and its members; therefore, it should be accurate. Minutes from one meeting are read at the following one for approval and are corrected if need be.

> **The Secretary stands to read:**
> *The Alumni Association*
> *July 15, 19—*
> *Tip Top Business School*
> *The President, Jane Block, called the meeting to order at 3:00 P.M. The Secretary called the roll. There were 17 (seventeen) present, one member absent and Lois Buelher was excused because of illness. The Secretary read the minutes taken at the Association meeting on June 15th. They were approved as read.*
> *The Treasurer, Margaret Reed, gave the treasurer's report. The balance in the Savings account was $50.00. The report was placed on file.*
> *The President reported that she had attended the Regional Trade Show and had been given some pamphlets on their newest electric typewriter. She distributed these to each member present.*
> *Madge Jones moved that a get-well card be sent to Lois Buelher. Sherry Badger moved that this be amended to limit the card to not more than .25 (twenty-five cents). This was seconded.*
> *The President put the motion up for a vote that a get-well card be sent to Lois Buelher that would not cost more than .25 (twenty-five cents). The motion was approved.*
> *The President directed the Secretary to send the card before the coming week-end.*
> *Judy and Lillian Cook sang a duet.*
> *The President announced that the next meeting would be held on August 15, at 3:00 P.M. in the classroom.*
> *The meeting was adjourned."*

After the secretary has read the minutes, the president says,

> *"Thank you, Miss Jones."*

Then she turns to the members and asks,

> *"Are there any corrections?"*

If no one makes a correction, the president says,

> *"The minutes stand approved as read."*

She pauses, then says, "The secretary has a letter to read to you."

HOW TO CONDUCT A MEETING

4. CORRESPONDING SECRETARY'S REPORT:

If there is no corresponding secretary then either the president or the recording secretary reads all communications.

The secretary stands to read the following:

> *"Southwest High School*
> *Miss Mary Brown, Dean of Girls*
>
> *Dear Miss Williams:*
>
> *When the Southwest High School conducted its Career Days, we had so many girls who showed an interest in a secretarial career that I'm sure a rather large group will want to take advantage of your Open House. Many of them have asked what training is necessary to qualify. I trust you will include a short lecture on the various requirements.*
>
> *Most of the students will come directly from school to your Open House. You can expect them to arrive about 4:00 P.M.*
>
> *I will take this opportunity to thank you for your help in guiding our young people toward a lucrative and satisfying career."*

Note: The sender's name is given first, it makes the contents of the letter more meaningful.

The secretary then adds,

> *"Miss Williams would like us to select two girls to show the high school group through the school. She has suggested that we take care of it today."*

The secretary sits down as the president arises. She thanks the secretary,

> *"Thank you, Miss Jones. We will take up this matter as soon as we hear the treasurer's report."*

Note: The treasurer's report is given first so that the members will know the financial standing of the organization before taking any action.

5. TREASURER'S REPORT

The treasurer reads,

> *"On July 15th, there was $50.00 in the treasury. It was agreed at the time that we spend twenty-five cents on a get-well card for Lois Buelher and this was done. There have been no other receipts or expenditures. The present balance is $49.75."*

At the end of the report, the president says,

> *"Thank you, Miss Green. Are there any questions?"*

She pauses for a response, then,

> *"The treasurer's report has been received and will be placed on file."*

6. THE PRESIDENT'S REPORT
None—

The president would report on her activities between meetings concerning the association.

7. COMMITTEE REPORT
None—

Had there been committees they would be heard from at this time.

8. UNFINISHED BUSINESS
None—

This would have been carried over from the last meeting.

9. NEW BUSINESS
The president says,

"We are to select two girls to accompany the high school students on a tour of the school at 4:00 P.M. during the Open House. How shall we choose them? Are there any suggestions?"

Member A arises and says,

"Madame President."

The president recognizes her by nodding her head.

Member A continues,

"I move that the teacher be allowed to decide which two students she would like to act as escorts for the high school group."

Member B says, without standing,

"I second the motion."

The president now states,

"It has been moved and seconded that our teacher, Miss Williams, choose for herself which two girls she would like to act as escorts for the high school group at the Open House. Is there any discussion?"

The president waits a moment and then says,

"Shall we take a vote? All in favor say "aye.""

Note: Everyone has an opportunity to vote. Those in favor say "aye" and those opposed say "no." A member may refrain from voting by keeping silent.

After listening to the response, the president says,

"All opposed say "no.""

If the "ayes" are in the majority, she says,

"The ayes have it. The motion is carried."

Note: The secretary will have been busy all this time recording the proceedings. She must put into the minutes the name of the person who stated the motion (the mover), but not the name of the person who seconded (the seconder).

The president then says,

> "As you know, the purpose of this meeting was to decide how we could help our school director with the Open House. He is holding the Open House as one of his activities during National Business School Week and has asked us to help. He has told me that he would like us to act as hostesses in greeting the guests, showing them through the school and serving them refreshments."

Member C arises and says,

> "Madame President."

The president recognizes her,

> "Yes, Miss Cook."

As soon as member C is recognized she may continue,

> "It seems to me that we better have a committee to handle each one of these three things. We will need, let's see, a reception committee, a guide committee and a refreshment committee."

The president replies,

> "That's right. Is there anyone who will volunteer for chairman of the reception committee?"

Note: The president has the right to select the chairmen of the committees to work under her unless this arrangement does not meet with the approval of the members. It is customary.

The president selects from among the volunteers those who are to "chair" the three committees. She then says,

> "Miss Wood is in charge of the reception committee. Miss Crawford is in charge of the guide committee. Miss McMann is the chairman of the refreshment committee. I delegate each of you to select a group of five to work with you on your committees."

10. PROGRAM

None—

11. ANNOUNCEMENTS

The president announces the date, time and place for the next meeting. For instance, she says,

> "Our next regularly scheduled meeting will be held here in the classroom on September 20th at 3:00 P.M. at which time we will hear from the committees and make final arrangements for the Open House."

12. CHAIR INSPIRES

President might say,

> "Let's show ————— (school director) that we can make the Open House on Friday, September 30th, the greatest ever."

13. ADJOURNMENT
President says,

"If there is no further business, the meeting will stand adjourned."

COMMITTEES

Nothing is more vital to the life blood of an organization than a group of active, energetic committees.

The committee chairmen are equivalent to the president's "cabinet." He appoints them and it is by their efforts that he is able to administer the club's affairs. It is through committee assignments that the club's various activities and projects can best be carried out.

THE COMMITTEE SETUP HAS THREE ADVANTAGES:
1. To divide responsibility for carrying out the club's objectives.
2. To give members an active interest in its program.
3. To provide a channel of direct communication with the president.

Following are a number of suggestions for committee assignments that work successfully for many clubs. From these, you can select the ones that may be necessary to run your organization successfully. Most of them are "standing committees"; that is, they operate continuously. Others are "special committees"; that is, committees that are appointed temporarily for some special projects as were the three committees—reception, guide and refreshment—in our dramatized exercise.

FUNCTION OF COMMITTEES

NOMINATING COMMITTEE This committee has a most important duty to perform. Upon its choice of officers depends the future success of the organization.

MEMBERSHIP COMMITTEE Its work consists of securing and maintaining a high level of membership in the association. It should carefully consider the approval of membership applications.

LEGISLATIVE COMMITTEE This committee watches city, state and federal legislation that may have an effect on the club or its activities. Even more important is its support of action taken to prevent passage of state legislation that would be harmful to the profession.

ETHICAL PRACTICES To promote high standards of ethical practice among members of the business community. To investigate complaints with regard to unethical practices and to bring such matters to the attention of the offender.

AFFILIATION CONTACT COMMITTEE This committee works in close cooperation with the headquarters office or Executive Secretary. It receives all bulletins and other information from the national headquarters and sees that it is brought to the attention of the club members.

PUBLICITY COMMITTEE This committee prepares advance notices of meetings as well as notices of special activities or accomplishments of the club. Its function is to publicize these events.

FINANCE COMMITTEE Provides ways and means of meeting club costs, collecting dues and initiation fees, and auditing accounts. This committee should work out a definite plan of financing and budgeting income and expense and see that it is carried through.

SPECIAL COMMITTEES

The Board of Directors may from time to time appoint such other committees as needed and grant them the powers with which to carry out their work. The following committees are typical examples:

PROGRAM AND ENTERTAINMENT COMMITTEE This committee obtains speakers and arranges programs for the club's meetings. It enables the club to prepare a calendar of meetings to promote club interest, attendance and new membership. Also responsible for the promotion of special social gatherings of the club, such as holiday parties.

WELFARE COMMITTEE Is formed to handle the sending of get-well cards, bridal gifts, etc. Had our dramatized exercise society had such a committee, it would not have been necessary to spend the meeting time in deciding to send out a card to Lois Buelher.

UNIT SEVEN
BODY PERFECTION

Introduction

For the young man or woman going into the business world, good health and vitality are essential to success. You cannot afford to feel ill, fatigued or in pain.

For you to attain the greatest amount of financial success of which you are capable, you must observe the rules for physical fitness.

These are:
1. Exercise
2. Deep breathing
3. Correct eating
4. Relaxation

Yes, exercise is important because it tones your muscles and encourages good posture and deep breathing. Actually, any physical fitness program should begin with proper body alignment—good posture.

CHAPTER 32

POSTURE FOR BODY PERFECTION

THE SPINE

The spine is divided into three sections. The first seven vertebrae, cervicals, are involved in the posture problem known as "kyphosis". The head is held forward, the shoulders droop and the chest is caved in. The middle twelve vertebrae, the thoracic, are involved in sway-back, "lordosis" "Scoliosis" is a combination of sway-back and hunch-back. It is the acme of confused posture. It confuses body functions, the impression you make upon others and the way your clothes *don't* fit. The lowest five vertebrae, the lumbar, hold your pelvis in balance.

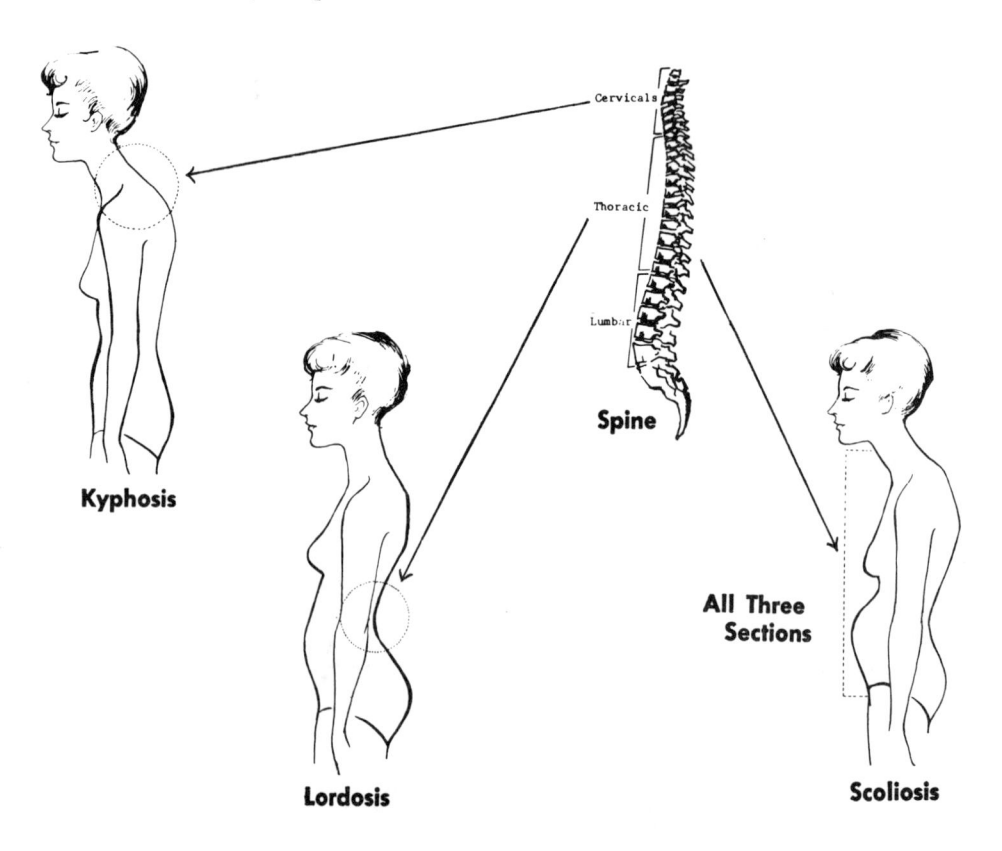

Kyphosis

Lordosis

Spine

All Three Sections

Scoliosis

GOOD POSTURE

Nothing will add more to the distinction of your appearance than beautiful posture and erect carriage. It seems that many people still believe that correct posture is military posture—stiff and tense. Nothing could be further from the truth. The good posture recommended here is relaxed and contributes to gracefulness and flexibility. It simply does away with exaggerated curves in the spine.

BENEFITS OF GOOD POSTURE
Some of the advantages of good posture are:
1. It gives an appearance of confidence. To be confident, you must act confident.
2. Good posture builds good health by allowing the inner organs room to function properly.
3. "Stretched up" posture helps to improve your speech by giving freedom to the power house of the voice, your diaphragm.
4. Proper body alignment makes for youthfulness both visually and physically.

POSTURE CHECK

Get into a pair of leotards (or your birthday suit if you have the privacy of your own room) and study your profile in a full length mirror. You will be able to get your head in profile too by holding a hand mirror in which to check your full length image.

CHECK THE FOLLOWING POINTS:
1. Is your head thrust forward on your shoulders?
   Actually, your ear lobe should be over your shoulder.
2. Are your shoulders hunched forward?
   The shoulder blades should form a *flat* surface behind the shoulders.
3. Is your chest caved-in? The bustline drooping?
   The chest should be lifted upward from the sternum.
4. Is your stomach protruding?
   This could be due to a sway-back or to fat over the stomach muscles. Check to see which. (Over an inch of pinch is fat.) A woman's breasts should lead—should be in front of the rest of her.
5. Are your buttocks protruding in back like a porch?
   When your pelvic bowl is even, your buttocks are minimized.
6. Are your knees straight and "locked" in position?
   The knees should be slightly flexed to avoid rigidity.
7. Are your feet pointing in any direction except straight ahead?
   When your feet are not used correctly, your posture cannot be "in balance."

POSTURE CORRECTION

After you have noted the defects that need to be corrected, get a friend or member of your family to assist you in assuming as nearly correct posture as you can manage. You may have to ask your assistant to actually push you into position. Here are the items to check to discover if your posture has improved.

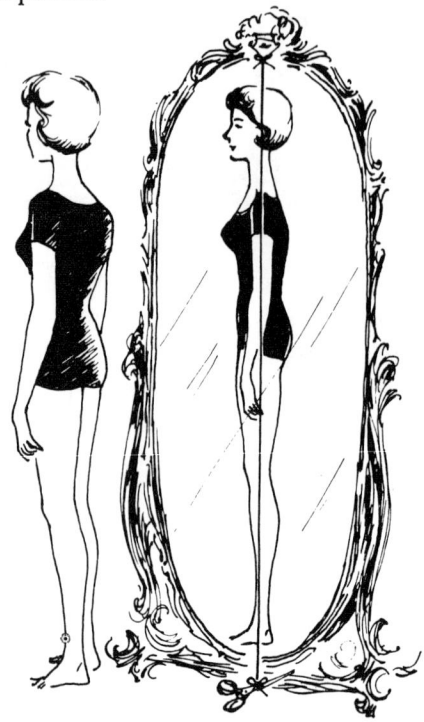

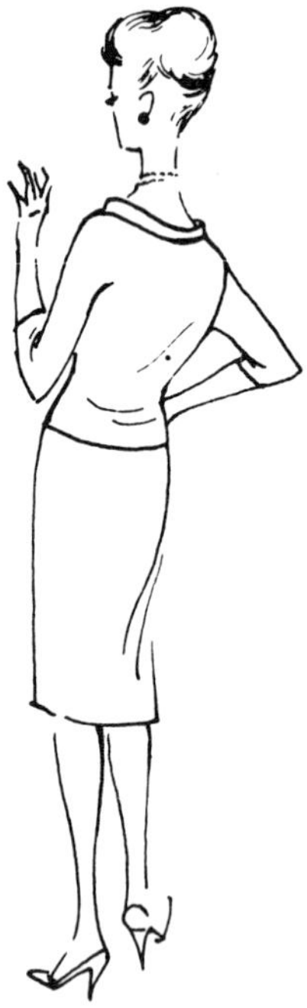

PERFECT POSTURE CALLS FOR:
1. The weight forward onto the balls of the feet.
2. The knees slightly flexed.
3. The pelvic bowl even.
4. The abdomen pulled flat.
5. The hips tucked under by the buttocks muscles.
6. The chest held high.
7. The shoulders stretched back and down.
8. The head lifted upward from the crown.
9. The chin at right angles to the neck.
10. The arms relaxed at the sides with the elbows slightly bent.

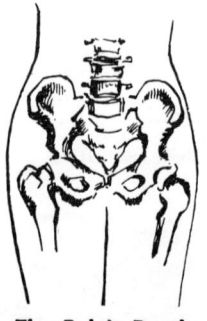

The Pelvic Bowl 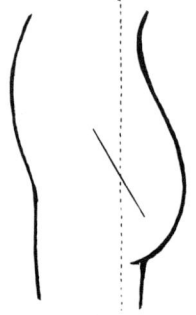   **Tilted** 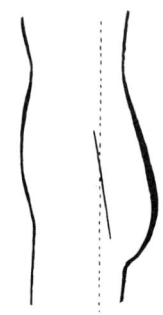   **Even**

POSTURE EXERCISES

Here are seven exercises that will help you attain better posture. They train the muscles so that the body position is controlled and fatigue reduced.

1. PLUMB LINE EXERCISE

Back up to the wall, place your feet about two inches away from the wall. Bend your knees and try to make the entire back, from buttocks to neck, touch. Push the small of your back against the wall until there is no space left. Get the shoulders flat. Stretch the head upward. Keep the chin parallel with the floor.

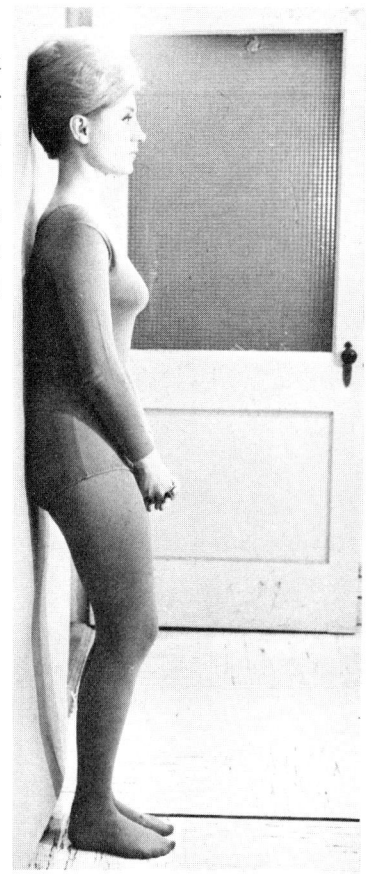

2. PELVIC TIPPING EXERCISE

Place your hands on your hip-thigh joints. Spread your feet about twenty-four inches apart. Ready! Bend your knees but keep the hip-thigh joint rigid. Hold it with your hands. Bend forward from the waistline with the upper body. If this exercise is done correctly, the pelvic bowl will tilt backward. The stomach will be pulled flat and the buttocks under. As you keep your knees bent, bounce by bending and slightly straightening your knees. Repeat three or four times.

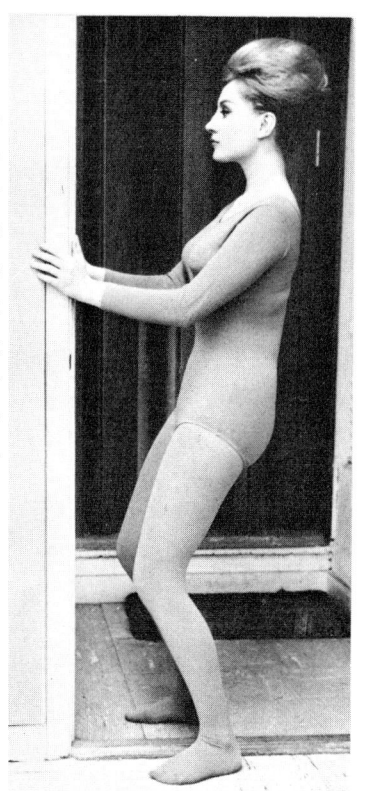

3. PELVIC ROCKING EXERCISE

This one will help to correct "lordosis" as did the foregoing one. Place your right hand on your lower abdomen and your left hand on the coccyx (tail bone). Now rock back and forth. If this seems a little like a primitive dance, it may be, but it will help you achieve the beautiful posture of a primitive woman and that would be good. You will notice that as the pelvic bowl is tilted backward, the gluteous muscles of the buttocks become firm and press together. This leads us into the beginning of the next exercise.

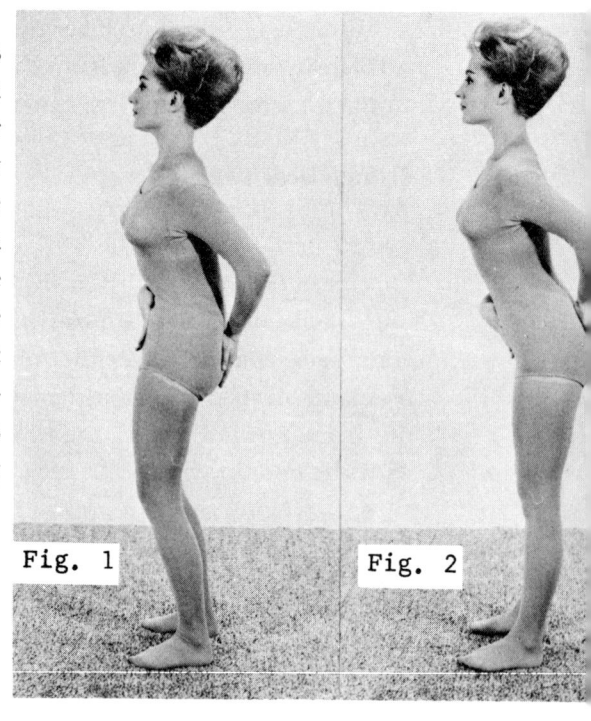

Fig. 1   Fig. 2

4. MUSCLE CONTROL EXERCISE

The tone of the gluteous muscles, the strength of the inner thigh muscles and the condition of the abdominal muscles — all these play a part in keeping the pelvic bowl in position, that is, not tipped either forward or backward.

Step One: Stand in a plumb line with your feet about two inches apart. Now tighten the buttocks muscles. Keep them contracted for the next two steps.

Step Two: Tighten your inner thigh muscles by attempting to pull the legs together. Hold the tension for step three.

Step Three: Tighten your stomach muscles. Lean forward from the waistline as though someone had just hit you in the solar plexus. The abdominal muscles should tighten from the groin up. These movements must be done slowly and with control.

Hold all three areas tensed for the count of three and then relax the muscles involved.

Repeat three times.

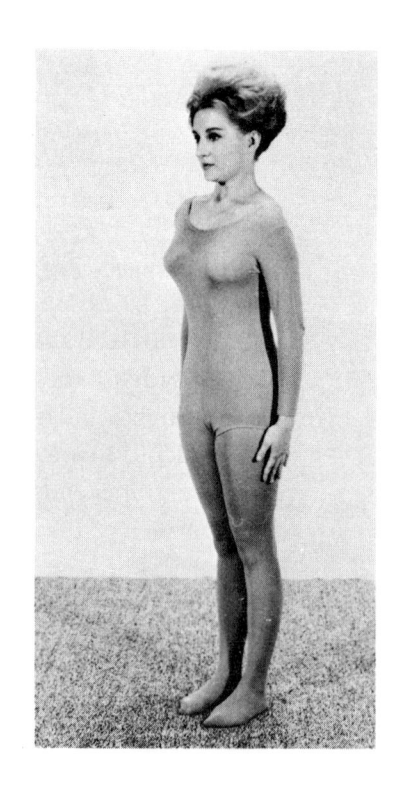

POSTURE FOR BODY PERFECTION

5. EXERCISE FOR SHOULDER BEAUTY

Place your hands in a fist with the arms shoulder high in front and the palms facing each other. Now swing the arms backward as far as you can. Keep the hands shoulder high. Repeat up to twenty times. This helps the shoulder muscles fore and aft.

By the way, watch breathing with all of these. The breath should flow easily in and out on all of them. The inhale is done as the arms swing backward, and the exhale as the arms come forward.

6. NECK & SPINE EXERCISE

Almost all of our daily work routine calls for us to keep the arms forward and the head down. This exercise will reverse this position. Stand with the feet about 18 inches apart and your hands resting on the back of the thighs. Now bend your head and spine as far back as you can. Can you see the wall behind you? Very good! Repeat five times.

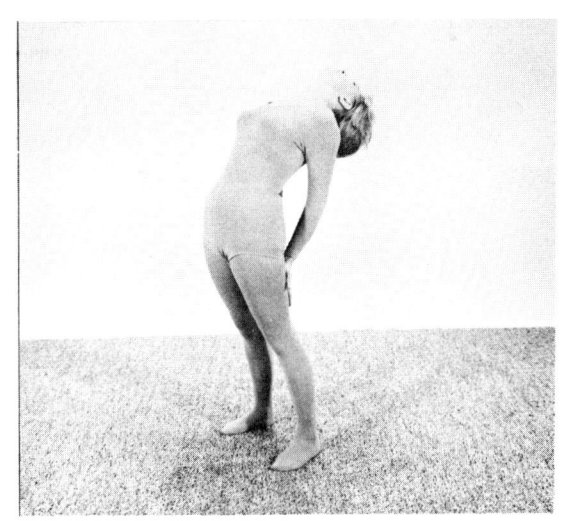

7. BACK FLATTENING EXERCISE

Lie on the floor, face up. Place your hands, with elbows bent, palms up by the ears. Bend your knees until heels are close to buttocks. *Try to make small of back touch.* Do not proceed until you can make your waistline touch the floor. Now, try to keep it touching as you straighten your knees and stretch your arms overhead. You must keep the small of your back touching, as well as your elbows and the backs of your hands. Start over from beginning position as soon as the small of your back comes off the floor.

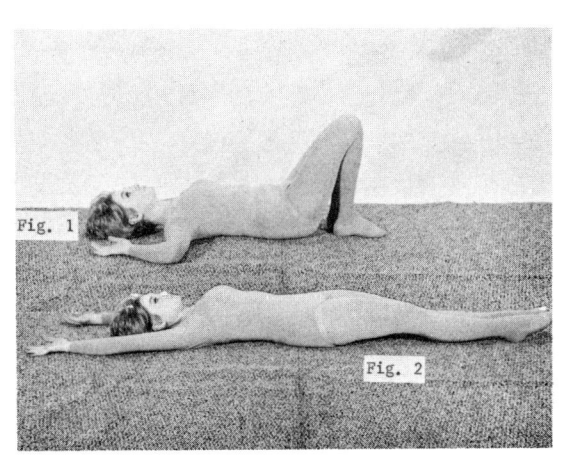

CAUSES OF BAD POSTURE

Most parents, as you know, attribute bad posture to "You're just too lazy to stand up straight." But aside from this, there are other causes. Our soft easy chairs, our mattresses, our brassieres, our girdles, our daily posture habits—all these contribute to muscles that are just too weak to do the job, or muscles that are trained and used in the wrong way.

Our day to day habits of standing, sitting and walking vitally influence our posture, not only while we are doing them, but for days, weeks and years. Therefore, it is important that you observe correct posture while working, standing or sitting.

CORRECT "IN BALANCE" STANDING POSTURE

You will find that by using the "basic stance" with one foot in front of and at an angle to the other, you will be able to stand on your feet for long periods without experiencing that "dead tired" feeling that comes from muscle tension. You will find it easy to shift your weight from one foot to the other which will allow your leg muscles to rest. Muscles can perform without cramping for many hours if they are used rhythmically without sustained periods of continuous effort.

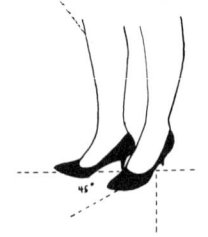

The Basic Stance

Another advantage of the "basic stance" is that body alignment can be maintained even while you work simply by placing the forward foot under the work surface. Keep your knees flexed, your back straight and your shoulders where they belong—back, down and relaxed.

From the viewpoint of body mechanics (making it easy for the body to work), the right height for a work surface is to have it even with your elbows. This is approximately waist high. At this height, your hands can be extended forward from the elbows at a ninety degree angle which is the least tiring position for them.

TO SUMMARIZE:
1. Use the basic foot position.
2. Place the forward foot under the work surface.
3. Alternate the forward foot from time to time.
4. Keep your body erect.
5. Keep your shoulders back, down and relaxed.
6. Have your work surface even with your elbows.

CORRECT "IN BALANCE" SITTING POSTURE

Just as there is a mechanically correct posture for standing, so there is one for sitting. It is highly important that you sit correctly, especially if your job keeps you in a chair for hours during the day. Learn to sit "in balance."

1. Place your feet on the floor directly under your knees.
2. Have the seat of the chair even with your knees. This will allow the upper and lower legs to form a ninety degree angle at the knees.
3. Allow your feet to carry the weight of your thighs.

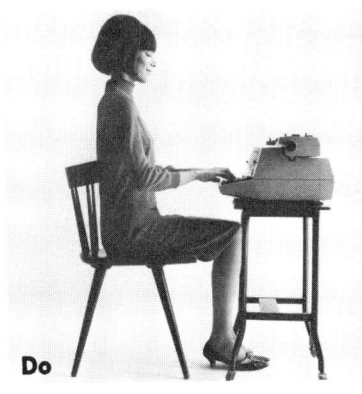

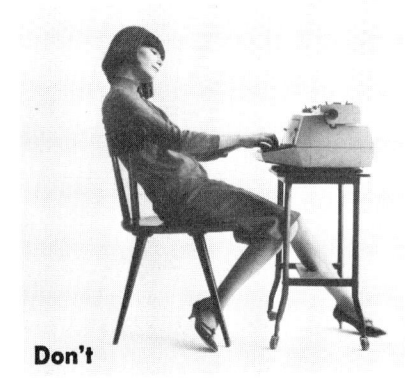

Do　　　　**Don't**

4. Rest the weight of your torso on the "sits" bones, not on the end of your spine.
5. Keep your torso erect.
6. Let your arms hang relaxed from the shoulders.
7. Never use the back of a chair unless it supports the small of your back. A secretary's chair should do this.

Note: For additional information on "Sitting," see Chapter 8 in the unit on visual poise.

CORRECT REACHING TECHNIQUE

An ideal work area would be so convenient that you would never have to stoop, reach or bend. But ideal situations practically never exist. Consequently, you can avoid much fatigue by learning the correct way to do these things.

When you reach, observe the following rules:

1. Reach forward by extending the body from the hip joint.
2. Keep your back straight, not hunched forward.
3. Balance yourself by placing one foot out in back. For instance, if you are reaching forward with your right hand, extend your left foot out in back.

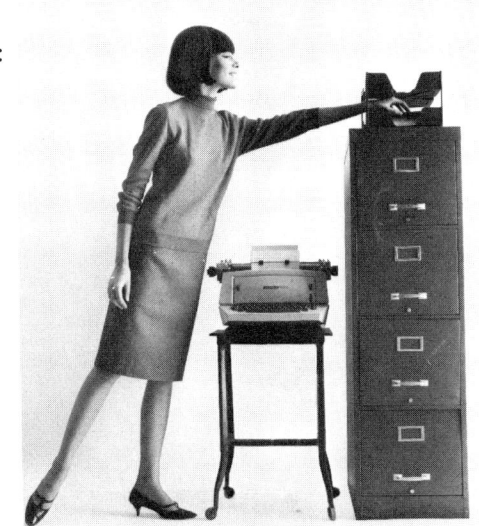

CORRECT STOOPING TECHNIQUE

If you wish to avoid back strain when picking up objects, or when stooping, observe the following:

1. Place your feet in the "basic stance."
2. Keep your back perpendicular as your knees bend.
3. Lift with the muscles of your legs and buttocks, not with your back.

The technique is very much like a deep knee bend exercise. It is the one you should use when getting into a file drawer, low cupboard, or when picking something up off the floor. It is interesting to note that many of your daily physical activities can be so performed as to create a healthful program of daily exercise.

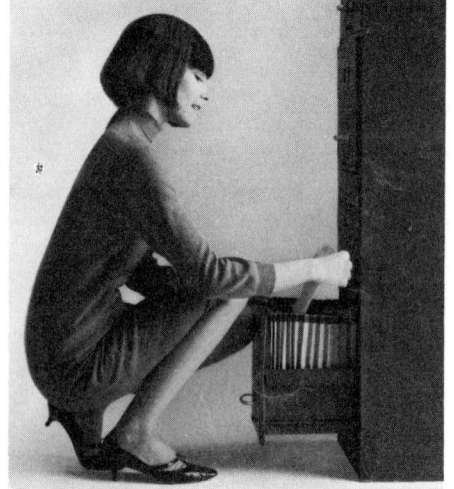

It is to be hoped that you are now well aware of the personal advantages of good posture which is the foundation of a beautiful body and vibrant good health.

You know the old saying about, "You can lead a horse to water but you can't make it drink." Well, you can be shown and told about good posture, but it is only your determination and your effort that will give you the type of posture you greatly admire in others.

If it's poor muscle tone, gain strength through exercise. If it's lack of confidence and a feeling that nothing is going to help, just try going around as though you are looking over the heads of a crowd for a few days. You'll soon hear comments about how your posture has improved.

And just remember, others take you at your own evaluation. Consider yourself inferior and they will agree with you. On the other hand, act as though you have a right to take up so much space and people will make way for you.

Try it and see!

CHAPTER 33

EXERCISES FOR BODY PERFECTION

Introduction

Experience has shown that there is only one road to body perfection and that is the road of exercise and balanced eating. Are you sold on this idea? If not, it is only because you have not tried it for yourself.

Exercise is the Hollywood stars' way to glamour. It can be yours. Within the limitations of bone structure, anyone can have a lovely figure that is devoid of both unsightly hollows and unruly fat. It is surprising how rapidly your body will respond to attention and care. Just fifteen minutes a day will work wonders to correct your figure faults.

It is assumed that you have a clean bill of health. Otherwise, you will not have the vitality and energy necessary. If you have had a physical checkup within the year, go to work and have fun!

TAKE YOUR MEASUREMENTS

The wrist bone measurement is taken first because it indicates the size of your bone structure. If your wrist is less than six inches, your frame is small. If your wrist is six inches, your frame is medium. If your wrist is over six inches, your frame is large.

Record on your measurement sheet found on page 360, what type of frame you have. You should measure just above the right wrist bone. Pull the tape tight. If you are overweight, don't be deceived into thinking that the fat is bone. Have someone to pull the tape very tight.

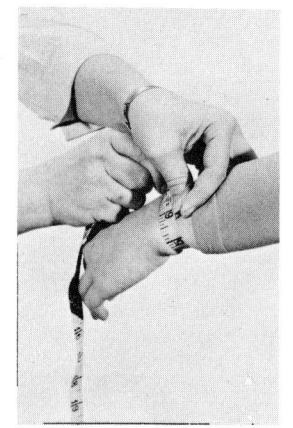

While you are writing down the size of your frame, also record what you should weigh according to the following chart. You are not advised to just blindly accept this weight as ideal for you. This is only an approximation.

Some weight charts make allowances for age, adding a few pounds every few years. But, obviously, if a woman is going to retain her youthful figure, her weight should be maintained at her "ideal" weight throughout her lifetime.

THE HEIGHT-WEIGHT CHART

Locate your height and then intersect your correct weight under your frame size.

Height	Small Frame	Medium Frame	Large Frame
5'	100	105	110
5'1"	105	110	115
5'2"	110	115	120
5'3"	115	120	125
5'4"	120	125	130
5'5"	125	130	135
5'6"	130	135	140
5'7"	135	140	145
5'8"	140	145	150
5'9"	145	150	155
5'10"	150	155	160
5'11"	155	160	165
6'	160	165	170

EXERCISES FOR BODY PERFECTION

FIGURE MEASUREMENTS When taking your figure measurements:
1. Measure with high heels on.
2. Measure the largest part of the bust.
3. Measure the smallest part of the waistline with the tape measure snug, but not pinching.
4. The hips are measured at the largest projections of the buttocks.
5. Measure the highest part of the thigh.
6. Always measure the knee just above the knee cap.
7. Measure the largest portion of the calf.
8. The ankle is measured just above the ankle bone.

**LOCATION OF
MAIN POINTS FOR FIGURE MEASUREMENT**

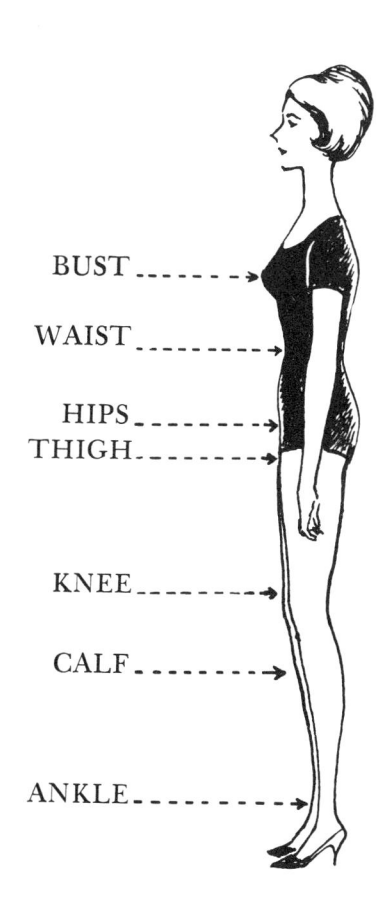

MEASUREMENT CHART

My frame is slender, medium, large. (Underline one.) My wrist measurement is _____. My height is _9′9″_. This is without heels, in bare feet. My ideal weight should be approximately _____. Interval between measurements _____.

Date measurements taken						Ideal Measurements
BUSTLINE						
WAISTLINE						
HIPLINE						
THIGH						
KNEE						
CALF						
ANKLE						
These measurements are optional, Neck—measure in middle						
Upper arm—measure four inches up from elbow.						
Diaphragm—measure just under the breasts.						
Abdomen—measure four inches below the waistline.						
Comments: Posture Firmness Special Conditions or Operations						

A BEAUTIFUL FIGURE

Here are some of the things you should look for in deciding which exercises will be best for you.

The chin and throat should be firm without rolls or wrinkles.

The bustline should be high and rounding with the nipples in a position half way between the shoulders and the elbows.

The back should be firm and flat with no shoulder blades protruding.
The waistline should cinch in from all sides, especially the front. There should be a slight rise to the diaphragm.
The stomach should be a slightly convex (outward) oval that is attached to the hip bones on either side, to the waistline above and the pubic bone below.
The buttocks should form a rounding hipline that stops high on the thigh. There should be no unsightly bulges to the hipline when viewed from front, back or side.
The legs should not be bowed with the knees turning inward. Rather they should be held with the knee caps straight forward.
Attractive legs look like this.

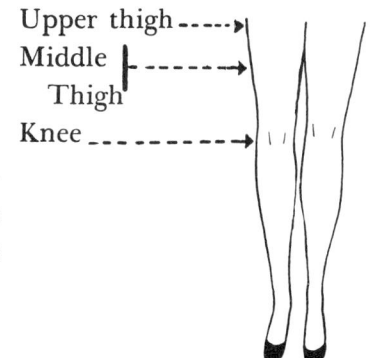

Upper thigh
Middle Thigh
Knee

There should be approximately 3 inches difference between the upper and the middle thigh measurement, and 7 inches difference between the upper thigh and knee measurement.

THE POWER OF EXERCISE The really wonderful and amazing thing about exercise is that it will reduce the overweight and build the underweight. It normalizes and beautifies. No matter what your weight or age, a certain amount of planned exercise is essential for muscle tone and general well-being.

THE IDEAL MEASUREMENTS

Here is a chart with which you can compare measurements. These measurements represent the general proportions of the ideal figure.

Height	Weight	Bust	Waist	Hips	Thigh	Calf	Ankle
5′	100-110	32	22	32	20	11½	7
5′2″	110-117	32½	22½	33	20	12	8
5′4″	115-122	34	24	35	21	12½	8
5′6″	125-135	35½	25½	36½	22	13½	8
5′8″	135-145	37½	27	38	22½	13½	8
5′10″	145-155	37½	27	38½	23¾	14½	9
6′	155-165	38	28	39	24	14½	9

It is important for you to remember that all charts are general and do no allow for individual differences. Therefore, when your figure is pleasing to the eye—to your eyes and the eyes of others—it has achieved the ultimate.

YOUR DAILY EXERCISE PROGRAM

Your daily program should include general exercises as well as those for specific figure problems. Where are your problems?

You will be able to improve your figure and push back your point of fatigue by keeping track, every day, of the number of times you can repeat each exercise. For instance, you may not be able to do more than two or three leg raises when you first start your program. By increasing the number of repetitions (times) you do this exercise, you will build strength and firmness in the stomach muscles in a relatively short period of time. On the other hand, if you are content to do this exercise only a few times, and not increase this number, it will be of relatively little value. To increase your strength and perfect your figure, you must have as your goal, the ability to do each exercise up to at least the number of repetitions recommended.

Your exercise program may be recorded in a workbook or on weekly cards similar to the following sample.

A TYPICAL WEEKLY EXERCISE RECORD CARD

Week of _____	Number of times I was able to do exercise on:							Measurements at:
No. & Name of Exercise	1st day	2nd	3rd	4th	5th	6th	7th	Beginning of Week: Wt._____ Bust_____ Waist_____ Hips_____ End of Wk. Wt._____ Bust_____ Waist_____ Hips_____
Warmup								
etc.								

ON YOUR MARK, GET SET, GO!
1. Start with the warm-up.
2. Do general exercises first, then specific ones.
3. Taper off with relaxing exercises that will help you "cool down".
4. Breathe in rhythm with the exercise—the faster the movements, the faster you breathe.
5. Inhale through the nose, exhale through the mouth unless you work so hard you have to "pant", then breathe entirely through the mouth.
6. Inhale on expansive movements, exhale on contracting movements. *Example:* On sit-ups—Exhale as you sit up.
   Inhale as you lie down.

EXERCISES FOR BODY PERFECTION

7. For reducing or building, use the same exercises; but *for building, use slow, deliberate, controlled movements; for reducing, use rapid, quick movements.*
8. Do about eight to ten different exercises each day.
9. Change your exercises every *two* weeks. This will make for more rapid progress and keep you from becoming bored with the same routines.
10. For bustline building, use *weights* in the hands. These can be books or cans of food or Glamour Belles.

THE EXERCISES

A beautiful body is supple, it moves with grace and rhythm. It is flexible and free. How long you exercise will depend upon how quickly you tire. Exercise should relax and exhilarate, not exhaust, so stop before you are fatigued.

It is important for you to concentrate on the results you wish to achieve so that you will do the exercises precisely and accurately. If at first you can't do them as well as you would like, keep trying.

8. WARM-UP EXERCISE
Stand with feet apart and arms spread. Keep the knees straight. Touch right hand to left toe. Alternate. Ten to twenty times.

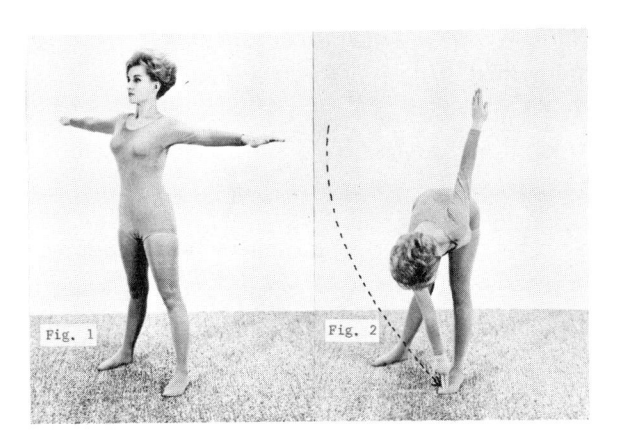

Breathe properly, exhale on contracting movements and inhale on expanding movements. Deep breathing has been of benefit to those who find it difficult to relax. It is wonderful for revitalizing the tissues with energy and oxygen.

9. BRAIN BREATHING
Feet together, arms relaxed at sides. Inhale. Bend forward, hold the breath. Return to starting position. Exhale. Three times.

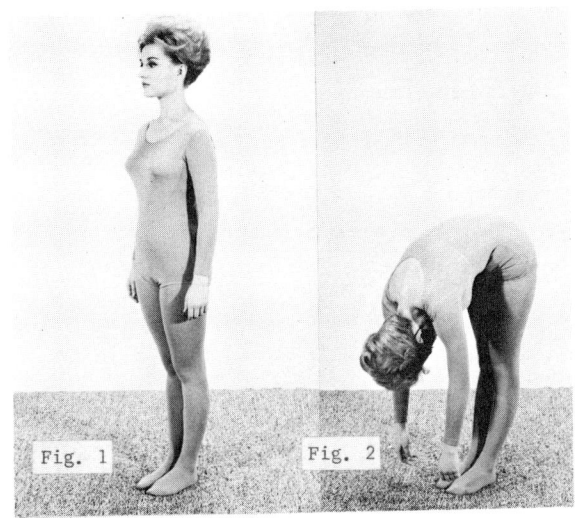

10. POSTURE BREATHING

Lie flat, arms at sides. Inhale, swing arms overhead, stretch feet downward. Tense, stretch. Touch waistline to floor. Return arms to sides. Exhale. Three times.

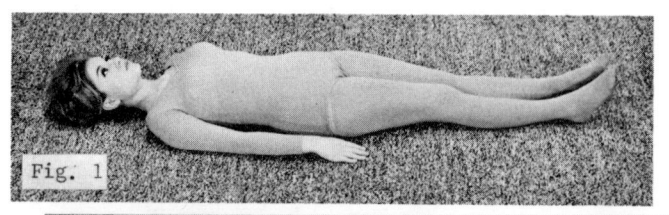

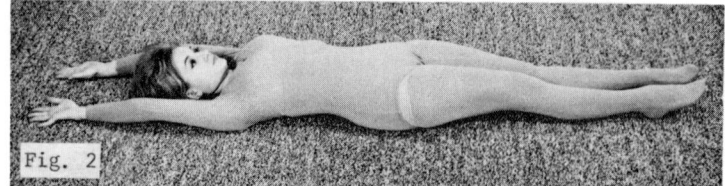

Note: Any dizziness that might occur on the breathing exercises is due to excess oxygen (hyperventilation) and will quickly pass.

Now, because grace and an appearance of youthfulness are dependent upon a supple spine, here are a couple of spine twisters and spine relaxers.

11. SPINE TWISTERS

a. Stretch arms up with palms of hands facing each other. Twist to right, then to left. Hold head between upper arms. Ten times.

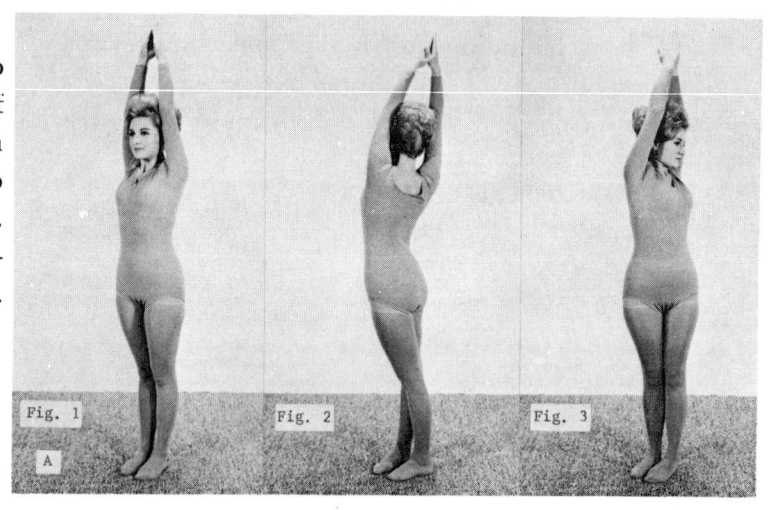

b. Spread feet. Touch right toes. Return. Now touch left toes. Ten times.

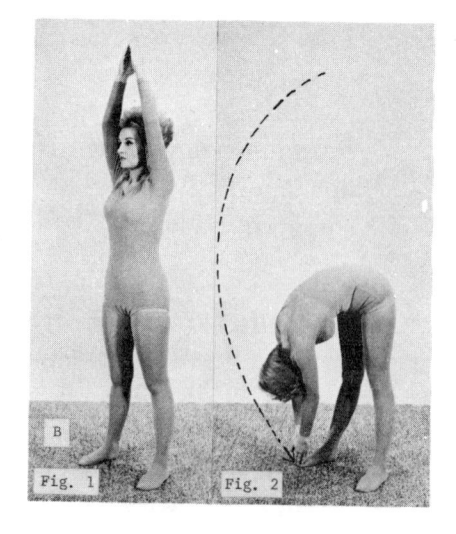

12. SPINE RELAXERS

a. Lie on stomach. Place hands behind head. Lift head and feet. Arch back. Hold five seconds. Repeat five times.

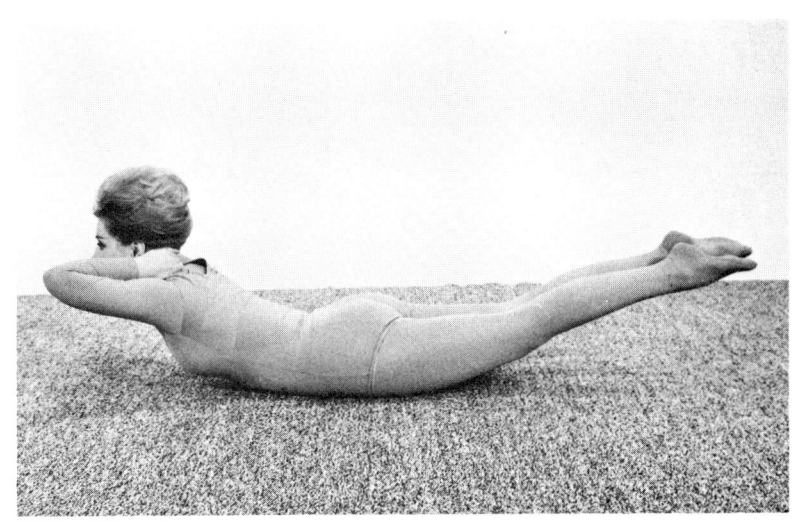

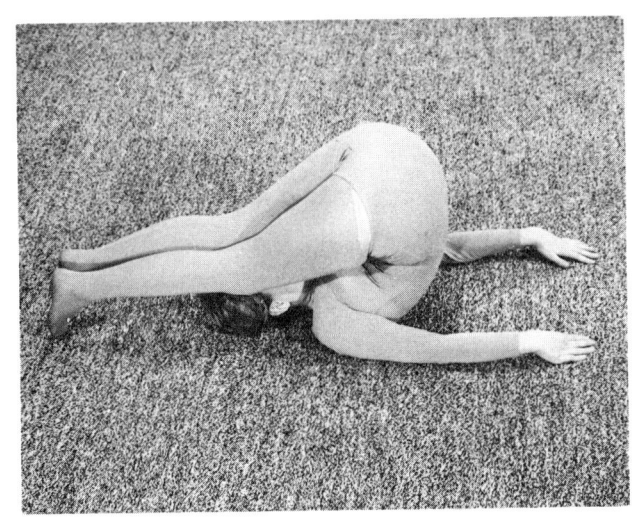

b. Roll over. Bring legs over head. Touch floor. Keep knees straight. Ten times.

GENERAL STRENGTH EXERCISES

In addition to the warm-up that you will do every day at the beginning of your exercise session, select one or two of these general exercises for well-being and strength. Do them immediately after the Warm Up before you do the more specific exercises for your own individual figure problems.

Don't forget to include in your exercise program any posture exercises you need from the previous chapter.

13. SIDE STRADDLE HOP

Feet together, hands at sides. Jump, extending feet sideways, fling arms overhead. Jump back. Bring arms to sides. Repeat ten times, more if you are able.

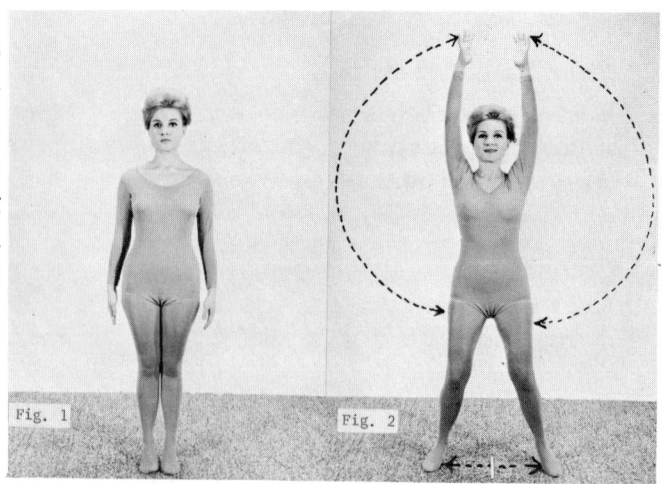

14. DEEP KNEE BENDS

Hold back of chair. Bend knees. Sit on haunches. Stand up. Repeat up to 25 times.

15. THE ARCH

Lie on stomach with pad under hip and pubic bones. See exercise #12.

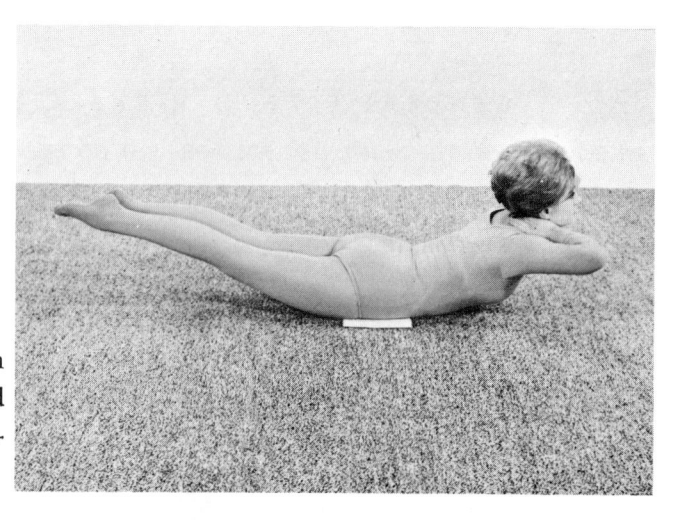

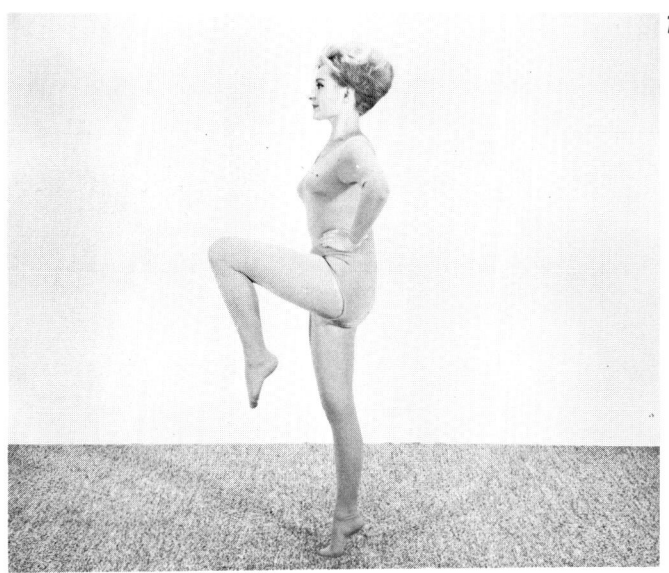

EXERCISES FOR BODY PERFECTION

16. PRANCING
Hands on hips. Run. Bring knees up high to chest. Stop if pain develops in side. 25 times.

17. STATIONERY TROT
Trot. Place one foot in front, then other. Keep weight on both feet. Faster! Stay on toes, hands at sides. Go! Up to 50 times.

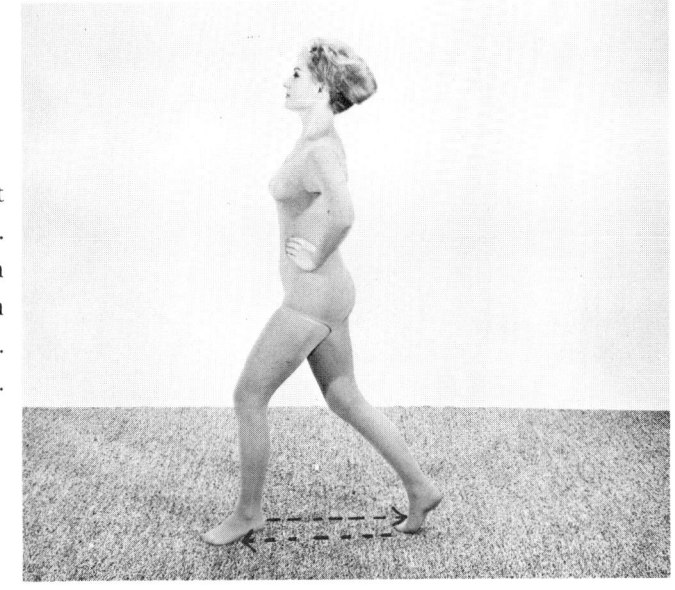

18. DEEP LEG PLUNGES
Feet together, hands at the sides. Extend right leg forward, bend right knee until left knee touches floor. Bounce back with feet together. Do not move left foot. Reverse. Use left leg to plunge forward. Repeat up to 10 times, each leg.

19. FROG JUMP

Crouch. Jump backward until legs are extended straight out. Lower hips to form a straight line. Jump back. Repeat no more than 10 times.

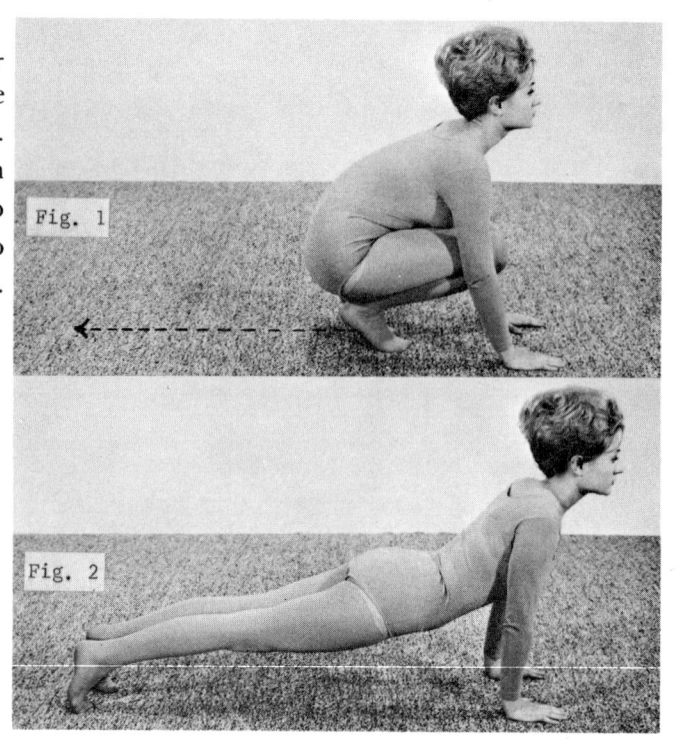

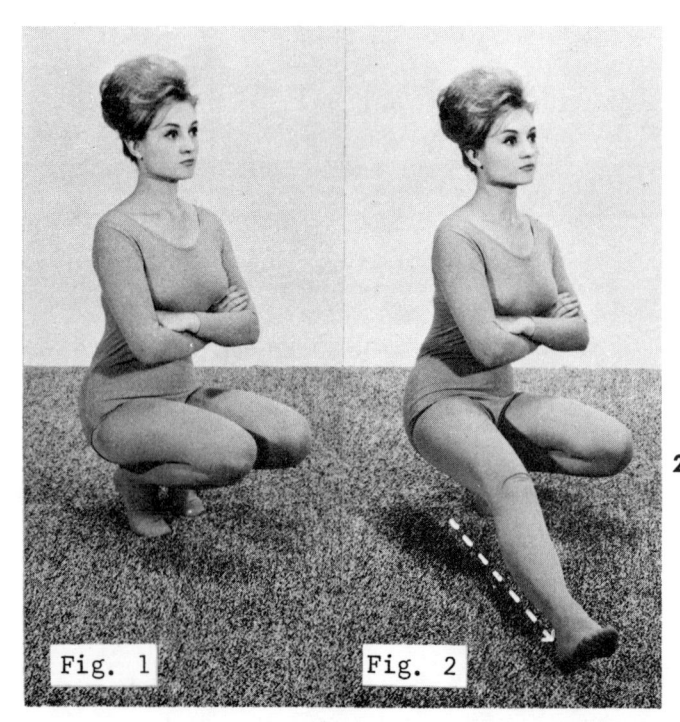

Fig. 1

Fig. 2

20. RUSSIAN DANCE

Squat, buttocks rest on heels. Fold arms. Extend first one leg and then other out in front. Try, try again. Up to 20 times.

Fig. 1

Fig. 2

21. SIDE LEG JUMP

Like Frog Jump except jump is alternately to each side rather than to back.

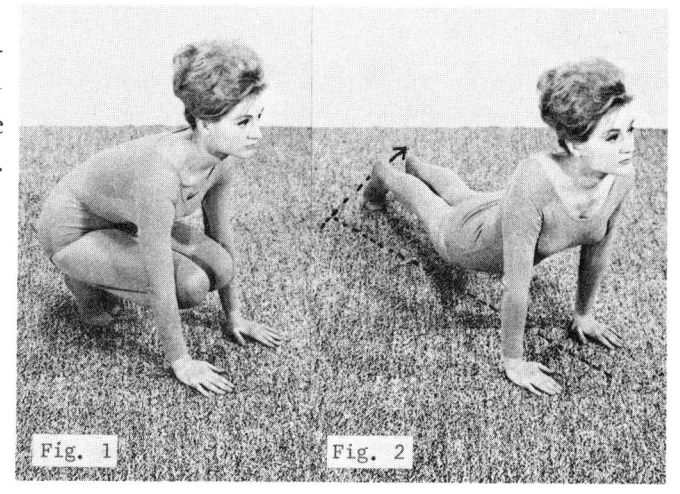

22. MULE KICK

Kneel on hands and knees. Extend right leg. Keep right knee straight. Kick up and down rapidly up to 20 times. Repeat with left leg. Good for hips, thighs and waistline.

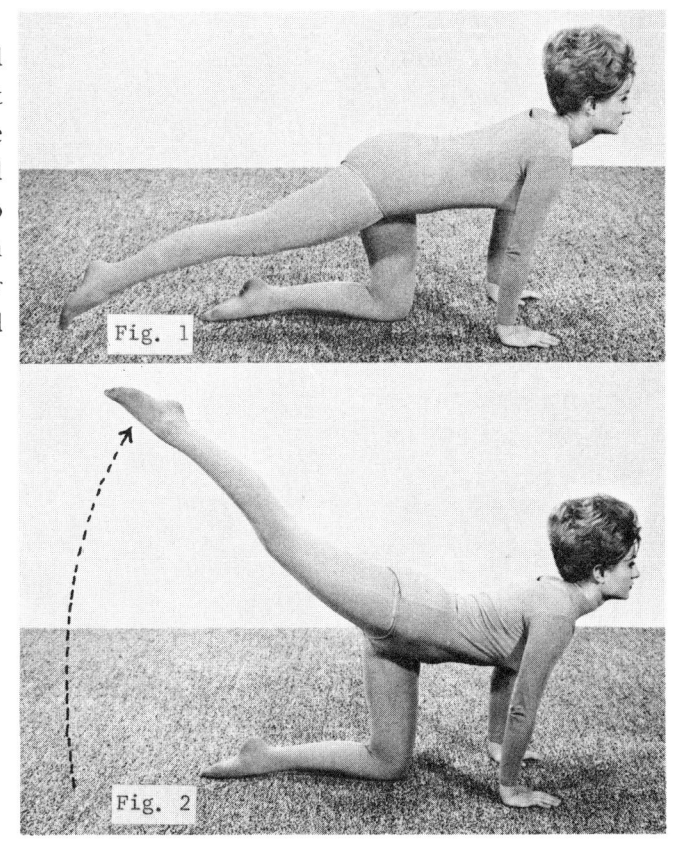

BUSTLINE BUILDING EXERCISES

Get a couple of books, tin food cans or Glamour Belles to use as weights in your hands before you begin. This weight places resistance on the muscles and will cause them to work harder; consequently, you will get faster results.
Do all Bustline Exercises slowly and breathe rhythmically.

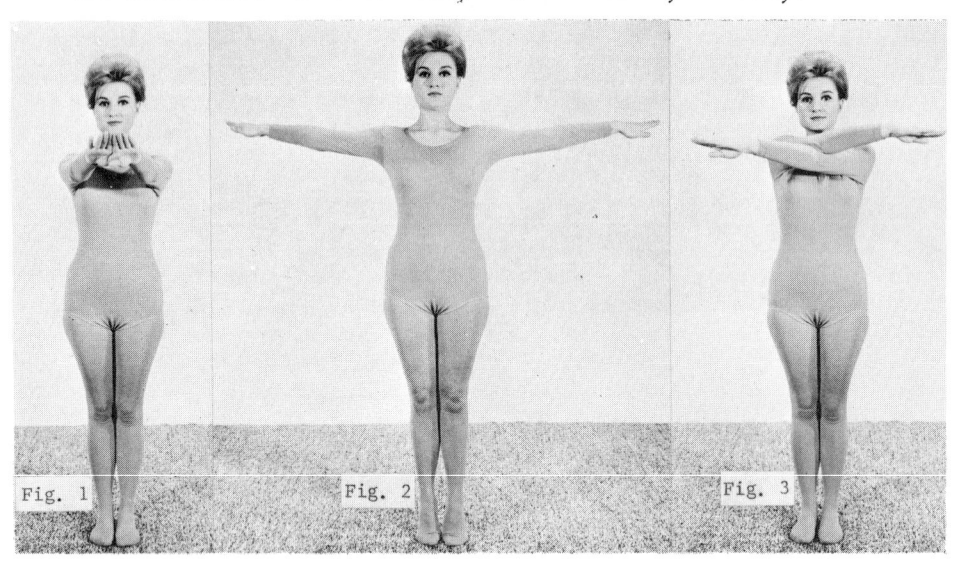

Fig. 1   Fig. 2   Fig. 3

23. FLY AWAY

Arms shoulder high, hands together in front, palms facing floor. Fling arms backward, shoulder high. Come onto toes. Inhale. Bring arms forward. Cross arms. Exhale and drop to heels. Repeat up to 30-40 times alternating one hand on top as they cross and then other.

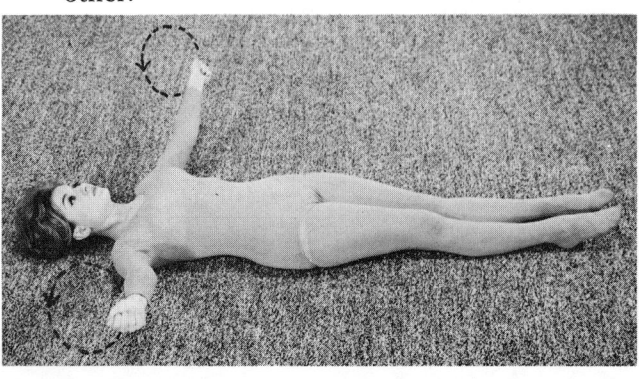

24. BUSTLINE CIRCLES

Lie face up, arms outstretched, palms facing ceiling. Keep elbows straight, circle hands backward toward head in circles twelve inches in diameter. Inhale and exhale with every circle. Repeat 30-60 times.

EXERCISES FOR BODY PERFECTION

Fig. 1

Fig. 2

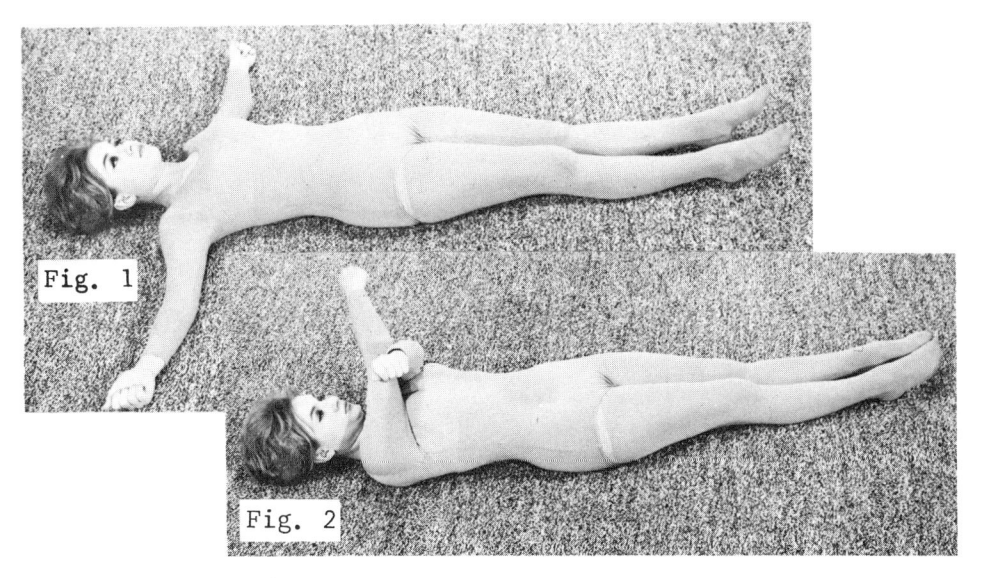

25. PECTORAL CRAMP
Palms face ceiling, bring arms upward across body. Place one arm closer to face, then other. Keep elbows straight. Exhale as arms come across chest, inhale as they return to floor. Repeat 30-60 times.

26. HEAD OVER EDGE OF BED
Arms are at sides, palms down. Go over head until hands nearly touch the floor. Inhale as hands go over, exhale as they return to sides. This raises, firms breasts. 20 times.

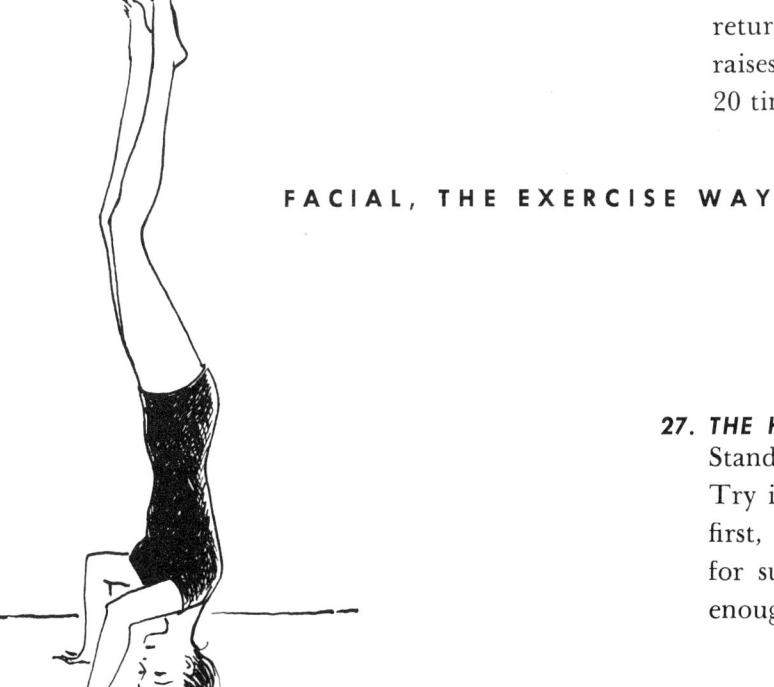

FACIAL, THE EXERCISE WAY

27. THE HEADSTAND
Stand on your head. Try it in a corner at first, using the walls for support. Once is enough in one day.

28. FACE AWAKENER
Say EEK then OH alternately fifteen times.

29. THE PUFFER
Stand in front of mirror. Puff out cheeks with air. Hold. Watch mouth lines disappear. Repeat 5 times.

30. THE LIP RELAXER
For softer mouth and lips, relax lips completely and blow through them. You should get a repeated putt-putt sound.

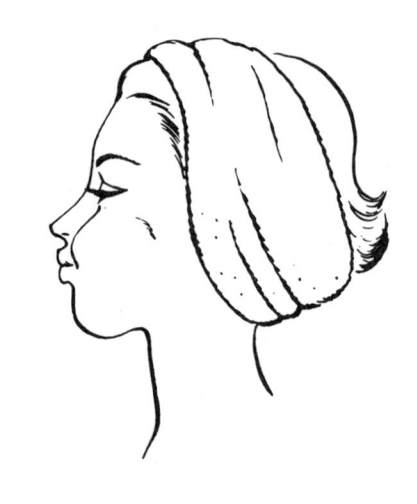

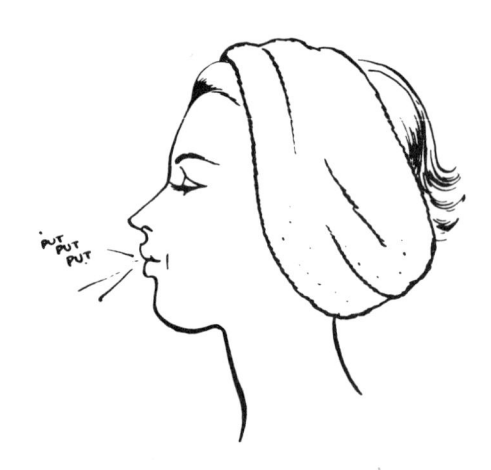

31. THE FACIAL SQUEEZE
Inhale, hold breath. Squeeze eyes shut. Squeeze features together. Pucker up for beauty, not for kissing. That comes later. Repeat 3 times.

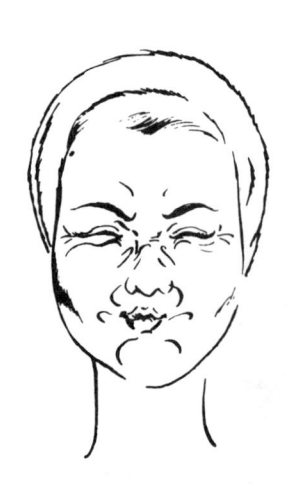

EXERCISES FOR A FIRM NECK AND CHIN

32. THE WALL STAND
Stand against wall, push neck close to wall. Neck beauty is ninety-five percent correct posture. Keep your ear lobe just above your shoulder bone. Once a day for the wall stand.

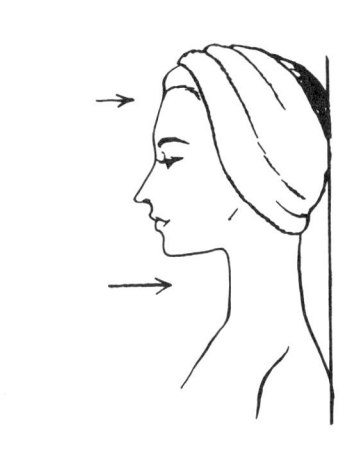

33. THE CHIN TONER
Throw head as far back as possible. Open mouth, thrust jaw forward. Close mouth. Feel pull on front neck muscles. Repeat 15 times.

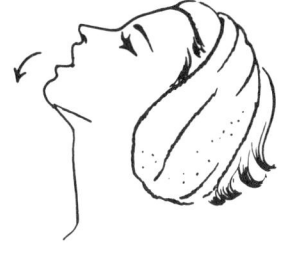

Fig. 1 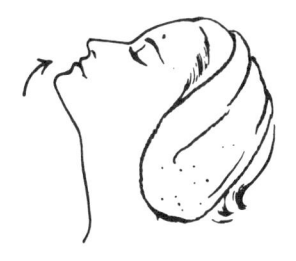 Fig. 2

34. THE HEAD NOD
Bend head forward to chest. Bend head back. Turn face to right side, touch chin to shoulder. Raise head up as far as you can. Repeat to left side. 5 times each direction.

Fig. 1 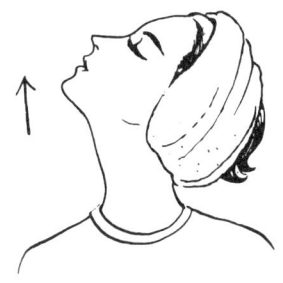 Fig. 2

35. THE INVERTED HEAD DIP
Tension in neck and shoulder muscles causes headaches. To relax these muscles, lie on bed, head hanging over edge. Raise to chest and lower slowly. 5 times.

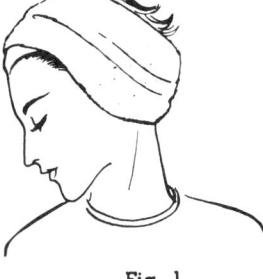

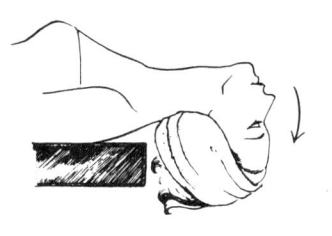

Fig. 1 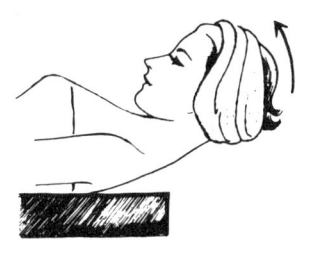 Fig. 2

374   EXERCISES FOR BODY PERFECTION

EXERCISES FOR BEAUTIFUL BACK, ARMS AND SHOULDERS

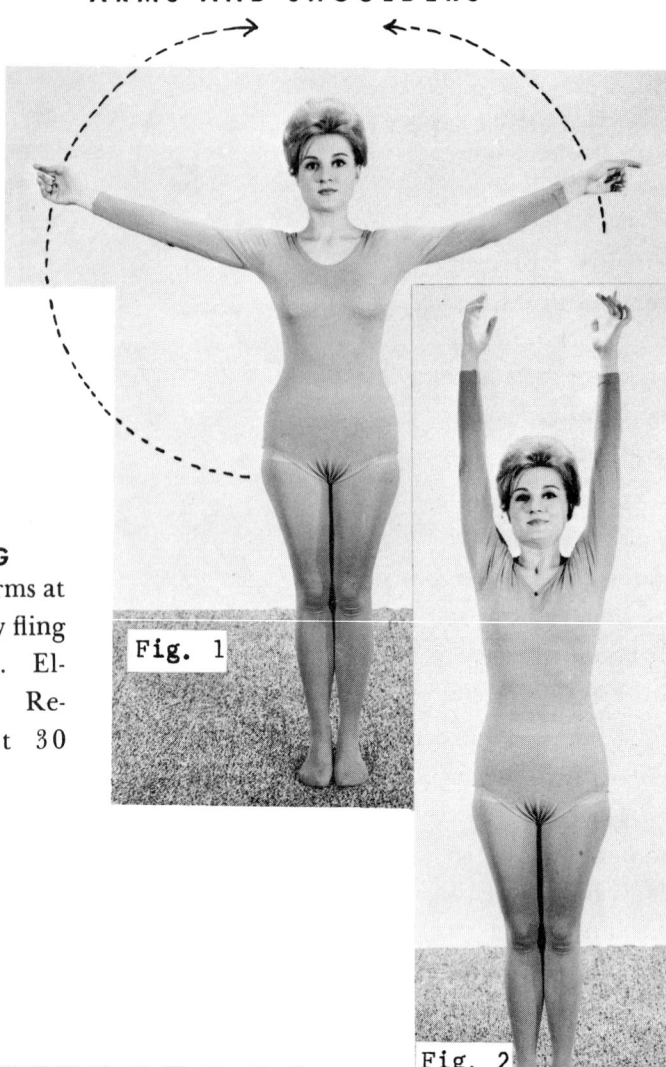

36. SIDE ARM FLING

Feet together, arms at sides. Vigorously fling arms overhead. Elbows straight. Return. Repeat 30 times.

Fig. 1

Fig. 2

37. SHADOW BOXING

Like to fight—pounds that is? Try punching. Give those pounds a left hook. Left fist to right, right fist to left. Flabby flesh is getting a beating. 30 times.

EXERCISES FOR BODY PERFECTION

38. THE ARM SWING

Feet together, hands at sides. Raise arms forward and up. Lower out to sides and down. Wonderful for winging away "dowagers hump."

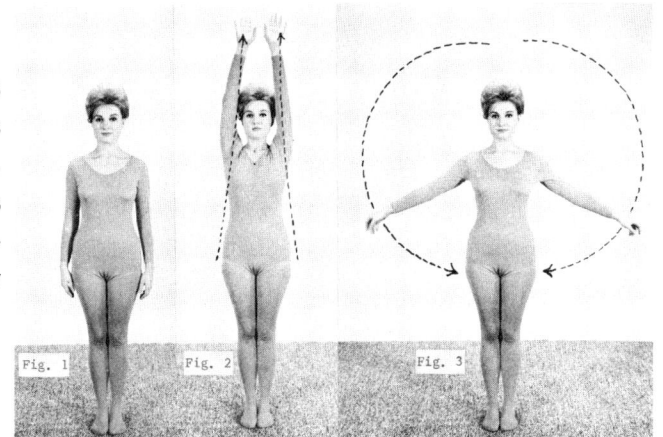

EXERCISES FOR DIAPHRAGM AND WAISTLINE

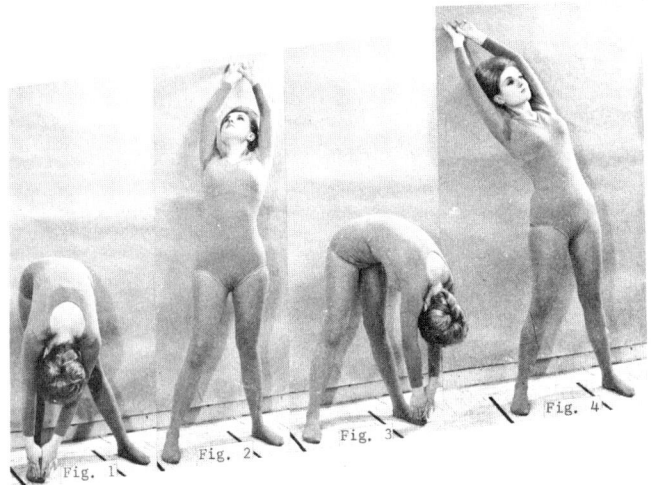

39. TOE TOUCH WALL REACH

Stand a foot away from wall. Place hands overhead. Clasp thumbs together. Ready! Bend, touch right foot with fingers. Come up, touch wall over your head and to left. R E A C H ! Reverse. Touch left toes and wall to right. Repeat 10 times.

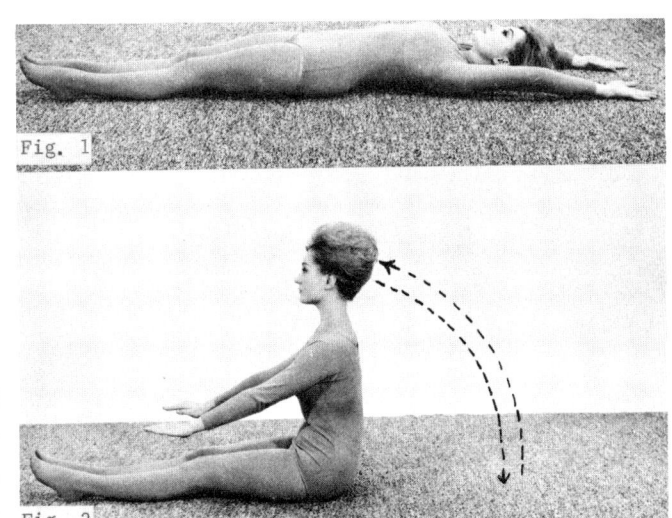

40. THE SIT-UP

Lie on your back, on the floor. Sit up to deflate your spare tire, and inflate your ego. 10 times.

41. THE WAISTLINE AROUND

Here's a terrific waistline cincher. Bend forward, bounce finger tips off floor four times. Come to upright position. Place left arm close to ear, hand overhead. Right arm relaxed at side. Bend to right side. Bounce four times. Place both hands on upper back thighs. Bend backward, bounce four times. Now to left side, right arm up. Around 10 times.

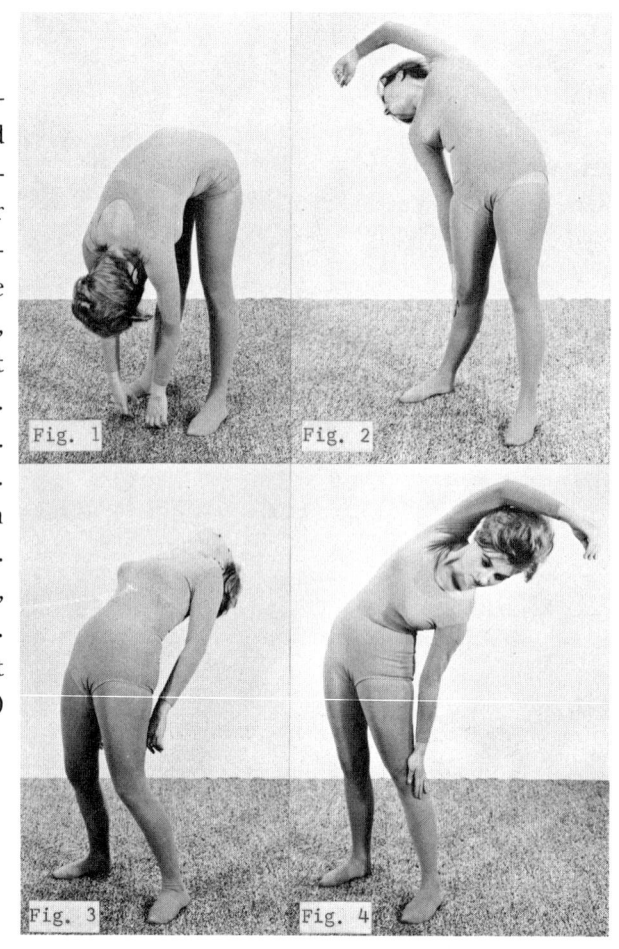

42. THE ELEPHANT SWING

Bend forward, keep upper torso parallel with floor. Let arms relax. Swing with arms. Slowly to right, then to left, farther and farther. Get your waistline into the act. See ceiling on each side? Good girl! 20 times.

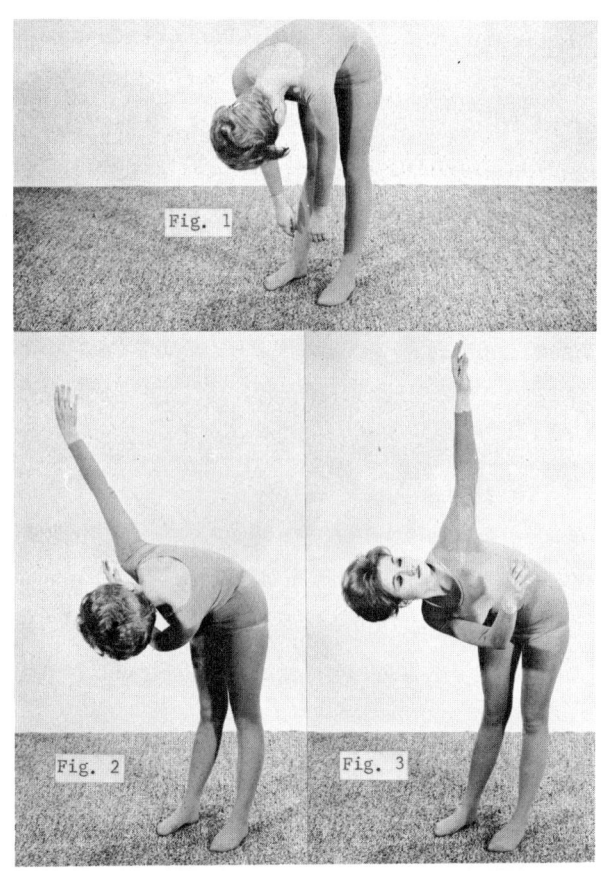

EXERCISES FOR BODY PERFECTION   377

HIPLINE TRIMMERS

If you're just plain too fat, the hipline exercises will give double duty for the waistline too. Let's roll it off! Where are you fighting the "Battle of the Bulge"?

43. KNEES TO CHEST ROLL
For fat on upper hips, lie on floor with arms spread. Bring both knees to chest and roll. First to right, then to left. Slap those thighs down hard. 40 times.

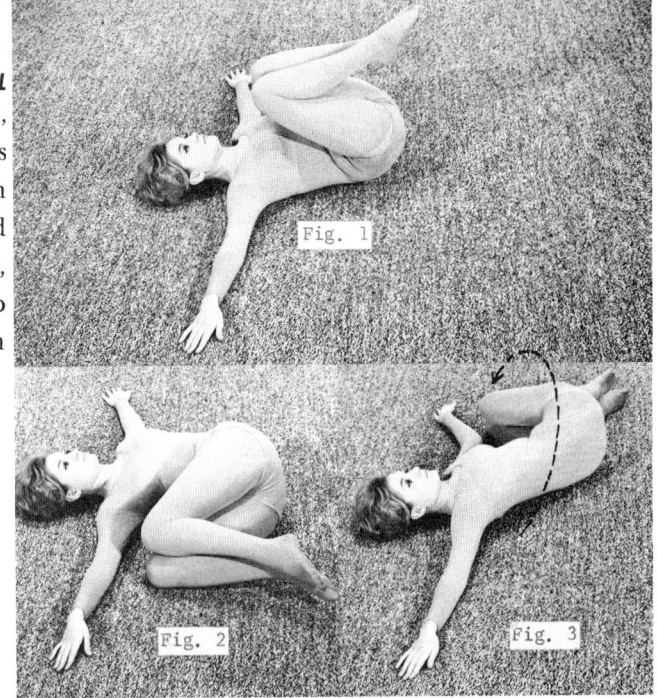

44. LEG OVER HIP ROLL
Lie flat, arms outspread. Bring right toes up to touch left hand. Keep knees straight. Alternate. 20 times.

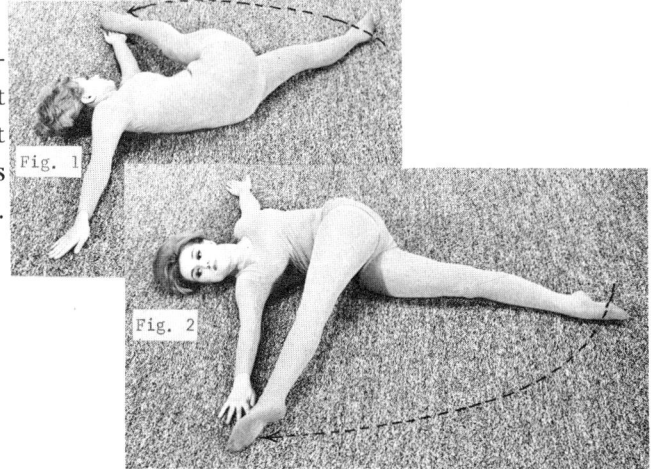

45. THE KNEE OVER HIP ROLL
Lie, arms outspread. Bend left knee, roll it to floor on right side. Alternate. 40 times.

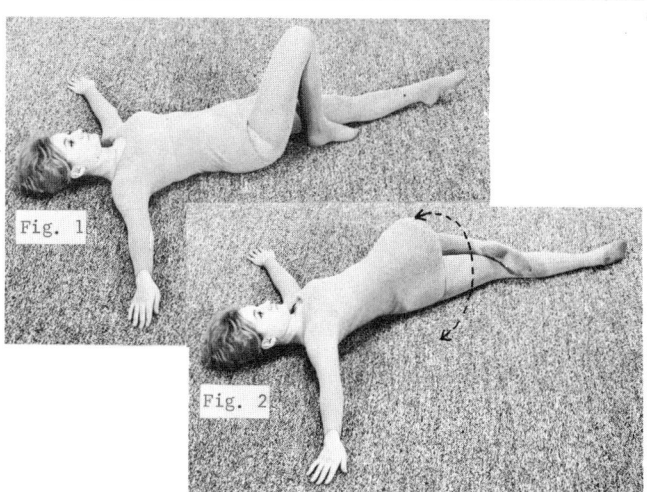

378   EXERCISES FOR BODY PERFECTION

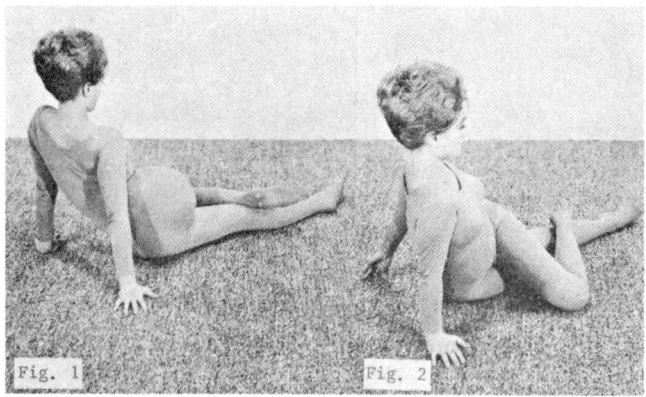

46. THE SITTING KNEE OVER

Rest on hands. Knee up and over as in previous exercise. Feel pressure on upper thighs? Alternate. 40 times.

47. THE "IN POSITION" HIP ROLL

Sit with left foot against right knee, right foot out to right side. Keep feet off floor as you swing legs to opposite side. Repeat. 20 times.

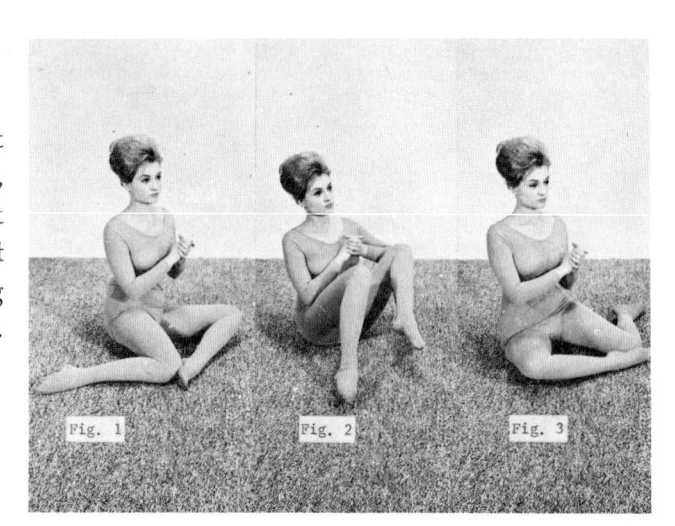

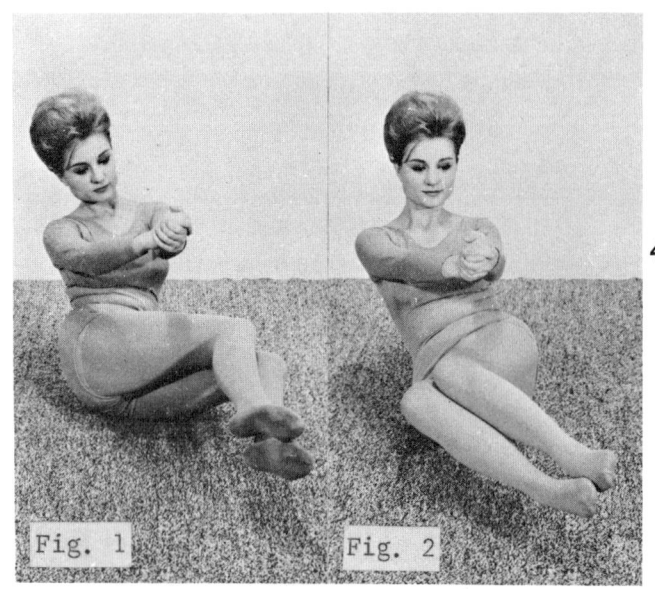

48. THE HIP ROCK

Put hands in front, arms straight. Bend knees, feet off floor. Roll on hips. As knees go to right, arms will go to left. Touch knees to floor on left, then right. 20 times.

EXERCISES FOR BODY PERFECTION

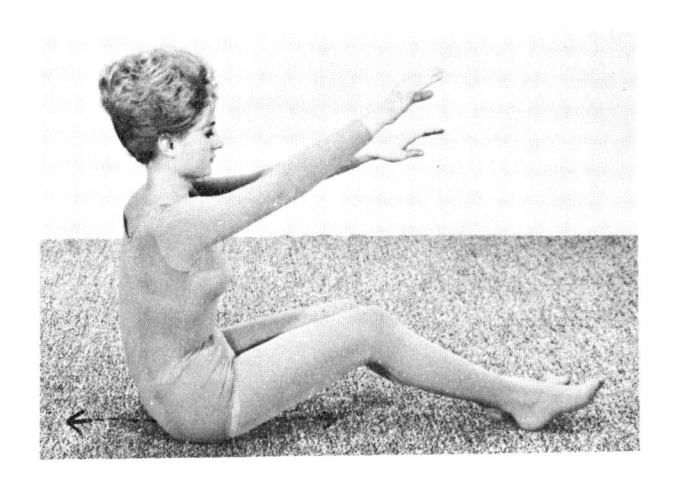

49. THE HIP WALK
Walk on hips, forward and back. Extend hands in front. 20 "steps".

50. THE JACK KNIFE
Good for hips and stomach. "Jack Knife" head and feet until all weight is on hips. Roll. 20 times.

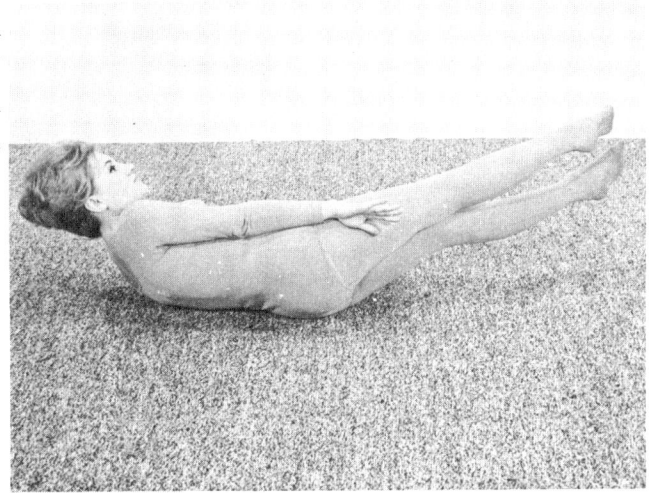

STOMACH EXERCISES FOR THE FLAT LOOK

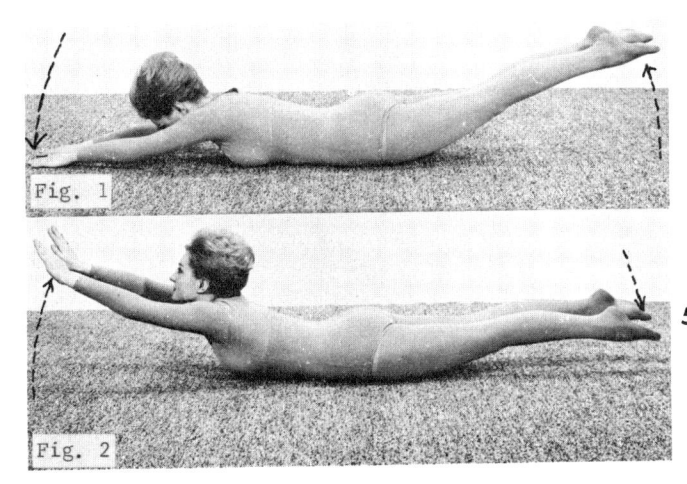

Fig. 1

Fig. 2

51. THE ROCKING HORSE
Lie on stomach. Extend arms. Arch and rock. 10 times.

52. LEG RAISES

Raise one leg at time, or both legs; slowly to a count of ten. Lower legs to six inches off floor, spread, place together, lower to floor and repeat from the beginning. 10 times.

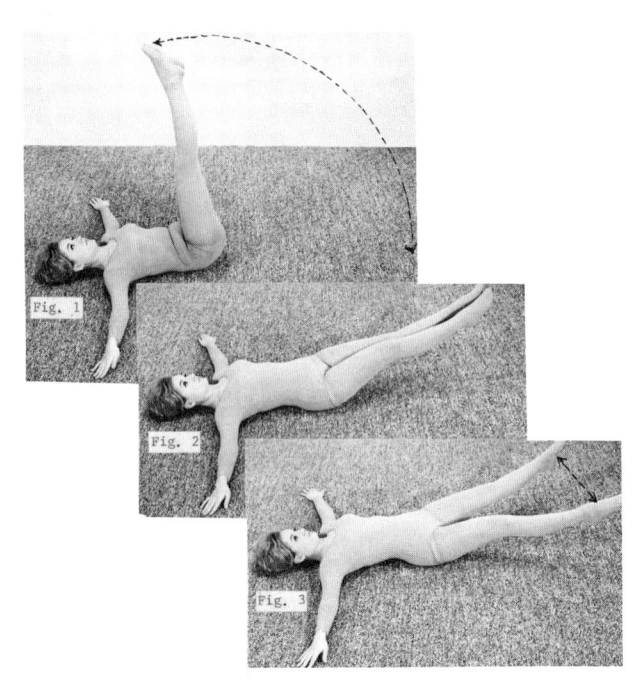

53. THE BOOK BOUNCE

Place book on tummy. Bounce it off by flexing stomach muscles. 20 times.

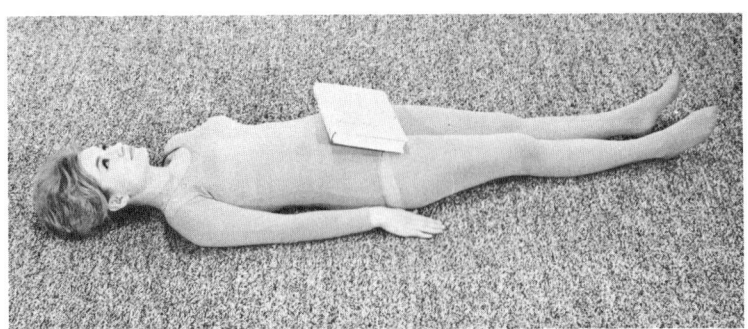

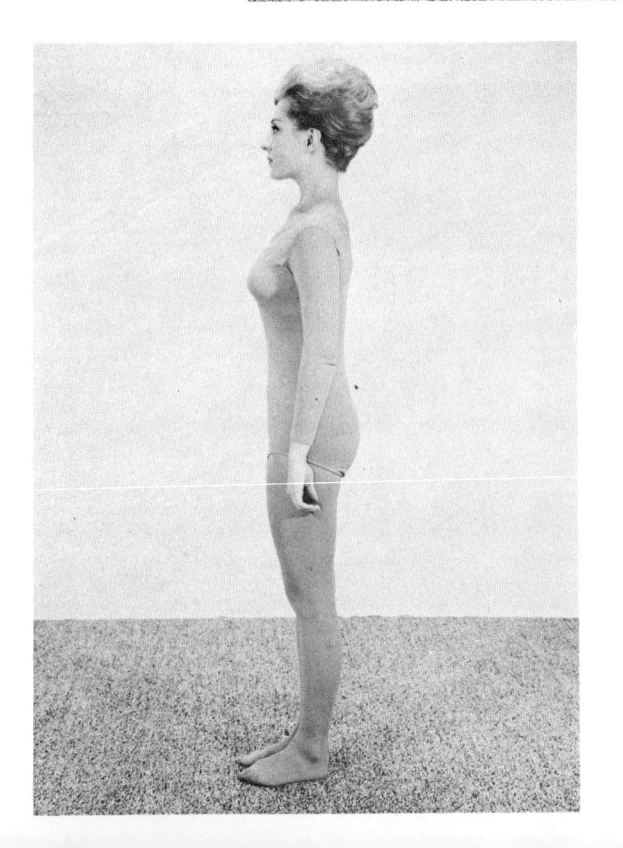

54. THE STOMACH FLATTENER

Pull stomach as flat as possible. Tense, relax. Muscle toning requires muscle tension. Hold tummy flat as a matter of habit. 10 times.

EXERCISES FOR BODY PERFECTION

LEGS

The contour and muscle tone of your legs have a great deal to do with your feminine attractiveness. They also have a great deal to do with how quickly you tire. Some women have unshapely legs because they are overweight, others because they have heavy muscles (these are rare), however, most unattractive legs are due to the lack of the right kind of muscle development.

When you realize that approximately 50% of your entire body is muscle tissue, you will come to understand the importance of good muscle tone and development. This is important not only to beauty, but also to stamina, health, and a feeling of well-being. Because your legs must carry you, literally, from the cradle to the grave you will want to do the following exercises daily. At least one or two to give those tired muscles a much needed change of pace and blood supply.

You have probably observed that men are instinctively attracted to a "well turned ankle"—and leg. Proper development will give you at least a two foot lead—you'll be out there in front—supported by good looking legs and feet, ahead in the race for social prestige, business success and feminine attractiveness.

Whether you are six or sixty, you can benefit. Just look at your favorite actresses and dancers, many of whom are over fifty, and they can still wear short shorts with pride. Can you?

Let's firm the muscles, revitalize the flesh, eliminate the bulges and fill in the hollows. Do yourself a good turn.

GAMS FOR GAPING AT AND GAMBOLING ON

55. THE LEG SWING

Hold onto back of chair. Swing outside leg back and forth. Ten times. Reverse. Ten times.

Fig. 1   Fig. 2

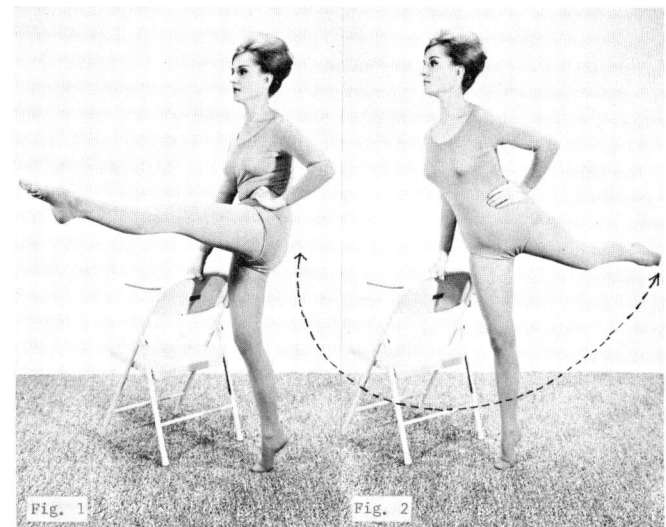

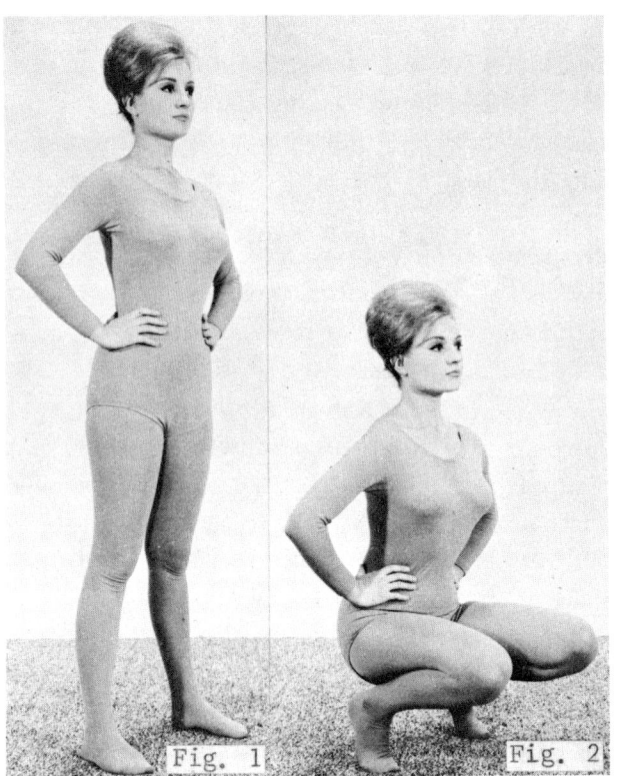

56. DEEP KNEE BENDS

Hands on hips, feet apart. Come onto toes, lower body to heels. Repeat. 25 times.

Fig. 1 Fig. 2

57. ARCH

Lie on tummy. Hands on hips. Hold ten counts. 10 times.

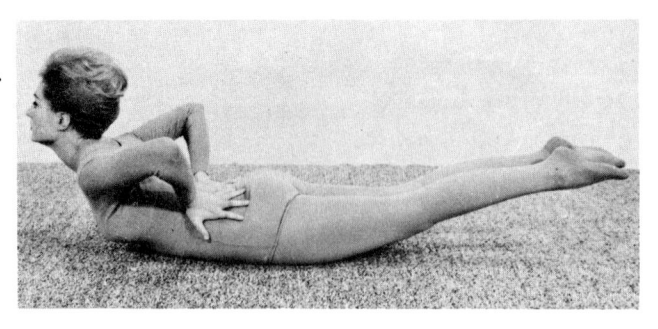

Note: The inner thigh is one of the first places to examine to find out if "the Old Gray Mare Ain't What She Used to Be." The following four exercises are for toning and building or reducing.

EXERCISES FOR BODY PERFECTION

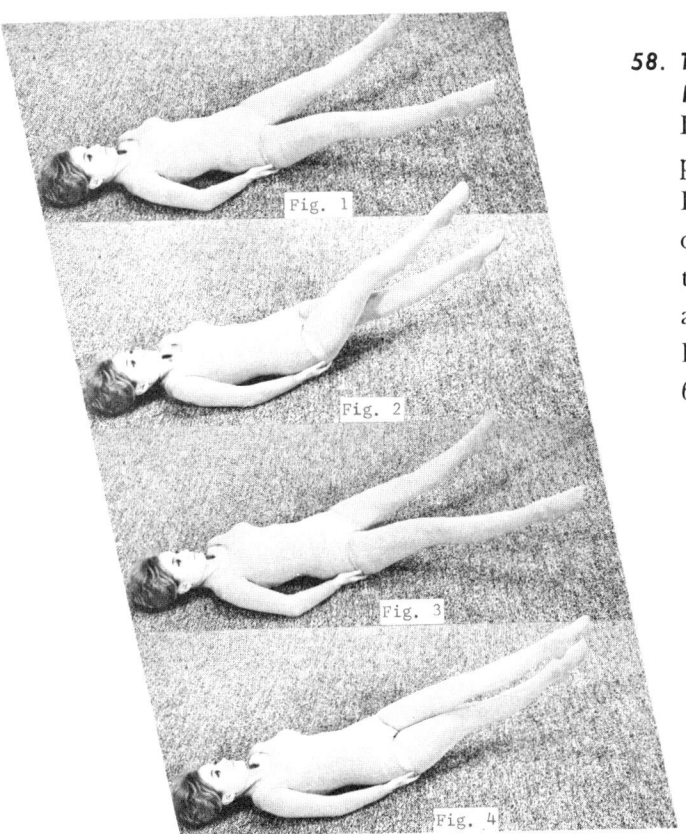

58. THE CROSS-OVER KICK

Lie with hands, palms up, under hips. Bring legs six inches off floor. Swing out, then across, out, then across. Alternate the leg on top. Try for 60 times.

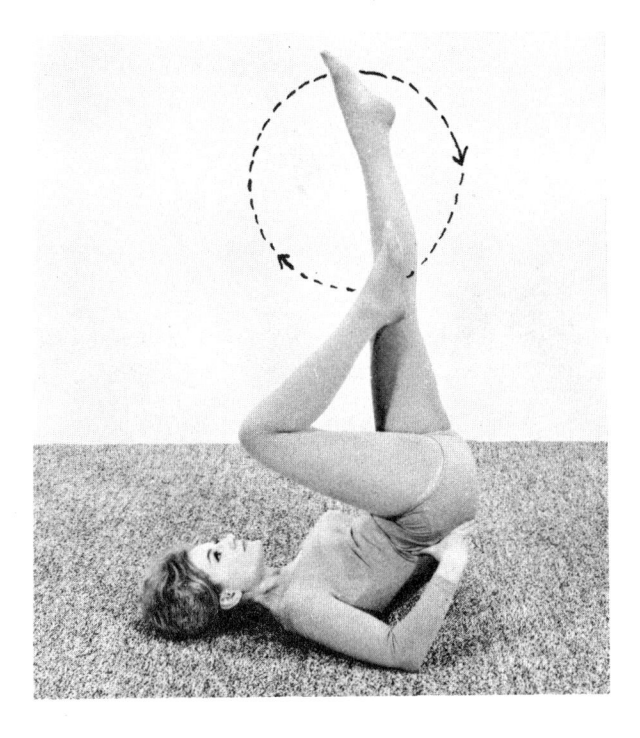

59. THE HIGH BICYCLE

Up on shoulders. Ride a bicycle—upside down. Go, go, go, faster, faster—100 times.

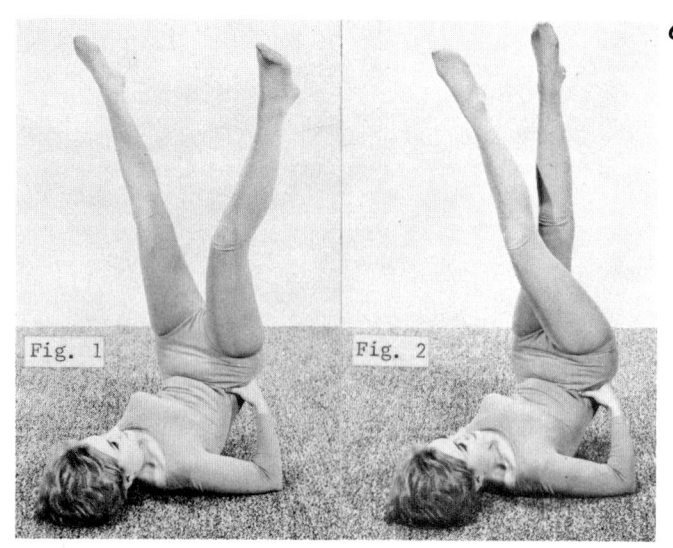

60. THE HIGH SCISSORS

Stay in bicycling position. Keep knees straight, extend sideways, out and across. Alternate crossover. 100 times.

61. SIDE LEG RAISES

Lie on side. Raise upper leg. Way up. Ten times. Roll over and repeat. Ten times.

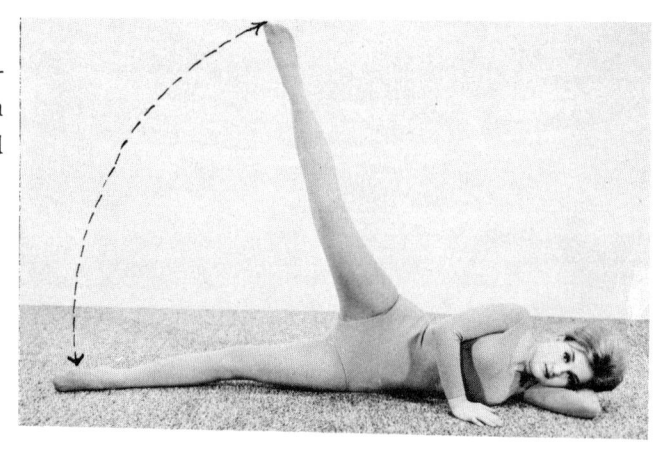

CALF BEAUTIFIERS

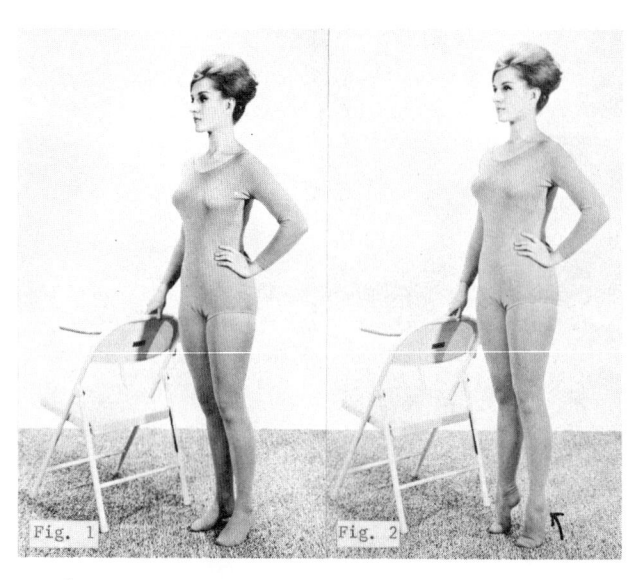

62. TOE RAISES

Bounce up and down on toes. Hold onto chair on floor or onto bannister on stairway. On stairway, let heels hang over edge of step. 20 times.

63. LEG CIRCLING

Lie on the back, raise one leg. Circle with foot ten times, circle with knee ten times, circle with hip ten times. Reverse direction of circles. Repeat. Now other leg. Same number of times. 10 each way.

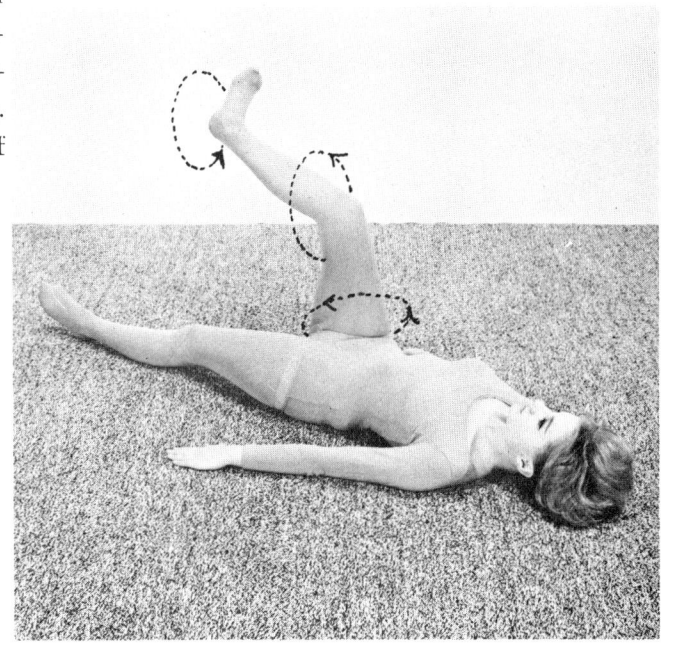

EXERCISES FOR THE UNDERWEIGHT

Thin, slender girls dream of having a figure that will look luscious in a bathing suit or in a dreamy dance dress with a decollete neckline. You can have just that, if you are willing to work for it.

To cover the bones of your chest, the pectoral muscles must be developed. The best exercises for this are the Bustline Exercises on page 370 Fortunately, these same exercises will fill out too thin arms too.

How long will it take? Well, this depends on how much energy you put into the exercises and how faithfully you do them. You must control the muscles involved by doing the exercises slowly and exactly. But it is worth it because after about three months, the unsightly hollows will be filled in.

Most underdeveloped girls, even with the best posture in the world, have a hollow between their shoulder blades. If you do, here is a cure-all for this figure problem.

64. THE CRANE

Note: Use weights in hands.

Bend forward. Keep back straight, parallel to floor. Palms face each other. Swing slowly outward and upward. Get arms up, keep elbows straight. Slowly return. Repeat until tired.

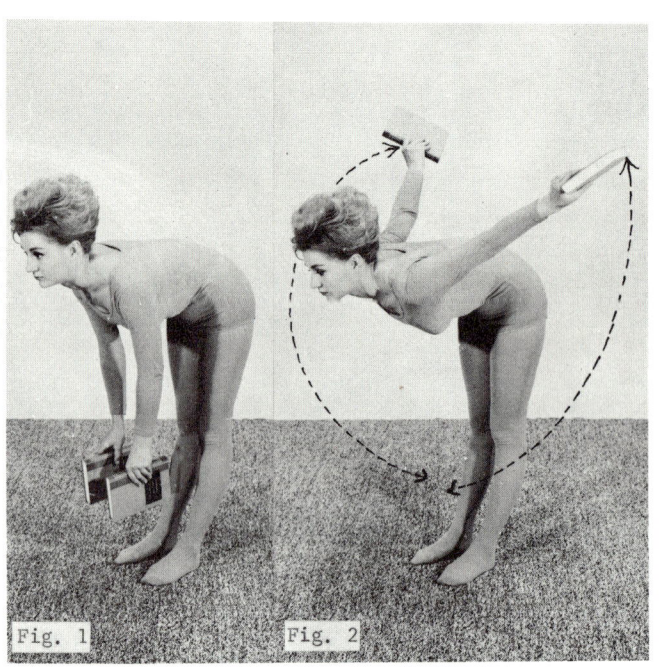

Fig. 1   Fig. 2

65-66-67

No girl is very happy with a pair of legs that look like two lollypop sticks. For curves, use exercises #52, #58, #61, and the following:

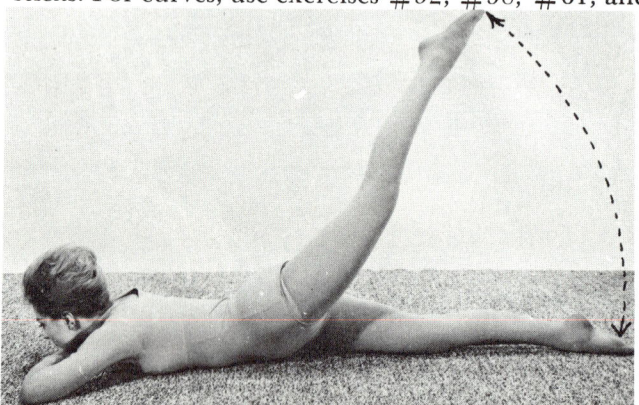

68. BACK LEG RAISES

Lie on stomach. Raise right leg slowly up and down ten times. Repeat with left leg. 10 times.

69. ELEVATOR RAISE

Lie on side. Keep both knees straight. Raise upper leg. Bring lower leg up to touch it. Return lower leg to floor. Repeat 10 times. Roll over to repeat with other leg. 10 times.

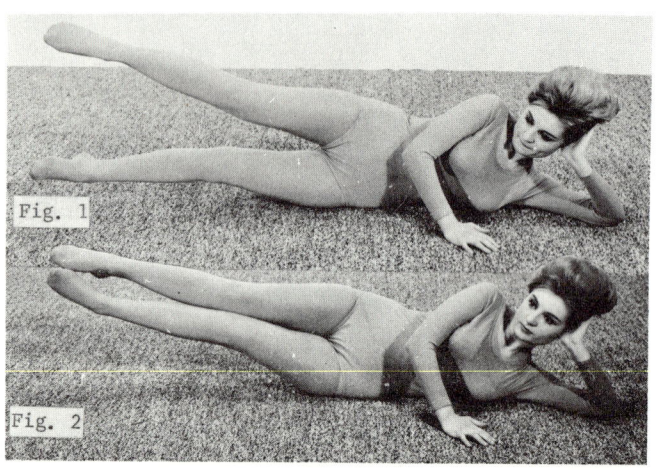

Fig. 1
Fig. 2

Just keep in mind that if you want to build bulk in muscles you must use slow, controlled movements.

EXERCISES FOR OVER-DEVELOPED CALVES

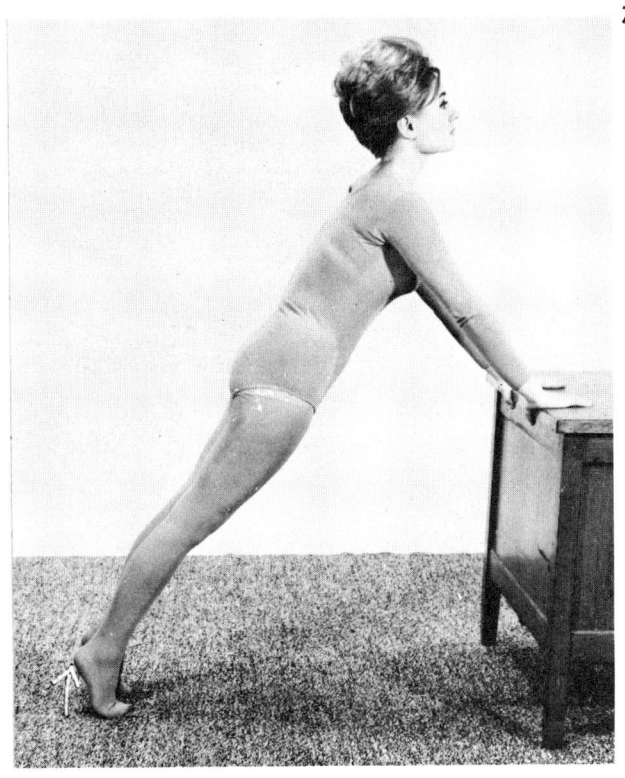

70. DIAGONAL CALF RAISES

Lean on table. Extend legs back, lower hips, raise onto toes. Lower and raise heels. Let it P-U-L-L 20 times.

71. THE TOE HOLD

Sit with knees straight. Lean forward. Grasp toes. Touch head to knees. Repeat up to 10 times.

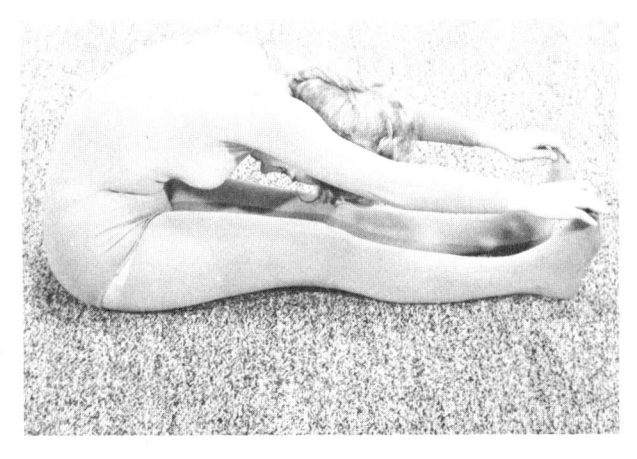

EXERCISES FOR BODY PERFECTION

EXERCISES FOR OVER FORTY

Whether you are forty by chronological age or body condition, you will find the following exercises wonderful for flabby, loose tissue. Go at 'em!

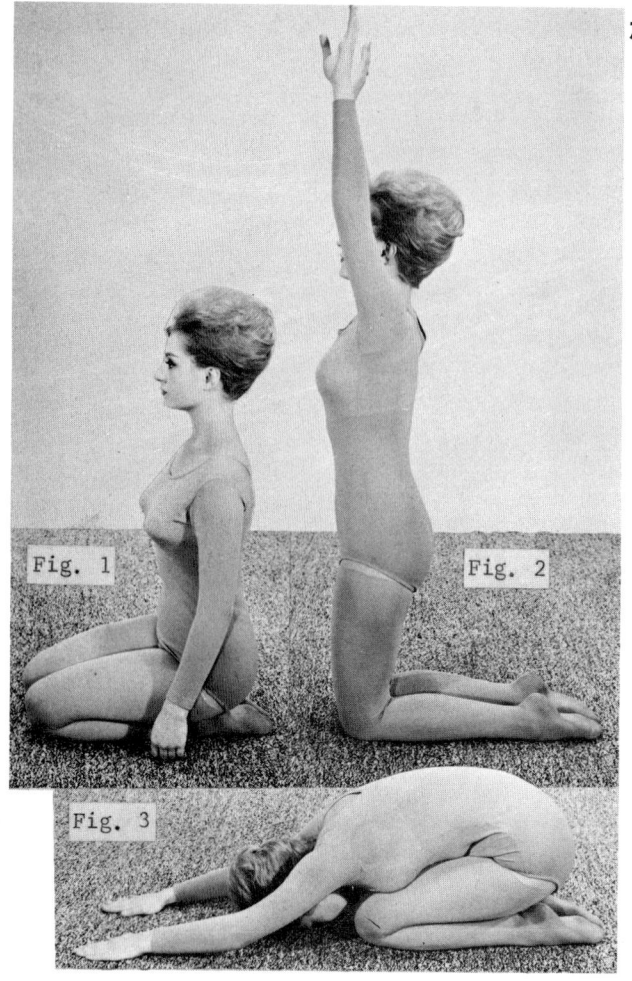

72. WARM-UP

Kneel, sit back. Inhale, bring arms overhead, come up to kneeling position. Exhale, drop forward to floor. Rest chin on it. Inhale, return to kneeling position. Exhale, drop to original position.

FOR FIRMING ARMS AND BACK

73. ROWING

Elbows shoulder high. Simulate rowing motion. Circle vigorously—up and out, back and down. Jiggle the flesh. Repeat until tired. The more the merrier.

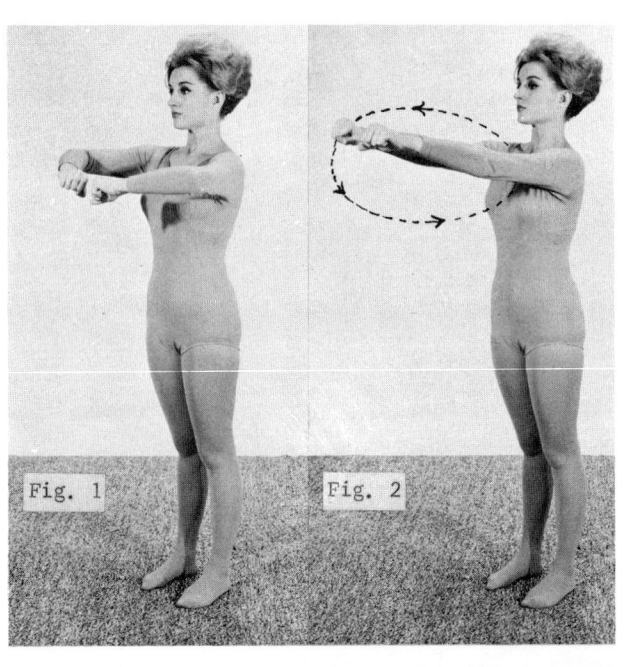

EXERCISES FOR BODY PERFECTION 389

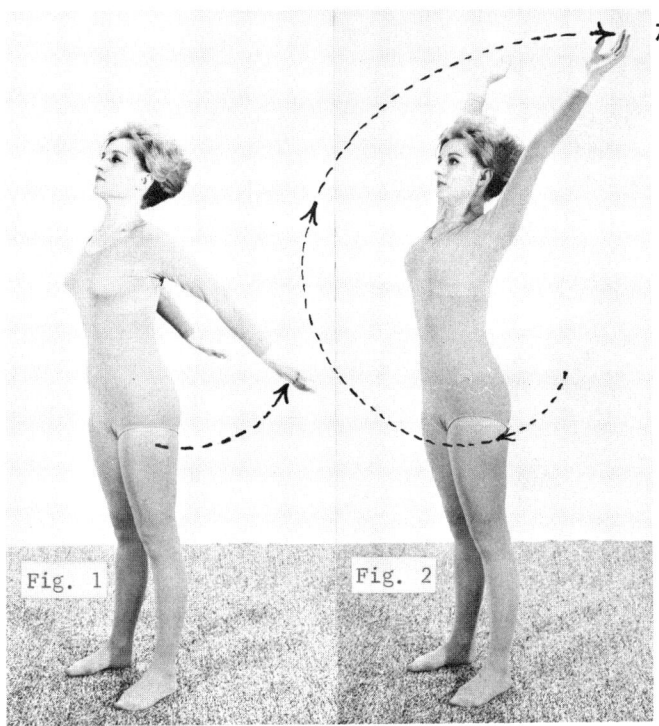

74. BACK PULLEYS

Feet slightly separated. Hands face backward. Swing arms back, then forward and up overhead. Swing back and forth Until tired. About 60 times.

FOR FIRMING THIGHS

75-76

Try numbers 59, HIGH BICYCLE; #60, HIGH CROSS-OVER SCISSORS; and the following:

77. SIDE BICYCLE

Lie on side. Raise feet slightly off floor. Bicycle vigorously 20 times. Repeat on other side. 20 times.

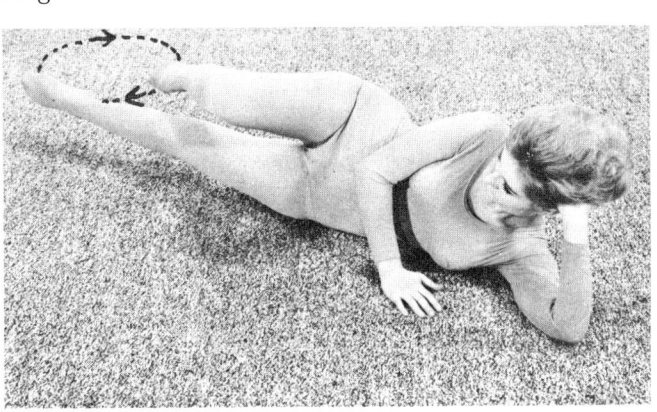

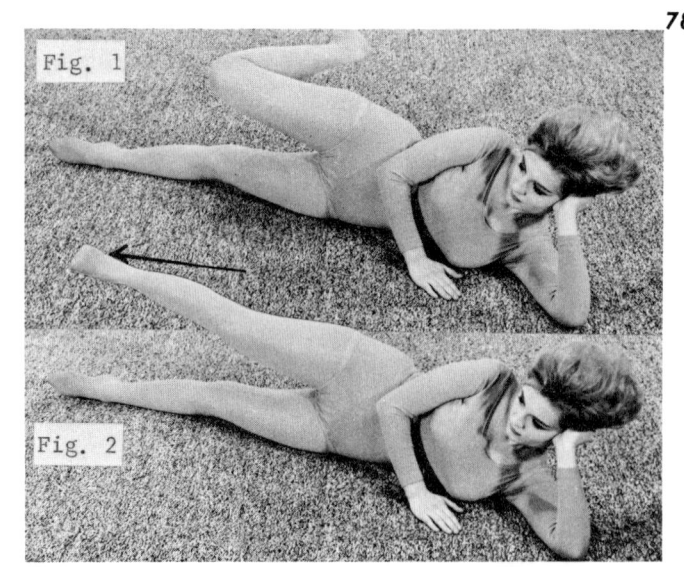

78. SIDE KNEE KICKS

Lie on side. Bend knee of top leg. Kick vigorously twenty times. Roll over, repeat with other leg. 20 times.

79. SIDE SCISSORS

Lie on side. Raise both legs slightly off floor. Keep knees straight as legs swing vigorously back and forth in opposite directions. 20 times each side.

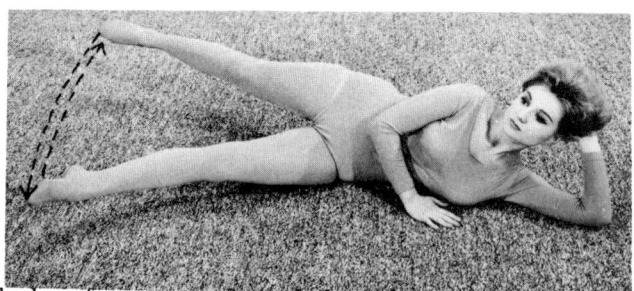

You will want to include, of course, some of the other exercises too. However, you will get faster and more satisfactory results if you will try to correct just one or two areas of your figure at a time. General calisthenics are not necessarily figure correcting exercises so concentrate on one figure fault at a time. When you see results, move on to another. Before too long, you will have taken years off your appearance.

Exercise can become a habit, and for those who have a sedentary way of life, it is a habit that pays off like money in the bank. It gives the continual dividend of better looks, more vitality and prolonged youthfulness.

CHAPTER 34

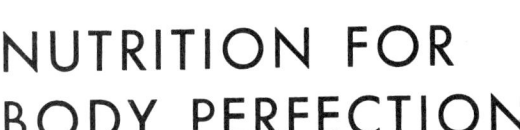

NUTRITION FOR BODY PERFECTION

Introduction

For you to get the most out of the Body Perfection program, you must follow the complete program. Each chapter is a vital part of the whole. This chapter on nutrition is designed to help make eating the pleasure it was intended to be, without fear of becoming overweight.

Suggestions are given on how to gain weight, how to lose weight, how to maintain normal weight. Why allow being overweight or underweight to stand in your way to success? You can, with patience and determination, reach your goal of physical perfection.

Every woman dreams of lasting beauty that does not fade with the passing of early womanhood. Yet, this lasting beauty can only be acquired by considering the body as a whole, the entire body from head to toe. This the author has attempted to do in a comprehensive, easy, do-it-yourself *WAY OF LIFE*.

Posture and exercise have already been discussed. Now it is time to study nutrition. We have in mind not faddish, foolish, calorie counting (everybody cheats) diets that are the roller-coaster (up again, down again) of so many women, but the safe, sane, sensible plan for balanced meals and good nutrition.

NUTRITION THROUGH BALANCED MEALS

A woman's beauty, your beauty, should not be left to the Fates. It is very important today to be physically attractive. You want the beauty that comes from the well-springs of good health. This means that you must be well nourished. It means that you must have balanced meals that provide the materials with which to make and maintain good bone, muscle, blood and other tissues. Sound tissues must be made from the food you eat, so in the truest sense of the word, you are what you eat.

BETTER FOODS MAKE BETTER TISSUES

Many nutrients contribute to the attractive appearance of your hair, skin, eyes and nails. Therefore, you should eat those foods that give the cells of your body the nutrients they need. Many of the nutrients in foods may be lost in various ways and in varying amounts. To help you to enjoy normal weight, lovely skin and a vibrant personality, you should choose your foods carefully.

FRESH FOODS It is desirable that we eat some fresh fruits and vegetables every day. Try to get an uncooked fresh food with each meal. For instance, at breakfast, in season, a citrus fruit or cantaloupe may be eaten; citrus juice also falls into this category. At lunch an apple or ripe pear and at dinner, a liberal helping of a dark green salad will add to the required daily quota of uncooked, fresh food.

The moment that a vegetable or fruit is harvested it begins to lose flavor and some nutritional value. When foods are promptly processed by canning and freezing, the loss in nutritional content is small and controlled. When fresh food is marketed, the conditions under which they are held directly affect the nutritional value. Therefore, buy only from markets which hold fresh foods under proper refrigeration and humidity control. Buy fresh foods as early in the day as possible. Wash, dry and refrigerate promptly at home until ready for use.

When foods are improperly stored, they decompose and may give off an objectionable odor. It is wise to discard any foods which have an "off" taste or odor.

COOKED FOODS Some of the vitamins and minerals are lost when foods are cooked. Careful preparation will help to preserve the nutritional value. Don't boil food and then throw the water away. It contains the water-soluble minerals. Rather, do as the nutrition experts suggest: just tenderize your food by the waterless method (just enough to cover the bottom of the pan) with the lid on.

GOOD DIGESTION—BETTER ABSORPTION —PROPER NUTRITION

Food can only nourish you if it is well digested and absorbed. All the care you may exercise in the selection and preparation of your food will be wasted unless it is properly digested.

Some underweight people claim they eat "enough to kill a horse". It may be that they are not digesting and absorbing the food they eat. Successful and complete digestion depends upon thorough mastication of the food into particles sufficiently divided so that they can be mixed with the gastric juice. The completeness of digestion depends upon the degree to which this is accomplished.

YOUR EMOTIONAL STATE affects the ability of your gastro-intestinal tract to manufacture sufficient quantities of digestive enzymes and to maintain normal muscle tone of its organs. Avoid tension at mealtime.

HARMFUL HABITS THAT IMPAIR DIGESTION

If you want to get the optimum nutritional value from the food you eat, then you must avoid the habits that impair digestion.

THE HURRY HABIT This is one of the chief offenders. It is better to skip a meal and take a liquid concentrated in nutritional value than bolt down a full lunch in jig-time.

OVER-EATING Habitual over-eating puts a burden on the digestive system. It is better to get up from the table feeling you can eat a little more rather than to leave the table stuffed like a Christmas goose.

SMOKING It can interfere with digestion by contracting the blood vessels.

EATING WHEN TIRED OR UPSET Emotional distress inhibits the digestive process. When you are angry or depressed, don't eat. If fatigued, rest for about a half-hour and eat lightly.

EXERCISING IMMEDIATELY AFTER MEALS Don't do any strenuous work or exercise for an hour after eating. Activity takes the blood away from the stomach to the muscles and slows down digestion.

DRINKING ICED OR VERY HOT DRINKS can impair digestion by temporarily deranging circulation of blood.

GOOD CIRCULATION—BETTER NUTRITION

Only when good blood flows freely to all the cells of your body can you have a healthy head of hair with lots of lustre, clear sparkling eyes, a smooth, soft, youthful skin, and a well proportioned body with plenty of vitality.

You can increase the amount of blood your heart pumps through your body by physical activity. You should schedule at least an hour of exercise daily; the remainder will be supplied in the course of your work. This will stimulate your circulation generally. Then you may stimulate circulation locally to any part of the body that is not functioning efficiently, *e. g.* to the feet by hot and cold baths or massage.

GOOD ELIMINATION—BETTER NUTRITION

Physical activity, such as walking briskly, hiking, swimming, golf, tennis, stimulates the flow of blood through the eliminative organs and stimulates their activity.

A thorough understanding of the function of each one of the eliminative organs—the lungs, skin, kidneys, liver and bowels, and what should be done to keep them functioning efficiently—is a very important part of your Body Perfection program.

THE LUNGS   From the lungs, oxygen is deployed to all the body cells; and carbon dioxide, the waste gas, is sent out of the body. Since foodstuffs cannot be utilized by the body unless oxygen is present, it is important to breathe deeply and exercise sufficiently to maintain good lung function.

THE SKIN   The skin is the largest of all the organs of elimination. It is one of the first to reflect body stress. It is highly sensitive to changes in temperature and humidity. Very few people realize how interdependent are feelings of well-being, the appearance of the complexion, and the function of the skin. To help maintain skin function at its best you should give it the care it deserves.

1. Take a daily bath. This cleanses the skin and removes the bacteria, perspiration and dirt.
2. Prevent dry skin by proper diet and wise external skin care.
3. Give your skin stimulation. Brisk rubbing of the skin with a rough terry-cloth towel or with a not too stiff brush removes the dead epidermis and stimulates circulation to the skin. Further, it helps to offset the bad effects on the skin brought on by the wearing of clothing. It also helps to stimulate more rapid regeneration of the skin which helps to keep it younger looking and free from premature flabbiness, lines and wrinkles.
4. Tone your skin. Through exercise and proper diet you can help to maintain firmness and elasticity of skin.

THE BOWELS   No person who has poor elimination through the bowels can possibly feel and look his best. Each individual has his own rhythm of bowel activity. To make this possible one should, therefore, cultivate the habit of

NUTRITION FOR BODY PERFECTION

setting aside time for evacuation. This, in combination with a few other good habits, will keep you regular.

1. Drink plenty of fluids each day. Plenty is approximately two quarts in the form of water, other beverages, fruit juices, soups and milk.
2. Get sufficient bulk into your diet from the ingestion of adequate amounts of fruits, vegetables and whole grain cereals and breads.
3. Strengthen the abdominal muscles with exercise.
4. Avoid emotional tension; practice good mental hygiene.

THE KIDNEYS The kidneys constitute a highly efficient filtering system which removes such waste products of protein metabolism as urea, uric acid and creatine. You can help them maintain peak efficiency by providing an ample volume of fluid and avoiding excessive use of irritants such as hot spices and alcohol.

THE LIVER The liver is the major organ of metabolism for the food you eat. It is also the depot for storage and distribution of food, and the center for detoxification of substances which exert toxic action in the body. Avoid overburdening the liver by moderation in the use of such fats as are found in fried foods, cream, butter, and alcohol. Eat a well-balanced diet rich in protein, vitamins and minerals.

BETTER NUTRITION—NORMAL WEIGHT

No physician will advise a "crash" diet for weight loss. People who go on "crash" diets usually regain the lost weight and acquire some extra poundage above their previous level. There is no particular food or group of foods with the unique power to cause weight loss. The only safe, dependable regimen for weight reduction is based on a manipulation of the kinds and amounts of foods to be eaten. Another essential goal of a good reducing diet is to help you acquire a set of eating habits which will prevent you from becoming overweight again. This means that you will eat regular, well balanced, nutritionally adequate meals that include proteins, fats, carbohydrates, vitamins and mineral-rich foods in sufficient planned amounts to cause loss of stored fat while vitality is maintained and improved.

TO LOSE WEIGHT

When dieting to lose weight, caloric intake is not the only consideration. Harmful effects can result if this is not understood. The objective is to burn off excess fat and not to interfere with the body chemistry. Otherwise unnecessary stress may cause irreversible damage.

A CALORIE

The standard unit measure of heat. One calorie, as used in human nutrition, is equal to the amount of heat required to raise the temperature of 1 kilogram of water one degree centigrade. Foods vary in caloric value. Fats are our most concentrated source of energy. One gram of fat yields 9 calories per gram. Carbohydrates, which include starches and sugars, yield 4 calories per gram. Hence, one can gain weight easily on excessive intakes of meat, cheese, poultry, fish and eggs as well as on starchy and sweet foods.

ORDINARY CALORIE REQUIREMENT

	Normally Active or Average	Caloric Requirement	To Reduce
Man	18-35	2900	1500
	35-55	2600	1500
	55-75	2200	1500
Woman	18-35	2100	1200
	35-55	1900	1200
	55-75	1600	1200

The more active you are, the more energy you will burn up. *The basis of reducing is that you supply less fuel than your body requires for its energy needs each day.* Thus the body will have to draw upon the stored-up fat for energy, and the excess fat will gradually be consumed.

For *you* this means that the food supply must be less than you use daily and that the rate at which you burn it should be speeded through exercise.

By now you realize that there is no easy, magic way to reduce. The only safe way is to:

   a. Balance your meals so that you get all the proteins, vitamins and minerals you need, but a decreased quantity of fat and carbohydrate.
   b. Step up your physical activity so that you accelerate the process of burning off excess fat.

CAUTION! Don't count on exercise alone to reduce. It takes far too much activity to burn off fat. The most convenient and easily regulated method is to eat your way down the scale.

NUTRITION FOR BODY PERFECTION

A SENSIBLE REDUCING DIET INCLUDES EACH DAY:

- 1 pint skim milk
- 6 ounces meat, fish, cheese or poultry
- 1 egg
- 1 citrus fruit
- 2 other fruits
- 1 cup (8 ounces) dark, leafy, green vegetables
- ½ cup deep yellow or green vegetable
- ½ cup whole grain or enriched cereal
- 2 other helpings of carbohydrate-rich foods, such as bread, potatoes, corn, rice or pasta (macaroni, noodles, etc.).

FOLLOW THESE RULES

1. Eat three regular meals as outlined in your diet.
2. Eat only the foods allowed in your diet in the amounts allowed.
3. Use a household measuring cup and measuring spoons to set up accurate helpings.
4. If you wish to have a snack, plan to subtract some foods from your meals for this purpose.
5. All fried foods are to be omitted. This means *nothing fried:* meat, potatoes, doughnuts, pancakes, fritters, etc.
6. No gravies, cream sauces, cream soups and rich casserole dishes.
7. No sugar, molasses, candy, jellies, jams, honey, syrups or preserves. You may use artificial sweeteners or artificially sweetened foods. The latter should be measured as part of the diet.
8. No carbonated beverages and tonics are to be used. Substitute artificially sweetened beverages for these.
9. Avoid the use of *all alcoholic* beverages.

THE 1200 CALORIE WEIGHT REDUCTION DIET

This will result in a regular weight loss of two pounds per week for most women, while maintaining good muscle and skin' tone, attractive hair, nails, teeth and improving general vitality.

For men, this diet is increased to 1500 calories per day to achieve the same results.

FOOD EXCHANGES

An exchange refers to a group of foods which have similar nutritive content. You may substitute one food for another if both belong to the same family or "exchange", provided that the listed amount is used. For example, if you have one fruit exchange, refer to the fruit list and choose any one from this list. This could be one small apple or ½ small banana or 2 dates or 12 large cherries or any other one which you may prefer. But your choice would be made from this list only and not from any other.

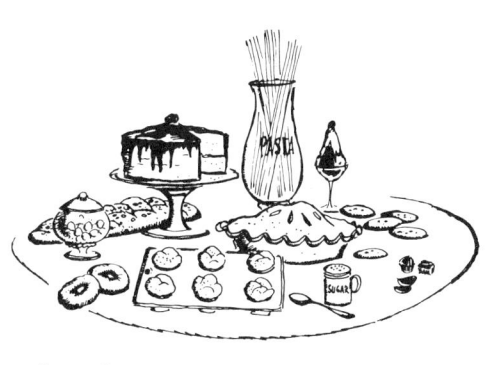

EXCHANGE LISTS FOR LOW CALORIE DIETS

1. MILK: Use only skim milk in the amount indicated 1 8 oz. cup = 1 skim milk exchange.

2. VEGETABLE A: Unless specified, eat as much as you desire of these.

Asparagus	Parsley
Beet Greens	Green pepper
Broccoli	Radish
Brussel sprouts	Rhubarb
Cabbage	Romaine
Cauliflower	Sauerkraut
Celery	Spinach
Chicory	Summer squash (Zucchini)
Cucumber	String beans
Eggplant	Swiss Chard
Escarole	Tomato (limit 1 at each meal)
Kale	Tomato (juice 4 oz. = 1 helping)
Lettuce	
Okra	Watercress
Mushrooms	

VEGETABLE B: 1 exchange = ½ cup

Beets	Pumpkin
Carrots	Rutabagas
Onions	Winter squash (Hubbard, Acorn, etc.)
Green Peas	Turnips

4. FRUITS: (must be fresh, frozen, canned without sugar)

apple—1 small	grapes—12
applesauce—½ cup	honeydew melon—⅛
apricots, canned—4 halves	nectarine—1 medium
banana—½ small	orange—medium
blackberries—1 cup	orange juice—½ cup
blueberries—⅔ cup	peach 1 medium
cantaloupe—1¼	pear—1 small
cherries—10 large	pineapple—2 slices
date—2	plum—2 medium
figs, dried—small	prunes—2 medium
figs, fresh—2 large	raspberries—1 cup
grapefruit—½ small	strawberries—1 cup
grapefruit juice—½ cup	tangerine—1
grape juice—¼ cup	watermelon—1 cup diced

5. BREAD EXCHANGES:

bread—1 slice
muffin—1 (2" in diameter)
cereals—½ cup cooked
cereals—dry ¾ cup

Crackers
graham—2
oyster—20 (½ cup)
saltines—5
soda—3
fruit ice—½ cup
macaroni—½ cup cooked
noodles—½ cup cooked
rice—½ cup cooked
spaghetti—½ cup cooked
sponge cake (no icing)—1½ inch cube

Vegetables used as bread exchanges
corn—⅓ cup, ½ ear
corn, popped—1 cup
parsnips—⅔ cup

Potatoes:
white, baked—1 small
white, boiled—1 small
white, mashed—½ cup
yam or sweet—¼ cup

6. MEAT EXCHANGES:

Meats (1 oz. = 1 exchange)

beef, fowl, ham (lean), lamb, liver, pork, veal	1 ounce
fish	1 ounce
cold cuts	1 ounce
cheese	1 ounce
cottage cheese	¼ cup
eggs	1

7. FAT EXCHANGES:

Fats
avocado—⅛
bacon, crisp—1 slice
butter—1 teaspoon
olives—5 small
cream cheese—1 tablespoon
cream, light—2 tablespoon
mayonnaise—1 teaspoon
nuts—6 small
oil or cooking fat—teaspoon

TYPES OF FATS

Fats not only cause overweight, but also affect the cholesterol level of the blood. There are two types of fats: saturated fats which tend to raise the cholesterol level—butter, ordinary margarines, hydrogenated shortenings, cream, animal fats except poultry, cocoanut and chocolate: poly-unsaturated fats which tend to lower the cholesterol level of the blood when it is too high—liquid vegetable oils (corn, cottonseed, soybean, sunflower and others), margarines containing substantial amounts of liquid vegetable oils, and peanut butter, fish oils and poultry fat.

Miscellaneous: use as desired—broth, coffee, gelatin unsweetened, lemon, parsley, saccharine, seasonings, tea, vanilla, vinegar, sour pickle.

MEAL PLAN FOR REDUCING

NOTE:

Consult exchange lists on pages 398 and 399 for information concerning amounts equal to 1 exchange.

BREAKFAST:

1 Fruit exchange, preferably citrus
1 Bread exchange
1 Meat exchange (1 ounce)
1 Fat exchange
½ Skim milk exchange
Clear coffee or tea as desired

LUNCH OR SUPPER:

3 Meat exchanges (1 exchange = 1 ounce, therefore 3 ounces)
1 Vegetable B exchange
Vegetable A as desired (at least 1 cup for nutrition and satiety)
1 Bread exchange
1 Fruit exchange
1 Skim milk exchange
0 Fat exchange
Clear coffee or tea as desired

DINNER:

Clear, fat-free consomme or broth as desired
3 Meat exchanges (3 ounces, total)
Vegetable A exchange as desired (at least 1 cup for nutrition and satiety)
0 Vegetable B exchanges
1 Fruit exchange
Clear coffee or tea as desired

FOR THE 1500 CALORIE DIET ADD THE FOLLOWING

Breakfast:
1 Bread exchange

Lunch:
1 Bread exchange

Dinner:
1 Meat exchange

NUTRITION FOR BODY PERFECTION

PROTEIN AND MINERAL EMPTY—CALORIED FOODS

The following foods offer calories chiefly in the form of carbohydrates (starches and sugars) and fats. The amount of protein, vitamins and minerals contained therein are minimal. Therefore, these foods should be avoided by those who wish to lose excess weight, maintain normal weight and enjoy optimum health. Optimum health means more than absence of disease. It means a state of mental health as evidenced by a cheerful, optimistic point of view, excellent physical health as demonstrated by a high degree of physical endurance, stamina and good resistance to infection, and a readily available fund of energy.

Food	Amount	Number of Calories
Apple Pie	1/6 Pie 9″ in diameter	387
Blintz	3″ section 3¼″ cake	152
Chocolate layer cake	1/6 cake, 2 layers, 6″ diameter	314
Milk Chocolate	Bar 5″ x 7″ x ⅛″	143
Chocolate Fudge	Square 1¼″ x 1¼″ x ½″	
Plain	1 oz.	66
With nuts	1 oz.	108
Hard candy	1 oz.	108
Jelly Beans	10—10 oz.	64
Marshmallows	1 med. 1¼″ diam.	24
Caramel	1 med.	42
Potato Chips	8-10 large 2″-3″ diam.	92
Chocolate Chip Cookie	1 2¼″ diam.	53
Pretzels	1 small—1⅞″ x 1″ OR 5 thin sticks	7
Ritz-type Crackers	2	35
Saltines	1 2″ sq.	17
Doughnuts	1—2¾″ diam.	136
Eclair, iced	1 4½″ long	78
Griddle Cake	1 4″ diam.	47
Syrup, maple	1 tablespoon	61
Molasses	1 tablespoon	46
Sugar	1 teaspoon	16
Cream, heavy whipped	1 tablespoon	49
Cream, light coffee	1 tablespoon	30
Coca Cola	1—6 oz. bottle	80
Jams, Marmalades, Preserves	1 tablespoon	55
Jellies	1 tablespoon	50

CONT.

Mince Pie	1/6 Pie 9" diam.	398
Cherry Pie	1/6 Pie 9" diam.	398
Pumpkin Pie	1/6 Pie—1 crust—9" diam.	307
Popcorn	1—8 oz. cup, no butter	54
Soda Pop	1—8 oz. cup	107
Waffles	1—6" diam.	240
Whip, commercial	¼ Cup	59

CALORIES WITH PROTEIN VALUES

Food	Caloric Value	Protein Value (Gms.)
Milk, Whole, 8 oz.	165	8
Milk, Skim, 8 oz.	85	8
Milk, Chocolate drink	185	8
Cheese, American or Swiss, 1 oz.	110	7
Cottage Cheese, creamed, 1 oz.	30	4
Butter, 1 tbsp.	100	0
Cream, heavy whipping, 1 tbsp.	50	0
Half and Half ¼ cup	80	2
Ice Cream, Vanilla ½ cup	150	2
1 medium scoop	125	2
Sherbet, ½ cup	145	2
3 oz. cooked meat, fish, poultry, lean to medium, fat, no bones	230	20
Liver, 3 oz.	180	20
Frankfurter, 1 med. 1¾ oz.	125	7
Luncheon meat 2 oz.	165	8
Tuna Fish, canned 2 oz. (⅓ cup)	105	14
Chicken ½ cup	210	18
Bacon, crisp 2 slices	100	4
Eggs 1 medium	75	6
Dried Beans ¾ cup cooked	150	10
Baked Beans with Pork ¾ cup	245	10
Peanuts, shelled, roasted, 30 (1 oz.)	150	7

GUIDELINES

1. *An adequate breakfast is a must in a reducing diet.* People who skip breakfast tend to overeat during other meals and indulge in unnecessary snacks.
2. *Chew your food thoroughly.* Eat slowly. Do two special reducing exercises at the table. One is to shake your head vigorously from side to side when offered second helpings and the other is to push your chair away from the table before you are full.

NUTRITION FOR BODY PERFECTION

3. *Watch your posture.* Be mindful of your abdominal muscles. Keep shoulders back. Hoist up your rib-cage.
4. Take plenty of fluid.
5. *Use salt cautiously.* Too much salt whets the appetite. This is the converse of what you are aiming for.
6. *Do your exercises faithfully.* It will help you to tighten up the skin while you are burning up the fat.
7. *Keep all your organs of elimination functioning efficiently.* This includes the skin, kidneys and bowels.
8. *No alcoholic drinks are allowed.* You will not lose weight unless you obey this rule. This applies to sweets, too.
9. *Weigh and measure yourself on the day you begin.* Wait one week before you repeat this procedure, preferably in the morning after elimination and before breakfast. Wear little or no clothes. There may be fluctuations but do not let these discourage you.
10. *Avoid abdominal distention.* Refrain from excessive use of carbonated beverages, even those artificially sweetened, due to likelihood of gas formation. Refrain from eating foods which cause distention or bloat. This mars your appearance.

MAINTAINING NORMAL WEIGHT AFTER REDUCING

It is very foolish to allow yourself to gain weight after you have reduced to your proper weight. To remain at your desired weight, follow this procedure: If you have been following the 1200 calorie diet, increase your intake to 1600 calories for one week. For the additions, choose high-vitamin, high-mineral, high protein foods rather than the high-caloried snacks with very little mineral and protein value. Therefore, add more fruits, vegetables, meat, fish or poultry and skim milk. Weigh in after one week. If you are still losing weight, although less than before, then add 200 calories more for a new daily total of 1800 calories. Weigh in one week later, If you are still losing weight, add 200 more calories to your diet. Once you hit 2000 calories it is more than likely that you are reaching the point of equilibrium.

THE EFFECT OF AGE

As we grow older, we need fewer calories. Therefore, people over 35 years of age need fewer calories and will reach equilibrium at a lower level of caloric intake than do younger people. This self-discipline will pay off in terms of increased health and well-being, an extended life-span, attractive figure and a stronger ego.

TO GAIN WEIGHT

To do any building, you must have a good foundation. This is equally true of weight-building. In this case the foundation is good health. Make sure you are free from infection or illness by getting a medical check-up.

If the physician recommends that you gain weight, make sure you know the specific number of pounds you should acquire. Remember that your weight gain should be a matter of increasing tissue as well as fat. People who find it difficult to gain weight should also evaluate their activity patterns, amount of time they take for rest and sleep and the foods they usually eat.

Many underweight persons are hyperactive. They need to slow down physically by having longer periods of sleep and choosing less strenuous means of recreation. Such individuals also benefit from eating smaller and more frequent meals with rest periods after each meal.

Eating to gain weight does not require stuffing yourself with food or straining the gastro-intestinal tract with rich, high-fat meals. Choosing your food wisely will result in a firm, lithe body while the mere acquisition of excess fat will result in a flabby, shapeless, aging appearance.

If capacity is your problem, then make your foods more concentrated in protein, vitamins and minerals without changing the visible quantity. Dry skim milk added to whole fresh milk will increase protein, calcium and riboflavin along with calories. Eggs added to chopped beef, milk beverages and puddings will contribute protein, iron, vitamin A along with its calories. Increase the consumption of lean meat and whole milk cheeses.

A DAY'S MEALS FOR THOSE WHO WISH TO GAIN WEIGHT

Breakfast:

6 oz. citrus fruit juice or 1 large fresh orange or large grapefruit half.
2 eggs, any style
1 slice of toast
1 pat of butter
1 tablespoon of jelly, honey or jam
1 cup hot cereal cooked in milk or cold cereal with added milk
8 oz. whole milk to which 3 tablespoons dry skim milk have been added
1 cup coffee or tea as desired

Mid-morning Snack:

1 Milk Shake containing 8 oz. whole milk, 1 egg and 3 tablespoons dry skim milk.
Flavor with ½ teaspoonful vanilla and 1 teaspoonful sugar

Lunch:
4 oz. tomato juice
Broiled lean hamburger on bun (4 oz. meat) or Meat Sandwich
Tossed Green Salad or Carrot Sticks
Fresh Fruit
8 oz. whole milk

Mid-afternoon Snack:
Fresh Fruit

Dinner:
Cream soup made with 4 oz. whole milk
4 oz. fish, poultry-baked, broiled or roasted
Starchy vegetable—potato, corn or enriched rice
Cooked yellow vegetable
Green Salad with dressing
Bread and butter
Ice cream or simple cake with fruit
Hot beverage as desired

TV or Bed-time Snack:
Sandwich of Peanut Butter, Cheese, Meat, Fish or Poultry
Milk with 3 tablespoons nonfat dry milk

THE NINE RULES FOR THOSE WHO WISH TO GAIN WEIGHT

1. Keep your bowels regular by including lots of leafy green vegetables and fresh fruit in your balanced eating program.
2. Eat more slowly and chew your food more thoroughly than you have done in the past. The digestion of starches and sugars begins in the mouth.
3. Rest before and after meals. This permits your food to be digested more easily. Don't rush out at lunchtime for a quick "ham on rye and a coke".
4. Eat an ample breakfast that includes a protein food (egg), a starch (toast), and a fruit.
5. Eat three meals a day with a mid-morning and mid-afternoon snack and a bed-time snack.
6. Plan your exercise routine so that you can do it at a leisurely tempo.
7. Keep warm in windy, wintry weather. Without ample clothing, your body will burn up too much fuel maintaining a normal temperature. Dress appropriately to avoid over-exposure.
8. Learn to take things more easily. Rushing spoils your poise and keeps your weight down.
9. Relax whenever you get a chance. This is particularly important after meals.

Remember that gaining weight is a slower process than losing it. But it is worth the effort because there is more than vanity involved in the matter of attaining normal weight. Primarily it is a matter of better health and increased vitality. A careful analysis of the living habits of underweight people usually reveals that their condition is due to their mental outlook and mode of living.

SOME OF THE CAUSES OF UNDERWEIGHT ARE:
 a. Poor digestion.
 b. Habitually eating too little or the wrong kind of food.
 c. Overactivity, producing excessive fatigue.
 d. Worry and mental strain.

When fretting, nervousness and worry are partially responsible for your condition, progress depends entirely upon your ability to overcome them. Learn to relax!

TO MAINTAIN NORMAL WEIGHT

What should your ideal weight be? The most recent weight charts account for differences in body frames and offer a range of weights for each frame. Certain firms publish weight tables for men and women of various ages. You should review these regularly in the light of the newest findings. These can be used as a guide.

POSTURE AND EXERCISE

Your appearance should correlate with your proper weight. Even if your weight is normal, you can improve your shape by toning up flabby muscles and improving posture. Sometimes a person looks fat because flabby tissues allow bulges to form where they shouldn't be.

SPOT REDUCING

A woman's muscle structure should be covered with a layer of fat. This layer makes you curvaceous; it makes the lines of your body oval and soft in appearance. Pinch with your thumb and forefinger, various parts of your body such as the thigh, the upper arm, the back and the stomach. If you have more than an "inch of pinch" between your fingers, you have discovered the fatty deposits that cause lumps and bulges. Even underweight and thin persons often have pockets of fat. Discover yours and outline a group of exercises that will eliminate them. Special spot reducing exercises that bring these parts into rapid action will tear down the fatty deposits and tone up muscles.

You not only want to maintain your normal weight as the years go by, but you also want to retain the look of youthfulness that is represented by a youthful tautness of the muscles, firmness of the flesh, and smoothness of the skin.

NUTRITION FOR BODY PERFECTION

BALANCED MEALS

Balanced meals are for you too—they are the foundation upon which you are going to build your lifetime beauty. They must include:

One pint milk—for those over 35, preferably skim

One egg—for those over 35, 3 to 4 per week

At least 1 per day of each—leafy green dark vegetables and citrus fruits

2 helpings of other vegetables including 1 small potato

2 helpings of other fruit

5 oz. meat, fish, poultry

1 whole grain or enriched cereal

2–4 slices whole grain or enriched bread, or sufficient quantities to maintain ideal weight.

TYPICAL DAILY MENUS FOR THOSE WHO WISH TO MAINTAIN IDEAL WEIGHT

Breakfast:

Orange juice

1 egg or 1 oz. meat, cheese or fish

1 slice whole grain or enriched bread

½ cup cooked or ready-to-eat whole grain or enriched cereal

1 cup whole or skim milk for cereal and hot beverage

Lunch:

Meat, Cheese, fish or poultry

Salad containing dark green leafy vegetables

Bread or Starchy Vegetable

Fruit

Milk

Dinner:

Meat, Fish or poultry

1 small potato or ½ cup cooked enriched rice or enriched pasta

½ cup (minimum) deep yellow or dark green cooked vegetables

1 green salad, containing dark green, leafy vegetables

Dessert: Gelatin, milk puddings, simple sweet-choice of one

Only occasional use of: ice cream, cake, cookies, pies, candy and other rich desserts. These should not be eaten every day.

VARIETY IN THE BALANCED MEAL

It is simple to obtain balanced meals if you follow a few principles of common sense nutrition. First, eat a variety of foods and a variety at each meal. Secondly, don't eat more than you can expend as energy. Thirdly, use protective, wholesome foods such as whole grain and enriched flours and breads, meat, fish, eggs, root and leafy vegetables, and fruits.

Eat a sensible amount of raw foods such as salads with meals, and fruit for dessert. Make an effort to stay away from heavy, sweet desserts. Think in terms of fruits and cheeses. Sweet desserts satisfy the appetite but are not likely to provide the necessary nutrition.

If it's variety you're aiming at, how about varying your usual coffee and tea break with fruit or vegetable juices?

What about food supplements? Your physician should be the one to decide whether you need a vitamin-mineral supplement. Taken as a supplement to a well-rounded diet, vitamins have their place. There is a certain danger in taking too many vitamins—so it's all a matter of common-sense.

Indeed, common-sense and moderation are your watchwords to greater beauty, vitality, productivity and longevity.

THE TEN RULES FOR THOSE WHO WISH TO MAINTAIN NORMAL WEIGHT

1. *Eat well balanced meals.* Get servings of each category of food every day. A well nourished body must have carbohydrates, fats, proteins, vitamins and minerals.
2. *Variety is the spice of life.* It will assure you that you are getting the proper amount of each food nutrient. What you don't get in one food, you will get in another.
3. *A good nourishing breakfast* will get you off to a good start.
4. *Regulate the time of your meals* to fit your way of life, but eat three times a day.
5. *Relax at mealtime.* This should be a pleasant time without hurry or worry.
6. *Drink water when you are thirsty.* Avoid the use of synthetic drinks such as those whose name ends with the suffix "ade" and carbonated beverages.
7. *Exercise regularly.* You should get from twenty minutes to a half hour of physical activity in addition to your job. Use spot reducing exercises in addition to general exercises to keep your body in top shape.
8. *Get eight hours of sleep a night.* Nothing robs beauty and vitality faster than insufficient rest.
9. *Keep bowels open.* Avoid constipation through sufficient consumption of fruits, vegetables and cereals.
10. For healthy attractive teeth free from cavities, *brush as frequently as you can,* avoid the use of chewing gum, carbonated beverages and sticky sweets. Remember that raw crisp vegetables such as carrots, green pepper and dark green leaves are nature's own toothbrushes.

FOR THOSE WHO ARE BOTHERED BY ACNE

1. Get medical help for control and management and follow doctor's orders.
2. Avoid high fat foods such as fried foods, nuts, chocolate, ice cream, olives and pastry.
3. Avoid iodine-rich foods such as shell fish and iodized salt.
4. Avoid spices and condiments such as prepared mustard, ketchup and pickles.
5. Follow the diet pattern as outlined on Page 407.
6. Keep calm.

CHAPTER 35

RELAXATION FOR BODY PERFECTION

Introduction

A balanced life gives a feeling of happiness and accomplishment because it fulfills the basic needs of the individual. Each day contains time for:

Vocation (earning a living)
Avocation (hobbies, cultural pursuits, etc.)
Social Activities (clubs, friends, get-togethers)
Physical Activities (keeping fit)

Doctors have found that some illnesses are not due to "germs" but are due to "stress". Some of the stresses placed upon us are physical. These would include:

1. Physical work done to the point of exhaustion.
2. Exposure to too much heat or cold.
3. Physical "shock", as that experienced in a car accident.

Some of the stresses are mental and some are emotional. These include:

1. Emotional upset due to the negative emotions of fear, hate, jealousy, etc.
2. Mental pressure because of illness in the family, financial problems, etc.
3. Mental or emotional "shock"—losing a loved one, losing our job, etc.

If we are going to feel fit as a fiddle and able to lick our weight in wildcats then we must eliminate, as much as possible, those circumstances and environmental factors that cause *stress* and spell *distress* to our well-being.

It seems one of the biggest physical and mental challenges facing the average American today is learning to *relax*. This is not an empty word that means trying to make your mind a vacuum and your body a non-entity. What it really means is: to make less firm, rigid or tense; to seek recreation or rest.

There are a number of ways to relax and you are going to explore in this chapter, some of the mental, emotional and physical disciplines that are roads leading to relaxation.

BARRIERS TO RELAXATION

Muscular tension is one of the main obstacles to be overcome. If we were all experienced Yogas with perfect control over our thoughts and actions, it would be one thing, but inasmuch as we are not, we must resort to hydrotherapy (water treatment), exercise and massage.

Let's learn the methods of relaxation starting with the feet where so much of our tiredness originates. Like the rest of the body, your feet will respond beautifully to a little care and attention.

If you have anything radically wrong with your feet, see a specialist (podiatrist).

To ease the tension caused by tired, aching feet here are several remedies.

FOR TIRED FEET

FOOT BATHS: Alternating hot and cold water will stimulate the circulation and relax tense muscles. You can use it for warming the feet in cold weather too. Never underestimate the efficacy of hydrotherapy for relaxation. It works.

FOOT MASSAGE: If you like the idea of a foot bath, you can use a rough towel for drying that will definitely massage the feet and stimulate surface circulation. While they are still slightly damp, rub off callouses with a pumice stone or emery board.

Use some of your cold cream or lanolized skin cream for your foot massage. Use both hands as you push the toes apart with the thumbs on top and the fingers underneath. It feels really wonderful! Now take each toe and give it individual attention rubbing from tip to base. Make a circle with each one, especially the great toe, get the toes out of their usual cramped position. Don't neglect the arches; they should be rubbed gently but firmly. You can use an old soda pop bottle for this if you wish. Massage from base of toes toward heel.

FOOT EXERCISES

Exercises to be done sitting. Shoes may be on.

1. Cross one leg over the opposite knee and circle the ankle, clockwise and then counter-clockwise. Twenty each way. Now the other ankle.
2. Raise both feet off the floor with the knees straight. Hold onto the seat of the chair with both hands for support. Rotate both feet in toward each other, then out, away from each other, then both to the right, then both to the left. Do ten rotations each way for a total of 40.
3. Leave the left foot on the floor directly under the knee, kick the right leg up straightening the knee and bringing the toes upward toward the knee as far as you can get them. Stretch those calf muscles by kicking the leg up high enough for the thigh to leave

the chair. Continue to kick it up and down with the knee straight, ten times. Now the left leg.

Shoes must be off!

4. By curling the toes under, attempt to pick up an imaginary pencil. Or you might try to pick up a towel or marbles.
5. Place the feet side by side under the knees with the heels touching. By rolling the toes under and turning the ankles out, scoop up a mound of imaginary sand between the feet. Repeat five times.

Exercises to be done standing.

6. Standing with feet side by side, about six inches apart and the hands on the hips, rock from the heels forward on the outside of the foot toward the little toe and then up onto the ball of the foot with most of the weight on the great toe. Rock back. Repeat five times.
7. Standing as above, rock back onto the heels bringing the rest of the foot off the floor and spreading the toes. Rock forward until the toes are on the floor, spread them as far apart as they will go. Repeat five times.

DON'T UNDERMINE YOUR UNDERPINNINGS

According to a survey, women who wear high heels around the house are more likely to get a divorce than women who wear low heels. This suggests that aching, tired feet ruin a woman's disposition. They deprive her of the joys of dancing, golfing, skiing and tennis too. How did they get that way?

Are you guilty of abusing your feet? You surely don't wear very high heels all day! Even if you don't, you may be guilty of equally grave sins against the health and comfort of your feet. Check these:

1. Are you guilty of wearing ill-fitting shoes and stockings?
    Do you have "hammer" toes, callouses, corns or bunions?
2. Are you neglecting a weekly pedicure?
    Do you have ingrown toenails?
3. Are you standing for long hours without resting occasionally?
    Do you use your ten minute break to relax—sitting?
4. Are you wearing too tight a girdle?
    Do your ankles swell?
5. Are you constipated?
    Do you have regular elimination?
6. Are you overweight from any cause?
    Do you watch your weight?
7. Are you troubled with itching, burning feet?
    Do you use a foot powder regularly?

8. Are you in the habit of changing your shoes during the day to rest your feet?

   Do you use old, sloppy house slippers with no support around the house?
9. Are you exercising your feet to keep them strong?

   Do you have weak arches?

CHECK YOUR ARCHES

Most weak arches are due to lack of exercise and incorrect use of the feet in standing and walking.

Wet both of your feet and place them on a piece of paper. Trace the outline of the damp imprints and compare them with the illustrations that follow.

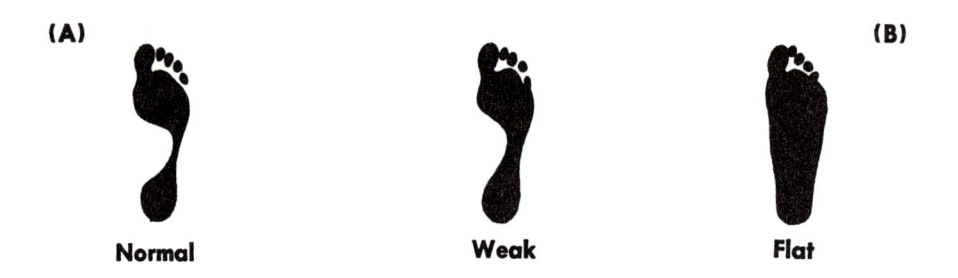

(A) Normal   Weak   **(B)** Flat

If the inner line of the foot curves away as in illustration "A" you have good healthy longitudinal arches; if the imprint of the middle of your foot is broader than in illustration "A", your arches are low; while if your feet are flat, the imprints will be like illustration "B". Special shoes are often necessary to relieve tensions caused by flat feet.

BUNIONS

MILD CORRECTIVE MEASURES Be sure to allow plenty of toe room in your shoes. For awhile, use the suggested toe circling foot massage, and place a small wad of cotton between the great toe and the next toe before you put your hose on.

FOR TIRED LEGS

In your opinion, what would make legs more tired, walking or standing still? Actually standing in one place is more tiring because blood is not stimulated to rush through the vessels to replenish the muscle cells. Standing has been accused of being the cause of varicose veins. If this is true, all women can benefit tremendously by following the simple ritual of. . . .

RELAXATION FOR BODY PERFECTION

THE TONING BATH Have you noticed, just under the skin, any delicate lacing of tiny blood vessels? Perhaps they seem to be getting too close to the surface, and, if you are older, they may seem to become more prominent each year. They probably are, but you can build up the minute muscles of the skin and keep it firm so that veins will stay where they belong, out of sight, by using the toning bath. Varicose veins require your physician's advice, although with his permission, you too can try the following:

Just before going to bed at night, get into a bath tub that has enough warm water in it to cover your legs. This is not to be your "get clean" tub, however. Now you can take advantage of your good bath brush or, if you prefer, a stiff hand brush. Start with the feet and ankles and scrub toward the thighs, up and up, right to the crotch. Yes, I did say "scrub." That's exactly what you should do. Gently at first perhaps, until your skin is pink and tingling. Turn on the cold water tap and sit until the water is cool enough to drive the blood from the surface. Quickly, out of the tub, blot yourself dry and hop into bed. You might want to use your pillows to prop your feet rather than your head. Wonderful feeling when the blood surges back into your legs. Keep them up—you're through for the night. One of the first benefits you will be able to notice will be the skin "you love to touch". But beyond that, you will be building a resistance to changes in temperature so that your resistance to colds will be higher. Also, you will be scrubbing off old, dead tissue and encouraging new, softer, more youthful cells to appear.

FOR TIRED SHOULDERS, NECK AND ARMS

Nowhere does tension show up so readily as in the shoulders and hands. Perhaps you can cover the frown and worry lines on your face with make-up, but it's impossible to hide muscular tension in the hands, unless you sit on them or otherwise keep them out of sight.

Relax means to make less firm, rigid, or tense; therefore, in order to relax we must first cause rigidity or tension. Sustained tension is not lovely or graceful.

Note: It takes one set of muscles to open your hand (these run up the back of the forearm) and it takes another set to close the hand (feel the muscles on the inside of the forearm as you make a fist). When both these sets of muscles are contracting at the same time . . . tension. Try it. It turns the fingers into claws. Not lovely, indeed.

To refer to a woman as a cat is insulting, but to allude to her as a feline is complimentary. It implies grace and femininity. Cats seem to have relaxing down to a fine art. A lesson can be learned from watching them stretch, yawn, relax, and s-t-r-e-t-c-h, an example for you to follow whenever you find it necessary to work in one position for long hours.

Scientific tests have conclusively proven that a person's efficiency is heightened by short rest periods. Use your ten-minute break for getting the kinks out of muscles, for deep breathing to renew your oxygen supply, for relaxation to relieve tension.

EXERCISES FOR SHOULDERS AND NECK

The following are interesting exercises for the shoulders, arms and hands. Exercises to give you the grace of a hula dancer and the litheness of a cat—without claws, that is.

1. Stretching is wonderful! Double the fists and pretend that you are Samson pushing down the pillars of the temple. One on the left and one on the right. Now start with fists over the shoulders and, like Atlas, lift the weight of the world off your shoulders. With tension, lift sky high.
2. Place the right hand on the right shoulder, the left hand on the left shoulder. Bring the shoulders forward as far as they will go, up to the ears, back, down, relax. Circle forward and around ten times. Hey, hey, the other way. Ten times.
3. Clasp the hands behind the head and pull those elbows back. Get them closer, pull. Relax. Inhale as your elbows go back and the chest lifts, exhale as you relax.
4. Nothing relieves muscle tension faster than gentle massage. Using both hands, work up the back of the shoulders, up the back of the neck to the base of the skull. This massage calls for a gentle circular motion with pressure applied with all four fingers.
5. Place both hands behind your back with the elbows straight and the palms up. Interlace the fingers, now turn the hands out away from the body and down, down, down. Push! Doesn't that feel good? Repeat the tension about five times.

Since anything that affects your shoulders will also affect your neck, it is important to guard against shoulder strain. To relieve neck strain, rotate the head slowly in a circle. Let your jaw droop open, relaxed.

If your neck is to retain vestiges of youthfulness, the flesh, tissue and muscles must be given the job nature intended them to have—the job of holding your head erect. It's no wonder our necks show age so early when we thrust our heads forward and carry them there. The front muscles become flabby, the skin looks crepey, our friends remark about our double chin. The cure? Pull the head back by straightening the spine and pulling up, up with the back of the ears. Remember, there has never been a lotion or cream invented that will do for your neck what good posture will do.

EXERCISES FOR THE ARMS

1. With the arms shoulder high in front and the hands in fists facing each other, swing the arms backward, bounce them three times. Inhale as the arms go back and bounce. Exhale as you return them to starting position in front of you. Three times.

   Repeat the above with the fists turned out away from each other.

2. With the arms spread eagle fashion and the hands in fists, turn the fingers up and then slowly, with tension in the entire arm, the fists down, back and up again. Imagine you are turning a rusty knob with much effort.
3. Place the right arm up with the elbow close to the ear. Hold it there with the left hand. Now bend and straighten the elbow about twenty times. Repeat with the left arm. When this is done correctly you can feel the triceps, on the underside of the arm, contracting and relaxing.
4. Place the arms in front shoulder high and stretch the fingers straight and apart from each other as far as possible. Keeping them tense, fling the arms to the sides, eagle fashion, and then over the head and back to starting position.

EXERCISES AND RELAXATION FOR THE HANDS
1. With the arms outstretched in front and the palms facing the floor, keep the fingers straight and let each finger become very active independently of the others. This is called the Hawaiian Rain Exercise. All together now!
2. Let's make a lazy figure 8. It's laying on its side, so tired and so relaxed. Your hands and wrists must be relaxed too if you are going to follow its contours. Right hand first with the palm facing the floor, bring the hand down and around in front of you, then as it comes up and over for the top of the first "o", let the hand turn over so it is palm up. It will then come down and up and over for the second half of the "o". As it rounds the curve coming up, the hand will turn face down again. This may sound complicated but is really very simple once you see how it's done. Try it with the left hand too and then with both hands together.
3. Shake the hands to relax them. Push each finger individually into the palm of the opposite hand. Oh, lovely.
4. Hold the right hand in front of you with the elbow almost straight. Turn the palm toward the floor then bend the wrist backward. Using the left hand, pull the fingers of the right, individually, back as far as they will go. Repeat with the left hand. You should be able to feel the tendons and muscles of the palm and lower arm stretching.
5. Now push each finger, individually, into the palm of the opposite hand.
6. Place both hands in front, shoulder high, arms straight, palms facing downward. Now pull the wrists down, the fingers in. Try to touch the wrists. You should be able to feel the muscles of the forearm stretching.
7. Shake the hands to relax them. Whenever your hands are tense, fling them until they feel like rubber.

8. Relax your hands by making them stay quiet. Stop:
   Biting your nails,
   Knotting your handkerchief,
   Fingering your face or hair,
   Chain-smoking nervously,
   Twiddling your jewelry,
   Clasping your hands.
9. If you feel more at ease holding something, hold one hand in the other, lightly and gently. Have one palm up and the other down, just below the waistline when you are standing and in the lap when you are sitting.

Hands should be beautiful. And they will be, no matter what their shape, when they are used with grace. Don't let your hands be just blobs of bone and muscle to lift and carry objects. Let them enhance your personality and dynamically add to the impression you make.

Ever see a concert pianist play the piano without "flair?" Take a lesson from him and discover how your dexterity and skill as a typist can be heightened through exercises that give strength, grace and coordination to your hands.

FOR TENSE AND TIRED TORSO!

Nothing will relax the body more than just letting it go limp all over. If you can lie down for a few minutes at any time during the day, you will be surprised how refreshing it will be. If this is next to impossible, go limp in a chair, leaning backward or folded forward. In either case, let the arms dangle loosely at the sides. If you can neither lie nor sit, try stooping.

STOOPING FOR RELAXATION:
1. Stand with the feet apart, the toes pointing outward, the hands dangling at the sides. Start going limp in the shoulders, let the head fall forward. Now let the torso slump forward as you bend your knees. Let the hands fall between the knees. Continue to go limp like a Raggedy Ann doll until the backs of the fingers are resting on the floor. Return to a standing position in three or four easy stages.
2. To stir up circulation after a long car ride, nothing can beat deep knee bends. This time place the hands on the hips, keep the back erect and stoop, as far as your clothing will allow.

FOR HEADACHE AND EYE STRAIN

You can sometimes stop a headache and relieve eye strain by gently massaging the temples with the three main fingers, allowing the thumbs to rest just under the cheek bones. The finger tips are rotated over a small area and then moved slightly until the whole area around the eyes has been massaged.

RELAXATION FOR BODY PERFECTION

The mind automatically tenses the muscles of the jaw as you think of words. The more emotionally tinged your thoughts, the tighter the jaw becomes. To relax these muscles, massage behind and just in front of the ear. Use a slight amount of pressure, not enough to cause discomfort.

Do you feel the tension ebbing?

EXERCISES FOR THE EYES AND FACE:

1. Hold the head erect. Place the chin in the heels of the palms—let your hands hold the head in place. Without moving the head, look away up; and then away down. Remember, it is the extra stretch and pull that will do the work. Now, slowly, steadily up and down. Close the eyes for a moment. This exercise stretches and strengthens the vertical muscles.

    Now exercise the horizontal ones by slowly looking from side to side. Farther to the right, farther to the left. Hold your head still. Now close the eyes for a moment.

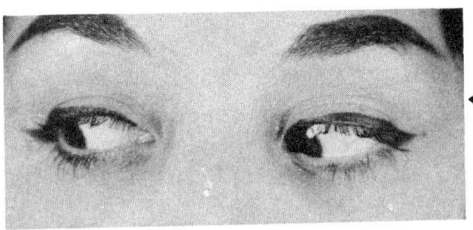

    ↑
    **From up . . .
    to
    Down**
    ↓

    **From
    ← Side
    to
    Side →**

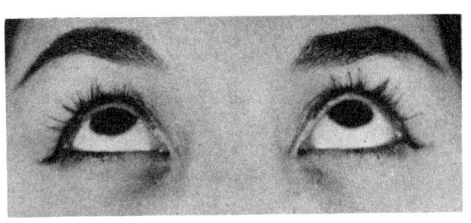

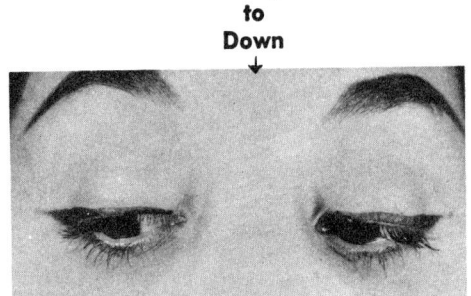

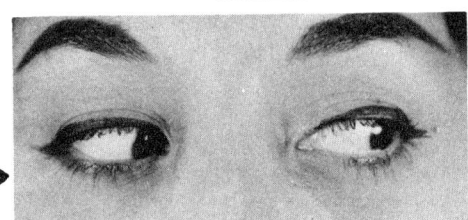

2. This next one is for the oblique or diagonal muscles. Look far up into the left-hand corner of the room. Steadily bring the eyes down on a diagonal line until you are looking way down in the right-hand corner. Up to the left, down to the right. Close the eyes for a moment and then reverse looking up to the right and down to the left. Be sure to turn your eyes neither to the side nor straight up, but in the direction between the two points.

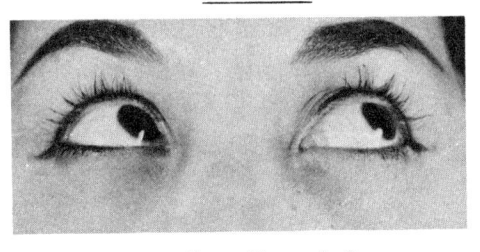

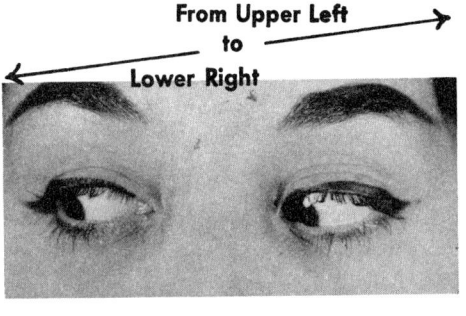

    **From Upper Left →
    to
    ← Lower Right**

3. Palm your eyes. Make a little cup with each hand, place the right hand over the right eye and the left hand over the left eye with the heel of each hand resting on the cheek bone just below the eyes. The cupping is formed over the eyes with the fingers resting on the forehead. Do not permit any pressure on the eye ball. Close the eyes.

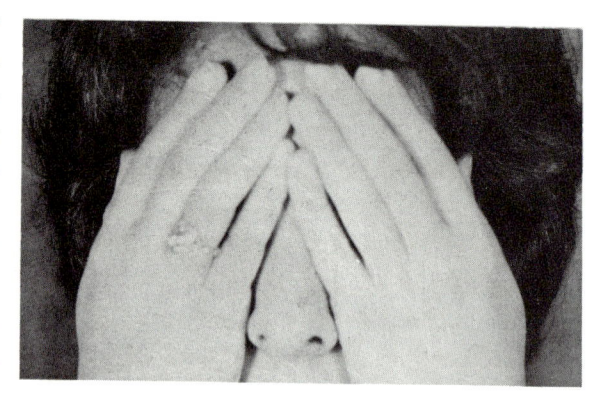

4. Holding the head erect with the hands holding the head still, look straight ahead and blink once. Don't grimace, just blink. Look straight up where 12 o'clock on a huge clock would be, blink five times, look straight ahead and blink once. Continue around the clock as shown in the diagram, to the right upper corner, the right side, the right lower corner, straight down, etc. Be sure to blink five times at each "numbers" position and then blink once as you look straight ahead between each position.

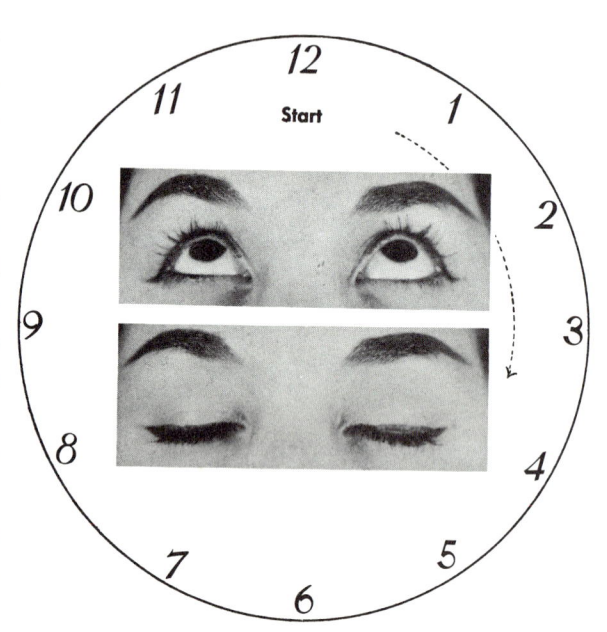

5. Squeeze the eyes shut, squeeze the mouth, squeeze the face, make it as small as you can. Now open the eyes, wide, open the mouth, raise the eyebrows. Repeat about five times.

If you need these exercises, they will pull the muscles and hurt while doing them, but afterwards your eyes will feel rested and relaxed. Just a few repetitions will do an eyesight of good.

MASSAGE FOR RELAXATION

Because massaging requires physical effort, it is for the more ambitious. There is nothing like it though for getting fast, fast results. There are several accepted techniques, each of which is supposed to produce a particular effect.

1. FOR KNEADING OFF UNNEEDED FAT.

Kneading is done with either one or both hands. Try it on your upper arm, for instance, using the right hand on the left arm. Use the heel of the thumb on top and the fingers underneath. Be sure to get enough flesh so that it fills the cup of the hand. Work from the elbow toward the shoulder, pushing down with the fingers and up with the thumb and palm. You'll have your skin pink in no time. With this one be sure not to rub the skin. Simply move the hand further up with each squeeze. You will be able to use both hands on the tummy or thighs. Keep the hands close together and press the flesh with the hands. Place the left hand on top and press down, the right hand under and press up.

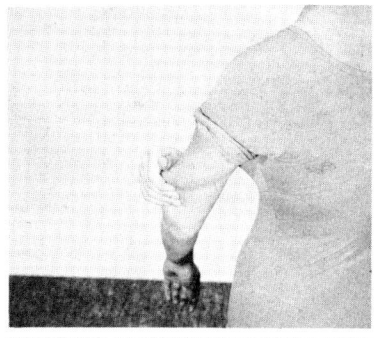

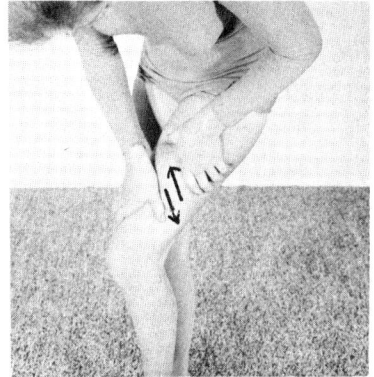

2. FOR WRINGING FLABBY FLESH.

Wringing is done with both hands and is especially helpful on the ankles and calves. You place the right hand with the thumb on top and the left beside it with thumb on top. Then you push the right hand counter-clockwise and the left hand clockwise. Yes, you are actually wringing out the fat and tightening the tissues. Be sure to work toward the heart.

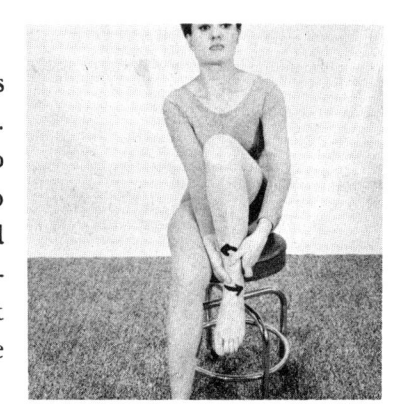

3. FOR RELIEVING MUSCLE SORENESS.

This must be a deep massage and should follow the contour of the muscle. You can use either your finger tips or the heel of your hand. Gently but firmly massage the muscle. Some of the smaller ones will benefit by your lifting them with thumb and fingers away from the bone. Easy does it. You'll be amazed at how quickly you can relieve muscular aches and pains with surface stimulation.

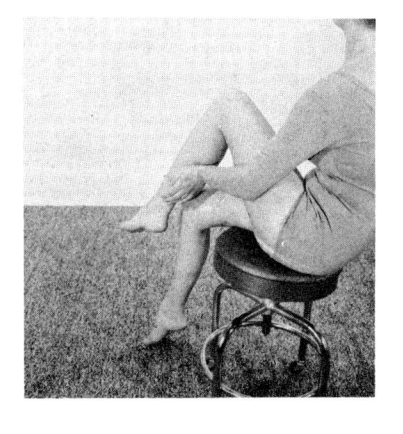

4. FOR FAT PADS AND TAUT MUSCLES.

You spank the body with the outside profile of each hand. The little fingers will do the actual work, but all the fingers will be pitching in. Be sure to keep them relaxed. It feels wonderful over tired muscles.

5. FOR STIMULATING CIRCULATION.

All of the various types of massage do stimulate the circulation. However, this can be done most effectively by brisk rubbing or slapping. We suggest this type of massage right after a warm bath or shower. Rub the entire body dry, then apply a generous amount of oil or skin cream to prevent chaffing. Now take your towel, one end in each hand and really rub. Across the back, buttocks, thighs. Now across the front—vigorously. The pink is blood close to the surface. Wonderful as a daily means for maintaining a youthful skin!

6. FOR RELIEVING TENSIONS.

With a slight amount of pressure, you slide over the skin working from the extremities toward the heart. You can use a skin lotion or body oil to facilitate the massage. This type of massage can be used at any time, but is most beneficial just at bedtime.

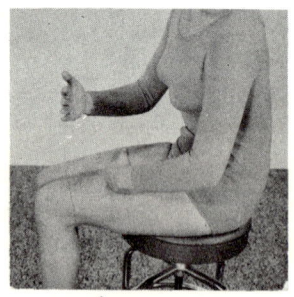

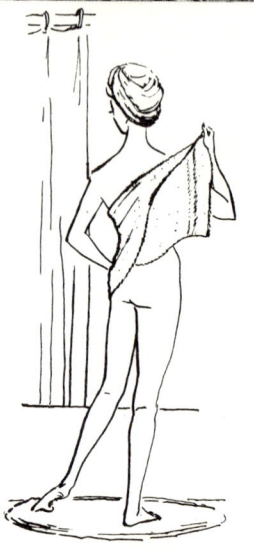

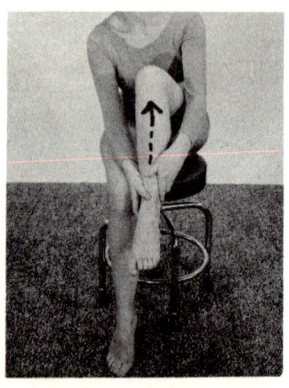

YOGA FOR BALANCE AND RELAXATION!

Yoga is a series of postures or positions that are controlled by mental concentration for maximum muscular control. A sort of mind over matter. Western culture has borrowed them from their point of origin, India, where they are practiced religiously with spiritual over-tones.

It is difficult for the Western mind to conceive of the mental value that is inherent in these exercises; but we are able to comprehend the physical value of learning better balance and muscle coordination.

As you know, the Eastern peoples are romantic and they give delightful names to each position, such as, the Lotus Pose, the Lion Posture, etc.

Just for fun, let's identify our Yoga exercises with names.

RELAXATION FOR BODY PERFECTION

YOGA FOR BALANCE

THE TREE:
Hold right foot against left thigh with left hand; raise right hand gracefully over head. Hold thirty seconds, reverse legs. Repeat three times with each leg.

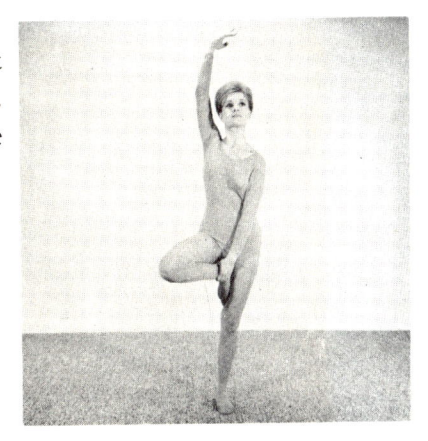

THE FISH:
Wrap right leg around left leg. Hold left arm in front with elbow bent, fingers facing away from the body. Place right elbow inside left with right hand facing body. Twist left palm into palm of right hand. Hold thirty seconds. Reverse. Repeat up to three times with each side.

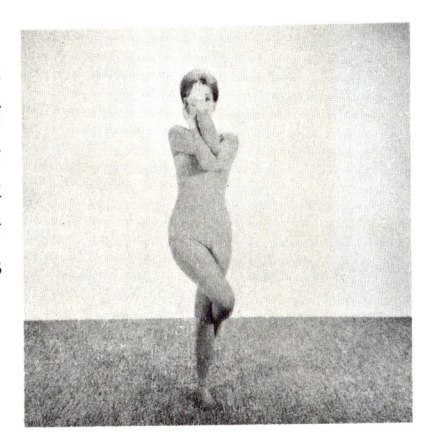

THE BLOSSOM:
Grasp left foot in left hand, bring it back to hip height. Slowly extend right hand till you feel maximum stretch in torso. Hold thirty seconds, reverse. Repeat up to three times with each leg.

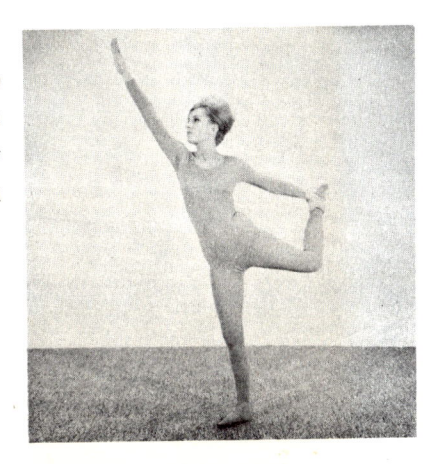

YOGA FOR STRETCHING

THE CAT:
Rise up on toes, raise arms overhead, interlocking thumbs. Pull upward, first with one thumb, then with the other, pulling head out of neck at the same time. Take relaxed breaths, inhaling through the nose, exhaling through the mouth. Fill the lungs with air.

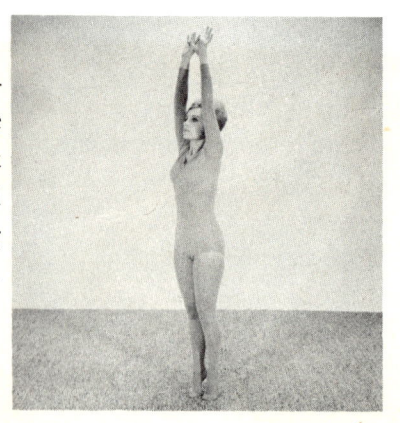

THE TWIST:
Feet apart, bring arms to shoulder level out at sides. Swing right arm forward, left arm back, turn head to left looking behind you. Exhale as you twist, inhale as you assume beginning posture. Repeat to other side, slowly. Continue six times.

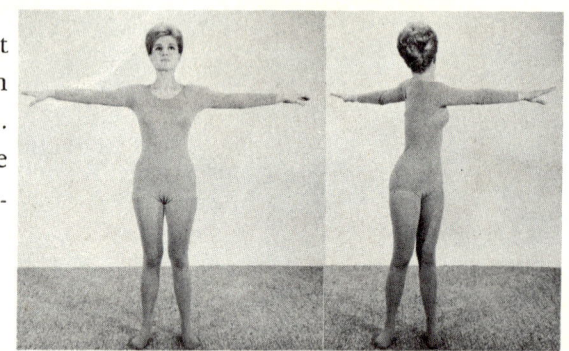

THE BELLOWS:
Feet apart, stand with arms out at shoulder height. Bend torso slowly to left until the left hand touches the left knee. The right arm is straight up. Slowly straighten, bend to the other side. Three times to each side. Exhale going down, inhale coming up.

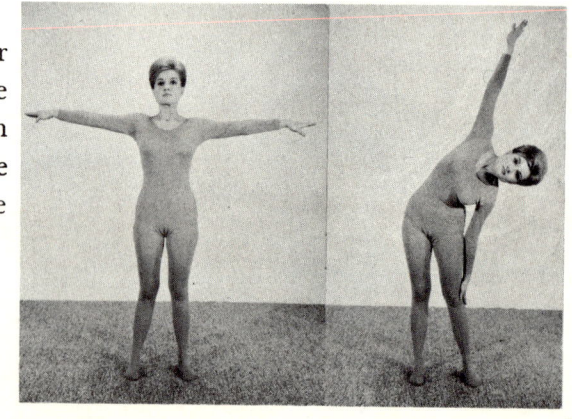

HOW NEVER TO BE TIRED! Boredom can make you tired, so vary whatever you are doing. Find a new way to perform an old act. Keep life interesting! *Unhappiness* can make you tired, so read the following:

RELAXATION FOR BODY PERFECTION

TEN COMMANDMENTS FOR HAPPINESS

1. Thou shalt not despise thy body, but shall consider it a vehicle most precious. Thou shalt eat nourishing food, exercise regularly and relax often.
2. Thou shalt look upon work as thy greatest source of happiness and find great satisfaction in thy accomplishments.
3. Thou shalt have a worthwhile purpose in thy life and allow nothing to deter thee from its fulfillment.
4. Thou shalt budget thy time, money, and energies so that thou art never without reserve.
5. Thou shalt not ignore the desires of thine heart, but shall supplement thy dreams with action.
6. Thou shalt renew the wellsprings of thy life by ever expanding horizons of achievement.
7. Thou shalt not covet thy neighbor's looks, possessions, or talents but shall do all in thy power to develop and make use of thine own.
8. Thou shalt develop a sense of values and be unperturbed by thine or others' follies.
9. Thou shalt have faith and believe in the, as yet, unseen and courage to face the, as yet, unknown future.
10. Thou shalt strive for a balanced life in which there is time for the enjoyment of THIS MOMENT.

TIME COUNTS!

Every minute you spend on yourself will pay dividends. It's important that you get into the habit *NOW* of spending a little time each day on those routines and activities that will make your life more worthwhile.

You have a date at eight! How can you revive yourself after a long day's work? You can:

1. Lie down for a short time.
2. Stretch taut muscles.
3. Take a cat nap.
4. Slump and let your mind go blank.
5. Massage tired areas.
6. Take a warm bath.
7. Assume the beauty angle.
8. Shut your eyes and palm them.
9. Go for a walk.
10. Think about the fun ahead.

And don't forget that eight hours sleep each night is the greatest beauty bonus you can get for nothing—except for the time it takes.

Yes, time counts, let it count for greater beauty and vitality!

INDEX

A

Adjustment, methods of, 289
Ageing skin, 14
American girl, 213
Appointments by telephone, 321
Arch in social postures, 98
Arms, clothing for, 173
    exercises for, 374, 388, 414
Athletic personality, 204

B

Back exercises, 374, 388
Beauty, illusion of, 16
Belongings, handling of, 105
Body perfection, 348-356
    exercises for, 357-390, 416
Boutonnieres, wearing of, 198-199
Boyish personality, 208
Brushing the hair, 57-58
Bust, clothes for, 173
Bustline exercises, 370-371
Buying (see purchases)

C

Calf exercises, 384, 387
Calorie, 396
Car, getting in and out of, 95-96
Chairman of meeting, 339
Charm training, importance of,
    (see foreword)
Chin exercises, 373
Chokers, wearing of, 193
Cleansers for skin, 5-7, 46-47
Cleopatra, 1, 202
Clothing
    accessories, 154, 185, 187
    care of, 135-137
    coats, 106-109, 152
    color selection, 185-186
    gloves, 114-115, 194
    hosiery, 142-143
    inventory of, 132
    seasonal, 157
    upkeep, 133-134
Coat,
    basic, 152
    checking of, 123
    wearing of, 106-109
Coiffure arrangements for
    facial shapes, 64-67
    hair colors, 59
Color,
    definitions, 27
    harmonies, 180
    magic, 177, 182
    nail polish, 54
    skin, 183-184
    wheel, 179
Colors of clothing
    accessories, 185-186
    effects of, 171
    matching of, 142
    significance of, 178
Combination skin, 4
Committees, 344-345
Complexion,
    make-up for, 26-32
    types of, 26-27
Conversational charm, 267
    leadership in, 273
    rules for, 268-272
Cooperation on job, 306
Cosmetic
    color in, 185
    inventory, 33-34
Courtesy on job, 308
Creams for skin, 14, 48
Customs, change in, 119-120

D

Dating after work, 315
Diamond-shaped face, 18
    eyeglasses for, 200
    hair style for, 67
    make-up for, 25
Diet (see Foods)
Digestion,
    good, 393
    impairment of, 393
Dinner,
    dancing at, 128
    eating at, 125-128
    going to, 123
    sitting at table, 124
Doorway, closed
    entering, 101
    leaving, 102
Doorway, open
    entering, 100

INDEX

leaving, 101
Dress (see clothes)
    changes, 159
    daytime, 152
    evening, 153, 160
    on the job, 314, 324
    optical illusions in, 161-162
    rainwear, 153
    shopping, 144
    special problems, 172-175
    sportswear, 153, 160
Dressing for personality types, 201-214
Dry skin, 4

E

Earrings, wearing of, 192
Ego motives, 287
Elimination, good, 394
Emotional stress, 409
Escort, coat assistance, 108-109
Escorting to the table, 123
Etiquette,
    eating, 128-129
    office, 300-305, 311-313
    smoking, 112-113
    telephone, 318
Eyebrow pencil, 36
Eyebrows, 35-37
    plucking of, 35
    shaping of, 35
Eyeglasses, 199-200
Eyes,
    colors for, 181
    make-up for, 45
Eye strain, 416
Exercises:
    body, 9, 363
    daily, 362
    face, 9, 371-372
    posture, 351-353
Exotic personality, 202-203

F

Fabrics,
    combinations, 160
    inferior, 138
    summer, 158
    synthetic, 137
    types of, 137-138
    winter, 158

Facial,
    exercise, 9, 371-372
    massage, 10
    packs, 10, 13
    treatment, 14
Facial features, improvement of, 37
Facial shapes, 16-18
    coiffure arrangements for, 64-67
Fashion, woman of, 206
Figure,
    basic, 168
    colors for, 181
    examination of, 168, 170
    lines, 161-175
    measurements, 358-361
    style selector for, 172-175
Foods, 392, 397-402
Foot care, 56, 410, 412
Foundation make-up, 41-42
Fragrance, 215-217
Friends, making of, 221, 225-227

G

Girdles, 147
Gloves,
    carrying of, 115
    wearing of, 114-115, 155, 194
Graciousness, art of, 231, 233
Greeting of people, 99
Grooming on job, 314
Grooming, personal, 1-68

H

Hair,
    brushing of, 57
    care of, 57-59
    grey, 184
    protection of, 59
    shampooing of, 58
Hair colors,
    coiffure arrangements for, 59
Hairstyle, selection of, 60
Handbags, 116-117, 155, 159, 195
Hand-hip positions in standing, 75-76
Handkerchief, 199
Hand positions in standing, 74-76
Hands,
    beauty tips for, 54, 77
    care of, 54, 415
Handshake, 99, 234-235

Happiness, 423
Hats,
    shapes of, 188-189
    wearing of, 157, 187
Headache, 416
Heart-shaped face, 17
    eyeglasses for, 200
    hairstyle for, 66
    make-up for, 23
Height, related to hairstyles, 60
Hip,
    clothes for, 174
    lines, 169
Hipline exercises, 377
Hosiery shopping, 142-143
Human relations, 221-224, 227-229

I

Ingenue personality, 203
Intellectual personality, 210
Interest in work, 255
Interview, job, 328
    acknowledgment of, 329
    manner during, 329
Introductions:
    group, 234
    office, 309
    people, 233-236

J

Jewelry, wearing of, 156, 190-191, 314
Job,
    application, 323
    dress for, 324-325
    interview, 324, 328
    qualifications, 324
    resumé, 326
    success, 285

L

Lanolin, 48
Leadership through conversation, 273
Legs,
    care of, 55, 412
    classification of, 71
    clothes for, 175
    exercises for, 381, 385
Lip line, correction of, 39
Lips, 38-39
Lipstick, 38, 41
Lotions for skin, 14

Loyalty on job, 303
Lubricating oils for skin, 7

M

Make-up,
    application of, 40-41
    corrective, 19-25, 41-42
    evening, 45-46
    lip line, 39
    nose, 37
Manicuring,
    equipment, 51
    procedure, 51-53
Manners,
    business, 311
    telephone, 322
    good, 237
    table, 129
    quiz, 238-247
Massage techniques for:
    body, 10
    chest, 11
    face, 10-12
    neck, 11
    relaxation, 419
    wrinkles, 12
Matron, 212
    young, 211
Meals, balanced, 392, 404, 407
Measurements, body, 358-361
Meeting,
    business, order of, 337-344
    committees, 344-345
    elections, 336
    officers, duties of, 335
    parliamentary procedure, 331-334
    people, 122
    voting at, 336
Members, rights of, 337
Motives, personal, 287, 292

N

Nail polish, 53-54
Nails, beauty tips for, 54
Names, remembering of, 236
Neck, as related to:
    clothes, 172
    exercises, 373, 414
    hairstyles, 61
Necklace, wearing of, 193

Normal
    eyebrows, 36
    skin, 4
    weight, 395, 406, 408
Nutrition for body perfection, 391-408
Nutrition of skin, 14

O

Oblong-shaped face, 17
    clothes for, 172
    eyeglasses for, 200
    hairstyle for, 66
    make-up for, 22
Office etiquette, 300-305
Oils for skin, 7
Oily skin, 4
Optical illusions in:
    beauty, 16
    dress, 161-162
    figure lines, 161-175
Oval-shaped face, 16
    clothes for, 172
    eyeglasses for, 200
    hairstyle for, 64
    make-up for, 19
Over-forty exercises, 388

P

Packs for face, 10, 13
Parliamentary procedure, 331-332
    definitions of, 333-334
Party, going to a, 121
Pedicuring, 56
Perfume, 215-217
Personality
    development, 219
    dimensions, 250-253
    interests, 254-255
    measurement, 249-250
    positive, 224
    potential, 293
    qualities, 293-295
    related to color, 181
    scientific approach to, 221
    telephone, 320
    traits, 221-224, 255-256
    types, 201-214
Persuasion, 231-232
Pin curls, setting of, 68

Planning of:
    clothing purchases, 139-140
    speeches, 277
    wardrobe, 131-132
Plastic surgery, 14
Platform technique in speaking, 275
Poise, visual, 69
Popularity,
    men, 228
    women, 227-228
Posing,
    before a group, 102
    picture, 100-101
Positions,
    arch, 98
    hand, 74, 76
    hand-hip, 75-76
Posture,
    bad posture, causes of, 354
    check of, 349
    correct postures, 354-356
    exercises for, 351-353
    good posture, 349-350
    social posture, 97-98
Problem skin, 5
Profiles, related to hairstyles, 62-63
Protection of skin, 13
Psychology of:
    color, 177-186
    success, 286-292
Public speaking, 258-266 (See Voice)
    body action in, 281-283
    developing the subject, 278-281
    facial expression, 283
    parts of speech, 276-277
    platform technique, 275-284
    success in, 283-284
Purchase,
    intelligent, 141-142
    order of, 140
Purchases:
    bras, 145-146
    foundation, 145
    girdle, 145, 147

R

Reaching posture, 355
Records, telephone, 321
Relaxation for body perfection, 409-423
Remembering names, 236

Romantic personality, 205
Rouge, application of, 43-44
Round-shaped face,
    clothes for, 172
    eyeglasses for, 200
    hairstyle for, 65
    make-up for, 20

S

Salesmanship, telephone, 317-322
Salt rub, 13
Scalp, dry, 58
Scarf, wearing of, 197-198
Sex appeal, 315
Shampooing the hair, 58
Shoes, wearing of, 154, 196
Shopping,
    dress for, 144
    habits, 143-144
    tour, 140
Short figure, what to wear, 165
Shoulders, clothes for, 172-173
    exercises for, 374-375, 414
Silhouette lines, 163
Sitting, 87-96
    chair position, 90
    correctly, 88
    position of extremities, 93-94
    posture, 355
    rules, 94
    "S" position, 92
    "T" position, 89, 91
Skin,
    ageing, 14
    care of, 3-14
    cleansers, 5-7, 46-47
    colors, 183-184
    conditions, 3-4
    creams, 14, 46-47
    lotions, 14, 46
    lubrication, 7-8
    massage, 10-12
    protection, 13
    stimulation, 12-13
    types, 4
Smoking etiquette, 112
Soap, cleansing, 47
Sociability, 249-256
Sophisticated personality, 209
Spine, 348
    exercises for, 364
Square-shaped face, 17
    clothes for, 172
    eyeglasses for, 200
    hairstyle for, 65
    make-up for, 21
Stage fright, 276
Stairs,
    rules, 103
    technique, 103
Stance,
    basic, 70
    pedestal, 73
    rules, 72-73
Standing, 70
    before a group, 102
    posture, 354
    review, 78
Stimulation for skin, 9-10
Stole, wearing of, 110-112
Stooping posture, 356
Stout figure, what to wear, 166
Strength exercises, 365-369
Success,
    barriers to, 287-288
    insurance, 285-292
    job, 285-292
Sun lamps, 12
Sunshine, 12

T

Tall figure, what to wear, 164
Telephone,
    answering the, 318
    appointments, 321
    business, 317-322
    complaint, handling of, 319
    etiquette, 318
    manners, 322
    personality, 320
    record keeping, 321
    speech habits, 319
    tools of, 321
Theatre, behavior in, 120-121
Thigh exercises, 389-390
Thin figure, what to wear, 167
Triangular-shaped face, 18
    eyeglasses for, 200
    hairstyle for, 67
    make-up for, 24

INDEX

U
Underweight, exercises for, 385-386

V
Visual poise, 69
    in social affairs, 119
Voice, 258-266 (see public speaking)
    expressions to avoid, 263-265
    improvement, 258-266
    qualities to develop, 261-263
    telephone, 319
Voluptuous personality, 207

W
Waist, clothes for, 173-174
Waistline exercises, 375-376
Walking, 79-86
    arm swing in, 84
    coordination of hands and feet, 84
    correctly, 80, 83
    five-step procedure, 81
    pivot, 82
    review, 84-85
    rules for, 85-86
    techniques of, 83
Wardrobe (see clothing)
    basic, 149-160
    planning of, 131-138
    purchase of, 151
Weight,
    gain of, 403, 405
    loss of, 396, 402
    normal, 395, 406, 408
Wraps, 105, 120
Wrinkles, 12
    overcoming of, 14

Y
Yoga exercises, 420-422